MR Contrast Agents

Editors

MARCO ESSIG
JUAN E. GUTIERREZ

MAGNETIC RESONANCE IMAGING CLINICS OF NORTH AMERICA

www.mri.theclinics.com

Consulting Editors
SURESH K. MUKHERJI
LYNNE STEINBACH

November 2012 • Volume 20 • Number 4

ELSEVIER

1600 John F. Kennedy Boulevard • Suite 1800 • Philadelphia, Pennsylvania 19103-2899

http://www.theclinics.com

MRI CLINICS OF NORTH AMERICA Volume 20, Number 4
November 2012 ISSN 1064-9689, ISBN 13: 978-1-4557-4700-9

Editor: Pamela Hetherington
Developmental Editor: Donald Mumford

Magnetic Resonance Imaging Clinics of North America (ISSN 1064-9689) is published quarterly by Elsevier Inc., 360 Park Avenue South, New York, NY 10010-1710. Months of issue are February, May, August, and November. Business and Editorial Offices: 1600 John F. Kennedy Blvd., Ste. 1800, Philadelphia, PA 19103-2899. Customer Service Office: 3251 Riverport Lane, Maryland Heights, MO 63043. Periodicals postage paid at New York, NY and additional mailing offices. Subscription prices are $337.00 per year (domestic individuals), $541.00 per year (domestic institutions), $172.00 per year (domestic students/residents), $376.00 per year (Canadian individuals), $678.00 per year (Canadian institutions), $488.00 per year (international individuals), $678.00 per year (international institutions), and $249.00 per year (international and Canadian students/residents). International air speed delivery is included in all *Clinics* subscription prices. All prices are subject to change without notice. **POSTMASTER:** Send address changes to *Magnetic Resonance Imaging Clinics*, Elsevier Health Sciences Division, Subscription Customer Service, 3251 Riverport Lane, Maryland Heights, MO 63043. Customer Service (orders, claims, online, change of address): Elsevier Health Sciences Division, Subscription Customer Service, 3251 Riverport Lane, Maryland Heights, MO 63043. Tel:1-800-654-2452 (U.S. and Canada); 314-447-8871 (outside U.S. and Canada). Fax: 314-447-8029. E-mail: journalscustomerservice-usa@elsevier.com (for print support); journalsonlinesupport-usa@elsevier.com (for online support).

Reprints. For copies of 100 or more of articles in this publication, please contact the Commercial Reprints Department, Elsevier Inc., 360 Park Avenue South, New York, NY 10010-1710. Tel.: 212-633-3812; Fax: 212-462-1935; E-mail: reprints@elsevier.com.

Magnetic Resonance Imaging Clinics of North America is covered in the *RSNA Index of Imaging Literature, MEDLINE/PubMed (Index Medicus),* and *EMBASE/Excerpta Medica.*

Printed and bound by CPI Group (UK) Ltd, Croydon, CR0 4YY

Transferred to digital print 2012

Contributors

CONSULTING EDITORS

SURESH K. MUKHERJI, MD, FACR
Department of Radiology, University of
Michigan Health System, Ann Arbor, Michigan

LYNNE STEINBACH, MD
Professor of Clinical Radiology and
Orthopaedic Surgery, University of California at
San Francisco, San Francisco, California

GUEST EDITORS

MARCO ESSIG, MD
Professor, Department of Neuroradiology,
University of Erlangen, Erlangen, Germany

JUAN E. GUTIERREZ, MD
Assistant Professor of Neuroradiology, Vice
Chair of Clinical Operations, Director of Clinical
Research, Department of Radiology, UHS
Director of Radiology, University of Texas
Health Science Center at San Antonio,
San Antonio, Texas

AUTHORS

TUSHAR CHANDRA, MD
Instructor, Department of Radiology,
Children's Hospital of Wisconsin, Milwaukee,
Wisconsin

JULIEN DINKEL, MD
Department of Radiology, Massachusetts
General Hospital, Massachusetts

MARCO ESSIG, MD
Professor, Department of Neuroradiology,
University of Erlangen, Erlangen, Germany

JEAN-CHRISTOPHE FERRÉ, MD, PhD
Division of Neuroradiology, Department of
Radiology, Keck Medical Center of University
of Southern California, Los Angeles, California;
CHU Rennes, Department of Radiology,
University Hospital, Rennes, France

THOMAS M. GRIST, MD, FACR
Department of Radiology, University of
Wisconsin–Madison, Madison, Wisconsin

JUAN E. GUTIERREZ, MD
Assistant Professor of Neuroradiology, Vice
Chair of Clinical Operations, Director of Clinical
Research, Department of Radiology, UHS
Director of Radiology, University of Texas
Health Science Center at San Antonio,
San Antonio, Texas

EMANUEL KANAL, MD, FACR, FISMRM
Director, Magnetic Resonance Services,
Professor of Radiology and Neuroradiology,
Department of Radiology, University of
Pittsburgh Medical Center, Pittsburgh,
Pennsylvania

BUM-SOO KIM, MD
Department of Radiology, Seoul St. Mary's
Hospital, The Catholic University of Korea,
Seoul, Korea

J. HARALD KRAMER, MD
Department of Radiology, University of
Wisconsin–Madison, Madison, Wisconsin;
Institute for Clinical Radiology, Ludwig-
Maximilians-University Hospital Munich,
Munich, Germany

MENG LAW, MD
Professor of Radiology and Neurological
Surgery, Division of Neuroradiology,
Department of Radiology, Keck Medical Center
of University of Southern California,
Los Angeles, California

CHRISTINA LEBEDIS, MD
Assistant Professor, Department of Radiology,
Boston University Medical Center, Boston,
Massachusetts

LAURIE A. LOEVNER, MD
Departments of the Neurosurgery and
Radiology, Hospital of the University of
Pennsylvania, Philadelphia, Pennsylvania

ANTONIO LUNA, MD
Submedical Director of Health Time Group,
Clinica Las Nieves, Jaén, Spain; Clinical
Assistant Professor, Department of Radiology,
Case Western Reserve University,
Cleveland, Ohio

ANDREW MAI, MD
Department of Radiology, Louisiana State
University Health Sciences Center,
New Orleans, Louisiana

ALEJANDRO MARMOL-VELEZ, MD
Division of Cardiology, Department of
Medicine, The University of Texas Health
Science Center at San Antonio, San Antonio,
Texas

ELIAS MELHEM, MD, PhD
Professor, Department of Radiology, Perelman
School of Medicine, University of
Pennsylvania, Philadelphia, Pennsylvania

IGOR MIKITYANSKY, MD, MPH
Windsong Radiology Group, Williamsville,
New York

SUYASH MOHAN, MD
Assistant Professor, Department of
Radiology, Perelman School of Medicine,
University of Pennsylvania, Philadelphia,
Pennsylvania

BROOKE MORRELL, MD
Department of Radiology, Louisiana State
University Health Sciences Center,
New Orleans, Louisiana

BRYAN PUKENAS, MD
Assistant Professor, Department of
Radiology, Perelman School of Medicine,
University of Pennsylvania, Philadelphia,
Pennsylvania

CARLOS S. RESTREPO, MD
Professor of Radiology, Director,
Cardiothoracic Radiology, The University of
Texas Health Science Center at San Antonio,
San Antonio, Texas

LUIS F. SERRANO, MD
Associate Professor of Radiology, Director
of Breast Imaging Sections, Department
of Radiology, Louisiana State University
Health Sciences Center, New Orleans,
Louisiana

MARK S. SHIROISHI, MD
Assistant Professor, Division of
Neuroradiology, Department of Radiology,
Keck Medical Center of University of Southern
California, Los Angeles, California

JORGE A. SOTO, MD
Professor, Department of Radiology, Boston
University Medical Center, Boston,
Massachusetts

SINA TAVAKOLI, MD
Radiology-PhD Resident, Department of
Radiology, The University of Texas Health
Science Center at San Antonio,
San Antonio, Texas

DAVID M. YOUSEM, MD, MBA
Department of Radiology, Johns Hopkins
University, Baltimore, Maryland

ERIC L. ZAGER, MD
Department of Neurosurgery, Hospital of the
University of Pennsylvania, Philadelphia,
Pennsylvania

Contents

> There has been much progress in contrast enhanced neuroradiologic magnetic resonance imaging in the almost 25 years since the first gadolinium-based contrast agent was approved in the United States. Much of this now focuses on the introduction of significantly higher relaxivity agents into our clinical armamentarium and the addition of T2*-weighted imaging sequences to hyperacute stroke or neoplastic evaluations. All 4 magnetic resonance contrast agents approved in the United States during the past decade have been higher relaxivity agents, suggesting a strong trend in our industry to continue to find more efficient, more powerful, more diagnostic means of increasing contrast on imaging studies.

> Since their introduction, gadolinium-based contrast media are routinely used in most CNS MR imaging indications. Due to their paramagnetic effect, they significantly shorten the T1 relaxation times of the tissue and are therefore applied to improve the sensitivity and specificity of CNS diseases and to allow a better treatment decision, planning, and follow-up. More recently, contrast media have also been used to allow the measurement of tissue perfusion and to follow the time course of enhancement in dynamic contrast-enhanced imaging studies. Routinely they are used to enhance MR angiography studies.

> MR imaging without and with gadolinium-based contrast agents (GBCAs) is an important imaging tool for defining normal anatomy and characteristics of lesions. GBCAs have been used in contrast-enhanced MR imaging in defining and characterizing lesions of the central nervous system for more than 20 years. The combination of unenhanced and GBCA-enhanced MR imaging is the clinical gold standard for the noninvasive detection and delineation of most intracranial and spinal lesions. MR imaging has a high predictive value that rules out neoplasm and most inflammatory and demyelinating processes of the central nervous system.

> Magnetic resonance (MR) angiography is a powerful tool for the evaluation of cervical and intracranial vasculature. Both noncontrast and contrast-enhanced MR

angiography can provide exquisite vascular contrast and detail without the use of ionizing radiation. More advanced techniques such as time-resolved MR angiography and parallel imaging provide dynamic information in rapid fashion. This article describes the basic principles and techniques of MR angiography image acquisition.

This article presents an overview of advanced magnetic resonance (MR) imaging techniques using contrast media in neuroimaging, focusing on T2*-weighted dynamic susceptibility contrast MR imaging and T1-weighted dynamic contrast-enhanced MR imaging. Image acquisition and data processing methods and their clinical application in brain tumors, stroke, dementia, and multiple sclerosis are discussed.

This article presents an overview of liver and biliary contrast agents including their mechanisms of action, dosage and elimination, current clinical indications, and potential future uses.

Cardiac magnetic resonance (CMR) imaging has significantly evolved in the past decade and is well established in the evaluation of coronary artery disease (CAD). The evaluation of cardiac anatomy and contractility by high-resolution CMR can be improved by using intravenous administration of gadolinium-based contrast agents. Delayed enhancement CMR imaging has become the gold standard for quantification of myocardial viability in CAD. Contrast-enhanced CMR imaging may circumvent the need for endomyocardial biopsy or localize the involved regions, thereby improving the diagnostic yield of this invasive procedure. The application of contrast-enhanced CMR as an advanced imaging technique for ischemic and non-ischemic diseases is reviewed.

Since the introduction of contrast-enhanced MR angiography (MRA), several different techniques for imaging the peripheral arteries have evolved. All of them provide good diagnostic image quality, whereas some older techniques suffer from drawbacks, such as long acquisition time, impaired image quality from venous enhancement, and limited spatial resolution. MRA provides the most comprehensive modality offering the ability to tailor the examination to the patient and the specific question to be answered. The drawbacks experienced at the introduction of MRA to clinical routine have largely been overcome or at least diminished, so that the benefits of MRA outbalance the limitations.

Although mammography is the standard imaging modality for detection of breast cancer, magnetic resonance (MR) imaging is a valuable adjunct and, in certain cases, is the imaging of choice. Contrast-enhanced breast MR imaging provides a noninvasive means of staging disease, assessing posttreatment response, and screening of high-risk patients with genetic predispositions. Additional indications for MR mammography include lesion characterization, contralateral breast evaluation in patients with proved malignancy, and identifying primary malignancy in patients with axillary nodal disease. There are several competing factors that influence the quality of the study. Finding the right balance is the key to providing high-quality images that can be accurately interpreted.

MR imaging of the brachial plexus assesses the continuity of the elements, relationship, and orientation of lesions, evaluates morphology, and reveals secondary features of plexopathies. The selection of sequences and imaging planes is guided by the history, clinical examination, and suspected type and location of the abnormality. Increased magnet strength and isotropic imaging with multiplanar reconstructions may allow for standardized imaging protocols and shorter examination time. This article discusses MR imaging evaluation of the brachial plexus, relevant anatomy, and common pathology with clinical and imaging details, indications for use of intravenous contrast, differential considerations, and diagnostic pitfalls.

MAGNETIC RESONANCE IMAGING CLINICS OF NORTH AMERICA

GOAL STATEMENT

The goal of *Magnetic Resonance Imaging Clinics of North America* is to keep practicing physicians up to date with current clinical practice by providing timely articles reviewing the state of the art in patient care.

ACCREDITATION

The *Magnetic Resonance Imaging Clinics of North America* is planned and implemented in accordance with the Essential Areas and Policies of the Accreditation Council for Continuing Medical Education (ACCME) through the joint sponsorship of the University of Virginia School of Medicine and Elsevier. The University of Virginia School of Medicine is accredited by the ACCME to provide continuing medical education for physicians.

The University of Virginia School of Medicine designates this enduring material activity for a maximum of 15 *AMA PRA Category 1 Credit*(s)™ for each issue, 60 credits per year. Physicians should claim only the credit commensurate with the extent of their participation in the activity.

The American Medical Association has determined that physicians not licensed in the US who participate in this CME enduring material activity are eligible for a maximum of *15 AMA PRA Category 1 Credit*(s)™ for each issue, 60 credits per year.

Credit can be earned by reading the text material, taking the CME examination online at http://www.theclinics.com/home/cme, and completing the evaluation. After taking the test, you will be required to review any and all incorrect answers. Following completion of the test and evaluation, your credit will be awarded and you may print your certificate.

FACULTY DISCLOSURE/CONFLICT OF INTEREST

The University of Virginia School of Medicine, as an ACCME accredited provider, endorses and strives to comply with the Accreditation Council for Continuing Medical Education (ACCME) Standards of Commercial Support, Commonwealth of Virginia statutes, University of Virginia policies and procedures, and associated federal and private regulations and guidelines on the need for disclosure and monitoring of proprietary and financial interests that may affect the scientific integrity and balance of content delivered in continuing medical education activities under our auspices.

The University of Virginia School of Medicine requires that all CME activities accredited through this institution be developed independently and be scientifically rigorous, balanced and objective in the presentation/discussion of its content, theories and practices.

All authors/editors participating in an accredited CME activity are expected to disclose to the readers relevant financial relationships with commercial entities occurring within the past 12 months (such as grants or research support, employee, consultant, stock holder, member of speakers bureau, etc.). The University of Virginia School of Medicine will employ appropriate mechanisms to resolve potential conflicts of interest to maintain the standards of fair and balanced education to the reader. Questions about specific strategies can be directed to the Office of Continuing Medical Education, University of Virginia School of Medicine, Charlottesville, Virginia.

The faculty and staff of the University of Virginia Office of Continuing Medical Education have no financial affiliations to disclose.

The authors/editors listed below have identified no professional or financial affiliations for themselves or their spouse/partner:
Tushar Chandra, MD; Julien Dinkel, MD; Eduard de Lange, MD (Test Author); Jean-Christophe Ferré, MD, PhD; Pamela Hetherington, (Acquisitions Editor); Bum-Soo Kim, MD; J. Harald Kramer, MD; Christina LeBedis, MD; Vivian S. Lee, MD, PhD, MBA (Consulting Editor); Antonio Luna, MD; Andrew Mai, MD; Alejandro Marmol-Velez, MD; Igor Mikityansky, MD, MPH; Suyash Mohan, MD; Brooke Morrell, MD; Bryan Pukenas, MD; Carlos S. Restrepo, MD; Luis F. Serrano, MD; Jorge A. Soto, MD; Sina Tavakoli, MD; David M. Yousem, MD, MBA; and Eric L. Zager, MD.

The authors/editors listed below identified the following professional or financial affiliations for themselves or their spouse/partner:
Marco Essig, MD (Guest Editor) is a consultant for Bayer Healthcare.
Thomas M. Grist, MD receives research support from GE Healthcare and Bracco Diagnostics, is on the Advisory Board for GE Healthcare and Bayer, owns stock in Novelos and Neuwave, is a consultant for Bayer and Guerbet, and owns a patent with Wisconsin Alumni Research Foundatio.
Juan E. Gutierrez, MD (Guest Editor) is on the Speakers' Bureau for Bayer Health Care.
Emanuel Kanal, MD, FACR is a consultant for Bracco Diagnostics and Guerbet Corporation, and is on the Speakers' Bureau for Bracco Diagnostics.
Meng Law, MD is on the Speakers' Bureau for Toshiba America Medical, is on the Advisory Board for Siemens Medical, iCAD Inc, and Fuji Inc, and receives research support from Bayer Healthcare.
Laurie A. Loevner, MD owns stock in GE.
Elias Melhem, MD, PhD is on the Speakers' Bureau for Bayer.
Suresh Mukherji, MD (Consulting Editor) is a consultant for Philips Medical Systems.
Mark S. Shiroishi, MD is a consultant for Bayer Healthcare.
Lynne Steinbach, MD (Consulting Editor) is a consultant for Pfizer, Inc.

Disclosure of Discussion of non-FDA approved uses for pharmaceutical products and/or medical devices:
The University of Virginia School of Medicine, as an ACCME provider, requires that all faculty presenters identify and disclose any "off label" uses for pharmaceutical and medical device products. The University of Virginia School of Medicine recommends that each physician fully review all the available data on new products or procedures prior to instituting them with patients.

TO ENROLL

To enroll in the Magnetic Resonance Imaging Clinics of North America Continuing Medical Education program, call customer service at 1-800-654-2452 or visit us online at www.theclinics.com/home/cme. The CME program is available to subscribers for an additional fee of $196.00.

Foreword

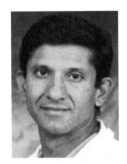

Suresh K. Mukherji, MD, FACR
Consulting Editor

Fortunately or unfortunately (!), I am old enough to have been present, the first time gadolinium was administered for a clinical study at Brigham and Women's Hospital at Harvard Medical School. I happened to be the first-year Neuroradiology resident on service as the group gathered around the MRI scanner to view the first post gadolinium images obtained in the sagittal plane. I had no clue what I was looking at and I was more amazed by the looks of awe on my attendings' faces as they commented on the sudden enhancement of the superior sagittal sinus. This really was the beginning of a new era and one that has revolutionized MR imaging.

One can make the argument that the most significant advancements in clinical MR over the last 15 years have been in the development of new contrast agents as opposed to inherent improvement in our magnets. There was a large time gap between the development of the 1.5 T and the 3 T. Some might even argue that the 3T has yet to be fully accepted for all clinical indications. However, during this period, we saw rapid acceptance and tremendous developments in MR contrast agents, which included fundamentally new compounds that were often organ-specific.

The challenge has been to keep up with these developments so that we can offer our patients the most up-to-date imaging. To help us meet these challenges, Drs Juan E. Gutierrez and Marco Essig graciously accepted our invitation to edit this issue of *Magnetic Resonance Imaging Clinics of North America*. Both are internationally recognized MR contrast experts who are also practicing radiologists. Thus, they bring the unique combination of clinical and corporate perspective. This important issue covers various different agents and clinical indications of the different classes of MR contrast agents. They also provide recommendations on the optimal use of MR contrast agents for better diagnostic quality while minimizing patient risk.

Drs Gutierrez and Essig have assembled an outstanding group of authors who are internationally recognized experts in their respective subject matter. I wish to personally thank Drs Gutierrez and Essig and the article authors for their commitment in creating such an outstanding edition that will serve as a state-of-the art reference on MR contrast agents for many years.

Suresh K. Mukherji, MD, FACR
Department of Radiology
University of Michigan Health System
1500 East Medical Center
Ann Arbor, MI 48109-0030, USA

E-mail address:
mukherji@med.umich.edu

Magn Reson Imaging Clin N Am 20 (2012) xi
http://dx.doi.org/10.1016/j.mric.2012.08.011
1064-9689/12/$ – see front matter

Preface

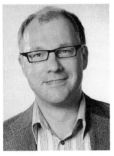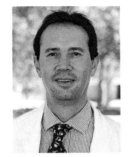

Marco Essig, MD   Juan E. Gutierrez, MD
Guest Editors

We were honored to be asked to edit this issue of the *Magnetic Resonance Imaging Clinics of North America*. Significant advances in the medical imaging world have occurred since the worldwide introduction of the first approved MRI contrast agent, gadopentetatedimeglumine (Magnevist; Gd-DTPA) in 1988. Although initially it provided a dramatic clinical contribution in the diagnosis of CNS conditions, based on clinical experience, its use extended rapidly to indications in other body areas. Also, the evolution of the gadolinium-based contrast agents (GBCA) has led to the development of other gadolinium complexes that show similar biodistribution with some differences in chemical structure, relaxivity, concentration, pharmacodynamics, and pharmacokinetics, which gives relevant advantages that can be applied to specific imaging indications. This has allowed the development of more sophisticated drugs such as the organ-specific and blood pool agents.

Radiologists, as well as any other physician, should well understand the clinical indications for the use of contrast agents as well as their mode of action, pharmacology, and efficacy. Most importantly, physicians should specifically understand the tolerance and risk of adverse events with GBCAs. It is important to reinforce this to our residents and fellows to reduce potential complications in our MR procedures. Since the link between Gadolinium and NSF was made, it is especially important to weigh the benefits and potential risks of GBCA administration for each patient.

The primary goals of this issue are to cover the different aspects and clinical indications of the different classes of MR contrast agents available as well as to provide some recommended techniques for use. Even more importantly, we wish to cover how to obtain an optimal use of GBCAs for better diagnostic quality and minimal patient safety risk. We have compiled comprehensive articles starting with an overview of the GBCAs followed by their clinical applications in the different body areas.

In the last 15 years, Marco and I have been involved in multiple development programs for most of the MR contrast agents at different stages and roles. Some of these agents have been successfully approved and marketed, while others have failed. During this experience, we have crossed roads and met many interesting colleagues and scientists, some with whom we share a good friendship. Based on the scope of this issue, we selected and invited an excellent group of professionals to be part of this project and we truly feel honored that they have agreed to share their knowledge and vast experience through the high-quality articles they provided. We wish to thank all authors for their valuable contribution.

It is our hope that this issue of the *Magnetic Resonance Imaging Clinics of North America* can

Magn Reson Imaging Clin N Am 20 (2012) xiii–xiv
http://dx.doi.org/10.1016/j.mric.2012.08.010

promote a better understanding and utilization of the MR contrast agents by all professionals in the imaging world for the ultimate benefit of our patients.

DEDICATION

"Every new step I take in my field I like to honor my beloved family, Catalina, Federico, Emilio, and Gabriel, for always being the inspiration in my endless search for professional evolution to inspire my three boys to do the same."

—J.E.G.

Marco Essig, MD
Department of Neuroradiology
University of Erlangen
Erlangen, Germany

Juan E. Gutierrez, MD
Department of Radiology
University of Texas Health Science Center
at San Antonio
San Antonio, TX, USA

E-mail addresses:
mediag@me.com (M. Essig)
gutierrezje@uthscsa.edu (J.E. Gutierrez)

Gadolinium-Based Magnetic Resonance Contrast Agents for Neuroradiology: An Overview

Emanuel Kanal, MD, FACR, FISMRM

KEYWORDS

• MR imaging • Gadolinium • Contrast agents • Relaxivity

KEY POINTS

- Because magnetic resonance (MR) imaging is intrinsically multiparametric (ie, it is able to image signal from tissues whose intensities are determined by any of multiple unrelated tissue properties), any agent that has the ability to modify or manipulate any of these variable tissue properties to which the MR imaging process is sensitive can be potentially used as an MR contrast agent.
- Due to its associated powerful magnetic field and safety profile (when appropriately bound to its ligand molecules), the vast majority of contrast enhanced studies in clinical MRI today is accomplished via the utilization of a chelated gadolinium ion, wherein the major differences between the various types available today is due to variations in the specific ligand molecule selected to which the gadolinium ion is to be chelated.
- The predominant mechanism of action clinically used for contrast enhancement in MR imaging today is that of T1 shortening.
- Certain clinical indications, such as hyperacute stroke and/or neoplastic evaluations, may benefit from T2* shortening capabilities of these gadolinium-based contrast agent in what have become known as (contrast-enhanced) perfusion-weighted imaging sequences.
- The relaxivity of an agent is that characteristic that describes and quantifies the degree to which a given dose/concentration of the agent shortens the T1 of the tissue(s) that takes it up. Tissue relaxivity properties can be quantified as r1 (describing the magnitude of T1 shortening potentiation relative to delivered dose/concentration in the tissue) and r2 (describing the magnitude of T2* shortening potentiation relative to gadolinium-based contrast agent delivered dose/concentration in the tissue).

INTRODUCTION

The first gadolinium-based contrast agent (GBCA) was approved by the Food and Drug Administration (FDA) for use in the United States on June 28, 1988. In the nearly 25 years that have transpired since that time, the magnetic resonance (MR) industry has seen marked growth in the use and applicability of GBCAs in neuroradiologic imaging. Among the numerous hospitals of the author's institution, the University of Pittsburgh Medical Center, GBCA administration varies from approximately 35% to 60% of all patients who pass through the doors of the MR suite. While early contrast enhanced MR imaging was essentially restricted to post contrast administration spin echo based 2D Fourier transform T1 weighted imaging sequences, we now commonly see contrast administration in conjunction with spin and gradient echo T1 weighted imaging sequences, T2 weighted post Fluid Attenuating Inversion Recovery (FLAIR) imaging, 2D as well as 3D imaging approaches, MR angiography, perfusion

Magnetic Resonance Services, Department of Radiology, University of Pittsburgh Medical Center, Presbyterian University Hospital, Presbyterian South Tower, Room 4776, Pittsburgh, PA 15213-2582, USA
E-mail address: ekanal@pitt.edu

Magn Reson Imaging Clin N Am 20 (2012) 625–631
http://dx.doi.org/10.1016/j.mric.2012.08.004
1064-9689/12/$ – see front matter © 2012 Published by Elsevier Inc.

weighted MR imaging sequences, and other newer, novel imaging techniques. Unlike computed tomography (CT)- and radiography-based contrast agents, whose only true capabilities essentially lie in producing modification of the linear attenuation coefficient of the tissue(s) taking up those agents, the multiparametric nature of MR imaging itself is ideally suited to taking best clinical advantage of the multifactorial, multiple magnetically active properties, or r1 and r2 relaxivities, of these unique and fascinating agents.

BACKGROUND

To more fully appreciate the unique nature of these agents as they interact with the magnetic fields used in the MR imaging process, a review of some of the imaging basics and physical properties at play is in order.

Radiography-based studies such as CT detect and differentiate tissues based on variations in their linear attenuation coefficients (LACs), which, in turn, is heavily based on the electron densities of the tissues through which the homogeneous x-ray beam will pass. The greater the electron density, the greater is the degree of attenuation of the x-ray beam and the whiter that tissue/object will appear on the resultant image. Two adjacent tissues with similar LAC values would therefore be difficult to differentiate on studies using x-ray–based technology. However, if these same 2 tissues differ in, for example, the rate at which an intravascularly administered electron dense contrast agent will reach or perfuse these tissues, one could time the x-ray irradiation event/exposure to coincide with a point in time when the relative electron densities, and therefore LAC values (induced by the variably perfusing contrast agent) of these 2 tissues would be markedly different. This would then produce images with greater densities and whiter depicted tissues from those which, at the time of irradiation, were being heavily perfused by this administered agent, and less from the adjacent and less-perfused, less–electron dense tissue. This is the basis of contrast agent use in CT and indeed all radiography-based studies. Note that with or without the use of an exogenously administered contrast agent, CT- and radiography-based physics remain essentially restricted to detecting and differentiating tissues based on—and only on—their LAC values. It is, in essence, a one-trick pony. It does indeed execute that "trick" astonishingly well, but it remains a one-trick pony nevertheless. If, in the end, the tissue LAC values are similar, then the CT (or other radiography-based) study will fail at contrasting and differentiating those 2 tissues from each other.

Because contrast between a target tissue and its background tissue(s) is a necessary basis for achieving diagnosis, having or creating tissues with significantly different LAC values de facto is a necessary step for CT/radiography–based technology to successfully diagnose that patient.

MR Contrast Agents

The technology for successfully creating diagnostic images in MR is similar, yet simultaneously dissimilar, to that discussed for radiography technology. It is similar in that here, too, the MR imaging system will be attempting to detect a characteristic property of a tissue, and attempting to contrast it against an adjacent tissue for which that same characteristic property at that same time has a significantly different value. Granted, the LAC value per se will not be the tissue characteristic or property that the MR imaging system will detect because today's MR imaging systems cannot detect or directly determine tissue LAC values. Nevertheless, it is still similar in that the MR imaging process will also rely on detecting differences in measured values of a given tissue property that the MR imaging system IS able to detect. The dissimilarities between MR-based technology on the one hand and CT- (and all radiogaphy-based) technology in the other, however, become especially fascinating. Whereas CT- and radiography-based studies have been shown to be one-trick ponies, limited in scope and sensitivity to the single tissue property known as LAC, the MR imaging system can be adjusted to provide sensitivity to any of various tissue properties–some of which are still being discovered and developed as this article is being written! Based on how the MR imaging parameters and variables are selected and adjusted, MR images can be acquired wherein the predominant mechanism of image contrast (that which determines whether a tissue is white, or dark, or anything in between) is dependent on such tissue properties known as T1, or T2, or T2*, or relative proton/hydrogen/spin density, or diffusion, or perfusion, or susceptibility, or gross coherent flow/motion, or "fat based," or "water based," "elasticity based," and so on. Since MR first became a clinical tool in the early 1980s, the industry has repeatedly continued to introduce new parameters for which the MR imaging system hardware/software could be made to be sensitive to detect.

To further strengthen—and complicate—the potential to generate image contrast in MR imaging, we have already noted that image contrast may be dependent on any of various tissue properties, as noted earlier. However, image contrast may also be manipulated to be determined not only by any of these various tissue properties in isolation, but modifying the imaging parameters selected in the MR imaging process can result in image contrast being determined by any combination and "weighting" of any/all the mentioned tissue properties *simultaneously*. These imaging parameters can even be manipulated in such a way as to result in *either* synergistically additive signal or competitively destructive and signal-negating outcomes! This increases the potential number of ways that image contrast could be produced by virtually a factorial of the number of tissue parameters to which the MR imaging system can be adjusted to be able to detect. By means of illustration, an image could be made to be T1-weighted, whereby the predominant mechanism of contrast is determined by the relative T1 values of the tissues being detected such that the shorter the tissue T1 value, the brighter it would be depicted on the image. In contrast to this, another set of MR imaging parameter selections might result in the production of a set of images that would be referred to as T2 weighted, whereby the longer the T2 of the imaged tissue, the brighter it would be depicted on the image. One might modify these choices yet again to this time produce an image that would be referred to as proton density weighted, whereby the higher the concentration per unit volume, or density, of hydrogen nuclei in the tissues being detected, the brighter it would be depicted on the image. If desired, however, one could modify the parameter selection further to produce images wherein its displayed contrast could be dependent on virtually any mathematical combination of these that are desired, such as an image that is partially T2 weighted and partially relative proton density weighted at the same time. There is thus quite literally virtually no end to the number and types of image contrast combinations and "weightings," as it were, that are available to the multiparametrically sensitive MR imaging system and its knowledgeable, experienced operator.

In this light, one can rapidly recognize that a contrast agent for an MR study would be any agent that has the ability to modify ANY of the tissue parameters to which MR imaging systems have been demonstrated to be sensitively able to detect—and/or any agent that can modify any combination of such tissue parameters.

Gadolinium-Based Contrast Agents: T1-Shortening Effects

This dizzying potential is brought under some modicum of clinical control by the early clinical availability of very few MR contrast agents. Indeed, at the initial FDA approval and clinical release of MR contrast agents in 1988 and for almost 2 decades thereafter, the clinically available MR contrast agents (at least those used for neuroradiologic imaging, which represented, and still represents, the extreme majority of all contrast-enhanced MR imaging to date) were based on the same "active ingredient," and therefore all functioned via the same mechanism of action. They all relied on the predominantly T1-shortening property of the gadolinium ion, which has resulted in these GBCAs being used predominantly the same way—as T1-shortening agents, which, when acquiring so-called T1-weighted images, enhanced the signal most from the tissues into which these intravenously administered contrast agents were able to rapidly perfuse and then leak into their extracellular fluid spaces. The higher the administered dose and, most important, the higher the concentration of the agent in the extracellular fluid space of the tissue at the time that it was being imaged, the greater was the T1 shortening and therefore signal intensity of that tissue on T1-weighted images. The various agents released and FDA approved did have some differences, but their similarities—including and especially in efficacies, reported safety profiles, biodistributions, and half-lives—far outweighed any clinically relevant differences between them.

Thus, after these GBCAs were first approved for use in humans, their clinical applicability was moderately simple and straightforward, given that the industry found itself implementing relatively few, fixed types of imaging sequences (ie, tissue parameter sensitivities) for which contrast has been clinically applied to date. Practically speaking, then, for years following the FDA approval of the first GBCA in 1988, MR contrast agents were used for, and only for, shortening the T1 values of tissues that might differentially take up these administered agents, such that the tissue that took up the agent would be depicted as brighter (because of its shortened T1 value and therefore faster longitudinal magnetization recovery rate) than other tissues that either did not take up the administered contrast agent or did so at a notably slower rate. This "T1 weighted imaging" enhancement served as the basis for clinical GBCA administration for almost 2 decades.

GBCAs: T2*-Shortening Effects

It was just a matter of time until the medical community recognized that there were also T2*-shortening properties inherent in these same magnetically active FDA-approved GBCAs. One could generate an MR imaging procedure that would be intentionally designed to emphasize the T2* properties of the imaged tissues, such that the shorter the T2* of the imaged tissue, the weaker was its signal and the darker it would appear on the resultant image, with longer T2* tissues appearing relatively brighter. On such imaging sequences, if these same GBCAs would be administered before image acquisition, their r2 (and therefore T2*-shortening) properties would produce signal *loss* from those tissues in whom these agents had achieved greatest concentration at time of imaging, with less signal loss and, therefore, greater relative signal from other tissues in which the GBCA concentration at time of imaging was lower. Further, as with the T1-shortening effect induced by the r1 properties of these agents, the greater the concentration of these agents in the tissues at the time of imaging, the greater was the T2*-shortening effect and, therefore, the greater was the induced signal loss in that tissue on the resultant image. This was found to be most clinically useful in assessing differences in macrovascularity and microvascularity and therefore rates of perfusion between tissues being images. By rapidly injecting a bolus of these GBCAs and ensuring that the image data acquisition transpired during the first passage, and therefore greatest concentration, of the administered GBCAs, the degree of signal loss was maximized in the tissue that perfused most rapidly. This was found to be of greatest clinical benefit in evaluating hyperacute ischemic events in which such perfusion-weighted studies can be rapidly performed and provide near real-time information as to tissue perfusion and, therefore, viability. Such perfusion-weighted imaging (ie, bolus GBCA administration coupled with carefully timed T2*-weighted imaging techniques) has also been successfully clinically applied to neoplastic processes, whereby the degree of vascularity often corresponds to clinically manifest aggressiveness of many malignancies.

Relaxivity

As noted earlier, the predominant application of a GBCA in the medical community was (and remains to this day) to provide T1 shortening and thus signal enhancement to the tissues that take up that agent. Practically speaking, the concept of "relaxivity" was neither discussed nor widely understood. This status quo first began to change around 2005. Again, a bit of introductory background information will prove useful.

Between June 1988 and November 2004, the 4 MR contrast agents for neuroradiologic application in the United States were gadopentetate dimeglumine (Magnevist, Bayer Healthcare, Germany), gadodiamide (Omniscan, General Electric Healthcare, USA), gadoversetamide (Optimark,

Covidien), and gadoteridol (Prohance, Bracco Diagnostics, Italy). We have discussed that the administration of any of these GBCAs results in shortening of the tissue T1 properties (for the tissues that take up the agent into their extracellular spaces) and produces faster longitudinal magnetization recovery and therefore greater signal intensity on T1-weighted images for these tissues than they would otherwise have displayed had these GBCAs not been administered. Also noted was that the greater the concentration of any of these GBCAs in the tissue's extracellular spaces (at the time imaging data are collected), the greater is the T1-shortening effect and, therefore, signal intensity on T1-weighted images. What has not been discussed, however, is the relative behavior of the approved agents. Put another way, if equal doses of these agents would be administered to the patient, would the degree of signal enhancement in that same tissue be expected to be the same—or different—among these agents?

Conceptually, what is being touched on can be thought of as the relative "potency," in a sense, of the T1-shortening abilities among these GBCAs. If one were to administer the identical dose of each of these GBCAs to the patient, would the resultant acquired T1-weighted images be indistinguishable from each other, or would the degree of signal enhancement produced by the presence of one or more of these agents yield significantly more T1 shortening, and therefore signal, from that tissue than it would from other FDA-approved neuroradiologic GBCAs?

The concept being discussed—namely, the magnitude of T1 shortening (and, most important, signal enhancement) relative to the administered dose—can be summarized by one word: Relaxivity. Specifically, the r1 relaxivity of a GBCA describes how efficiently a GBCA shortens the tissue/sample T1 at a given concentration. Measured in units of per millimoles per second, the greater the r1, the greater is the T1 shortening and, therefore, the greater is the produced signal intensity on T1-weighted images for any given concentration of the agent.

Returning to the original discussion, the reason that relaxivity was an almost unknown quantity among radiologists for nearly 20 years of clinical use of 4 different FDA-approved neuroradiologic GBCAs is because the relative relaxivities of these agents was found to be, from a clinical point of view, interchangeable. Put another way, the degree of clinically observed signal enhancement from similar administered doses of gadopentetate dimeglumine, gadodiamide, gadoversetamide, and gadoteridol was thought to be essentially the same. No claims of competitive signal intensity advantages or increases in diagnostic accuracy from using one of these agents relative to another were made. There are reported differences in the measured relaxivities among the various FDA-approved neuroradiologic GBCAs, to be sure.[1,2] However, the clinical impact of these reported different relative r1 relaxivities proved to be sufficiently similar such that any differences that might mathematically exist among their measured r1 relaxivities did not reach clinically detectable or significant levels.

In 2004, however, the FDA approved the first GBCA for neuroradiologic application that had a significantly and clinically detectable higher r1 relaxivity than did the others that had been FDA approved to that date. When released, gadobenate dimeglumine (Multihance, Bracco Diagnostics, Italy) reported an r1 relaxivity that was substantially higher at practical clinically commonly used static MR imaging field strengths than the other available GBCAs that had been used to that time. Further, numerous comparative studies began to appear in the peer-reviewed literature that bore out the clinically detectable impact of this more potent T1-shortening ability per unit of administered dose of this agent in the form of increased sensitivity to lesion detection, increased ratio of lesion to background contrast, and improved diagnostic performance for various diseases compared to identical administered doses of lower relaxivity GBCAs.

Since the FDA approval of gadobenate dimeglumine in 2004, all new GBCAs approved by the FDA have been higher relaxivity agents. These include gadofosveset (Ablavar; for contrast-enhanced MR angiographic indications), gadoxetate disodium (Eovist; for hepatic imaging indications), and gadobutrol (Gadavist (Bayer Healthcare, Germany); for neuroradiologic indications). Comparative human studies for neuroradiologic imaging have just started to appear for the more recently approved gadobutrol. Interestingly, despite its higher reported relaxivity in human blood plasma than the 4 lower relaxivity agents just noted (1.5T r1 values of 5.2 L/mmol/s for gadobutrol relative to 4.1 for gadopentetate dimeglumine and 6.3 for gadobenate dimeglumine as reported by Pintaske and colleagues[1] when measured in human blood plasma, or 1.5T r1 values of 4.7 L/mmol/s for gadobutrol relative to 3.9 for gadopentetate dimeglumine and 7.9 for gadobenate dimeglumine as reported by Rohrer and colleagues[2] when measured in bovine plasma), it is reported to have an essential interchangeable diagnostic accuracy compared with gadoteridol, one of the lower relaxivity agents (65.1% accuracy of diagnosis for gadobutrol versus 65.5% for gadoteridol in 229 patients).[3] This seems to document that despite mathematically higher r1 values

for gadobutrol than the lower relaxivity agents such as gadoteridol, the magnitude of any r1 differences between gadobutrol and gadoteridol was not sufficiently higher to be of clinical diagnostic accuracy relevance. In a more recent direct comparison of gadobutrol to gadobenate dimeglumine when the same subjects were administered each agent at identical and clinically indicated doses and reexamined a few days apart,[4] significantly increased lesion enhancement and contrast-to-noise ratio was observed between the enhancing pathology/lesion and the nonenhancing brain for the higher r1 relaxivity gadobenate dimeglumine than for the lower r1 relaxivity gadobutrol despite both being labeled as high relaxivity agents.

It should be noted that GBCA relaxivites are not constant and, in fact, may vary considerably under certain conditions, including and especially by field strength. In general, for most GBCAs, relaxivities decrease with increasing static magnetic field strengths. However, as documented so well by Laurent and colleagues[5] and as explained further by Giesel and colleagues,[6] because of the known protein binding property of gadobenate dimeglumine with human serum albumin (HSA) and the lack of significant protein binding for gadopentetate dimeglumine, Dotarem (Guerbet Corporation, France), gadodiamide, gadoteridol, and gadobutrol, this agent specifically exhibits increased r1 relaxivities at all tested field strengths, and especially so from the 0.3T to 1.5T range, compared with that which it would have been predicted to exhibit had there been no significant interactions and protein binding between gadobenate dimeglumine and HSA. The measured increased r1 relaxivities for gadobenate dimeglumine with increasing concentrations of HSA and the lack of significant increased r1 relaxivities with increasing concentrations of HSA for gadopentetate dimeglumine and gadobutrol further confirm the role of protein binding for specifically this agent in creating its higher r1 relaxivity values. Rohrer and colleagues'[2] observation of a relative decrease in r1 relaxivity advantage of gadobenate dimeglumine relative to gadobutrol or gadopentetate dimeglumine in water as opposed to plasma (4.0 for gadobenate dimeglumine, 3.3 for gadobutrol, 3.3 for gadopentetate dimeglumine at 1.5T) is further evidence of the clinical role that HSA binding plays with this, and only this, neuroradiologic GBCA.

Finally, it should be pointed out that all the arguments presented here explaining and demonstrating the advantages provided by higher r1 relaxivity agents for T1-weighted imaging applications apply in parallel to higher r2 relaxivity agents on T2*-weighted imaging. In such circumstances, at identical administered doses (technically, at higher concentrations in the extracellular spaces of the tissues being studied), the higher the r2, the greater is the signal loss on the same T2*-weighted imaging sequence and thus the greater the signal *loss* from these tissues. Although not clinically used as much as is postcontrast T1-weighted imaging today, higher r2 relaxivity agents would be expected to demonstrate similar clinical contrast-to-noise ratio advantages relative to lower r2 GBCAs at equivalent administered doses in more powerfully darkening the signal from the tissues that take up these agents compared with lower r2 GBCAs on T2*-weighted MR imaging examinations. This may well be even more evident at higher fields in which the clinical effects of shortening T2* are markedly more pronounced than they are at lower static magnetic field strength MR imaging systems. Further, higher concentrations of GBCA should also prove advantageous in providing for increased signal loss from those tissues taking up the agent compared to those agents with lower gadolinium concentrations. Of all the FDA approved neuroradiologic GBCA today, only gadobutrol is distributed at 1.0 molar concentrations, which is twice that of the 0.5 molar concentration found in each of the other FDA-approved neuroradiologic GBCAs available today.

Dose Versus Volume

One final point that should be stressed is that of the GBCAs FDA approved for neuroradiologic indications today, all but one are distributed in the same concentration, and all but one are approved to be administered at the same, standard dose. Specifically, gadopentetate dimeglumine, gadobenate dimeglumine, gadodiamide, gadoversetamide, and gadoteridol are all distributed as 0.5 Molar solutions. Gadobutrol is distributed at twice that concentration, namely, at 1.0 Molar. However, note that all 6 of these FDA-approved neuroradiologic GBCAs are approved to be administered to humans at 0.1 mmol/kg doses (with the additional exception that under certain specific situations, gadoteridol is also FDA approved to be administered at a total of triple dose, or a total administered dose of 0.3 mmol/kg for 1 MR imaging examination (this will be discussed in greater detail momentarily)). Thus, because all are approved to be administered to humans at the same delivered dose (ie, the same amount of gadolinium ions per patient mass) and because the concentration of gadolinium ions in gadobutrol is twice that of all the other 5 FDA-approved neuroradiologic GBCAs, this would mean that the *volume* of gadobutrol to

be administered to patients for standard-dose administration should be half of that which it would be for any of the other 5 neuroradiologic GBCAs. For example, a 70-kg patient receiving 0.1 mmol/kg of a 0.5 Molar concentration of gadopentetate dimeglumine, gadobenate dimeglumine, gadodiamide, gadoversetamide, or gadoteridol would receive 0.2 mL/kg or 14 mL of any of these agents as a standard-dose administration. At twice the concentration, or 1.0 mol/L concentration of gadobutrol, that same patient, to receive the same approved standard dose, would receive 0.1 mL/kg, or 7 mL, of gadobutrol. Thus, 7 mL of gadobutrol is precisely the equivalent delivered gadolinium dose to the patient as 14 mL of gadopentetate dimeglumine, gadobenate dimeglumine, gadodiamide, gadoversetamide, or gadoteridol, and would all constitute a standard dose for a 70-kg patient.

Note, however, that today the only agent that carries an FDA labeling approving a higher than standard dose administration is gadoteridol, which under specific circumstances is FDA approved to be administered at a total of triple dose, or 0.3 mmol/kg (which is the same as a delivered volume of 0.6 mL/kg of this half molar concentration solution).

SUMMARY

There has been much progress in contrast enhanced neuroradiologic MR imaging in the almost 25 years since the first GBCA was FDA approved in the United States. Much of this now focuses on the introduction of significantly higher relaxivity agents into the clinical armamentarium and the addition of T2*-weighted imaging sequences (eg, perfusion-weighted imaging) to hyperacute stroke or neoplastic evaluations. All 4 MR contrast agents that are FDA approved in the United States during the past decade have been higher relaxivity agents than what had been previously available, suggesting a strong trend in our industry to continue to find more efficient, more powerful, more diagnostic means of increasing contrast on MR imaging studies between pathologic conditions and the more normal background tissue against which it is being detected and differentiated.

REFERENCES

1. Pintaske J, Martirosian P, Graf H, et al. Relaxivity of gadopentetate dimeglumine (Magnevist), gadobutrol (Gadovist), and gadobenate dimeglumine (MultiHance) in human blood plasma at 0.2, 1.5, and 3 Tesla. Invest Radiol 2006;41(3):213–21.

2. Rohrer M, Bauer H, Mintorovitch J, et al. Comparison of magnetic properties of MRI contrast media solutions at different magnetic field strengths. Invest Radiol 2005;40:715–24.

3. Text, Table 10, Briefing Document for Gadobutrol Injection, NDA 201,277, Bayer HealthCare Pharmaceuticals, as submitted to the FDA Peripheral & Central Nervous System Drugs Advisory Committee, January 21, 2011.

4. Seidl Z, Vymazal J, Mechl M, et al. Does higher gadolinium concentration play a role in the morphologic assessment of brain tumors? Results of a multicenter intraindividual crossover comparison of gadobutrol versus gadobenate dimeglumine (the MERIT study). Am J Neuroradiol 2012;33(6):1050–8.

5. Laurent S, Elst LV, Muller RN. Comparative study of the physicochemical properties of six clinical low molecular weight gadolinium contrast agents. Contrast Media Mol Imaging 2006;1:128–37.

6. Giesel FL, von Tengg-Kobligk H, Wilkinson ID, et al. Influence of human serum albumin on longitudinal and transverse relaxation rates (R1 and R2) of magnetic resonance contrast agents. Invest Radiol 2006;41(3):222–8.

Use of Contrast Media in Neuroimaging

Marco Essig, MD[a],*, Julien Dinkel, MD[b],
Juan E. Gutierrez, MD[c]

KEYWORDS

- CNS imaging • Contrast media • DSC-perfusion MRI • Dynamic contrast enhanced MRI

KEY POINTS

- Gadolinium-based contrast media are routinely used in most CNS MR imaging indications, including assessment of CNS tumors, vascular pathologies, infections, degenerative diseases, and posttreatment imaging.
- Contrast media is applied to improve the sensitivity and specificity of CNS diseases and to allow a better treatment decision, planning, and follow-up.
- The standard dose used is 0.1 mmol/kg of body weight, with some exceptions that allow injection of up to a triple dose.
- More recently, contrast media have also been used to allow the measurement of tissue perfusion and to follow the time course of enhancement in dynamic contrast-enhanced imaging or dynamic MR angiography studies.
- With the presence of the BBB, contrast media does not leak into the tissue. Only vascular structures and areas of the brain that have no BBB (choroid plexus, pineal and anterior lobe of pituitary gland) physiologically enhance after contrast injection. The mechanisms of tissue enhancement in the brain are related to a higher vascularity of the pathology or a disruption of the BBB.
- Tissue enhancement is, besides the degree of BBB, disruption further dependent on the applied magnetic field strength, with higher field providing a better enhancement and the applied dose of contrast media.

INTRODUCTION

The goals and indications of central nervous (CNS) or neuroimaging are multiple and involve detection of pathologies, including making a precise diagnosis and a differential diagnosis, and detection of disease complications that require an immediate intervention and proved to be an essential part of the decision-making process for therapy. In the case of neoplastic disorders, for example, neuroimaging can precisely define the location and accurately delineate the lesion before intervention. In the case of radiation oncology, it should precisely define and demarcate the margins for targeted intervention. Neuroimaging is also mandatory after any therapeutic intervention for monitoring of disease and for detection and monitoring of possible side effects.

In emergency medicine, computed tomography (CT) assumes a critical role for the evaluation of traumatic and nontraumatic evaluations.[1] CT scanners are fast and widely available, which makes CT a great choice for assessment of neurologic or

Disclosures: M.E.: Consultant Bayer Healthcare, Speaker for Bayer Healthcare and Bracco; J.D.: None; J.E.G.: Speaker Bureau Bayer Healthcare.
[a] Department of Neuroradiology, University of Erlangen-Nuremberg, Schwabachanlage 6, Erlangen 91054, Germany; [b] Department of Radiology, Massachusetts General Hospital, MA, USA; [c] Department of Radiology, University of Texas Health Science Center, San Antonio, TX, USA
* Corresponding author.
E-mail address: marco.essig@uk-erlangen.de

Magn Reson Imaging Clin N Am 20 (2012) 633–648
http://dx.doi.org/10.1016/j.mric.2012.08.001
1064-9689/12/$ – see front matter © 2012 Elsevier Inc. All rights reserved.

neurosurgical emergencies. Usually, a conventional noncontrast brain CT is performed in an emergency to detect, for example, fractures and intracranial bleeding, and also to exclude tumors and subdural/extradural hematomas. Nevertheless, the intrinsic tissue contrast is limited in the CT images. Neuroimaging with CT relies, therefore, deeply on contrast media to improve lesion detection (sensitivity) and characterization (specificity).[2] Furthermore, contrast agents can be used for functional assessment of physiologic process: the blood perfusion and for the depiction of the vessel compartment (angiography/venography). In CT angiography, the images are obtained a few seconds after high-flow contrast injection and most of the observed enhancement is intravascular. When CT acquisition is delayed for 10 to 15 minutes after contrast agent injection, most of the observed enhancement is interstitial. When CT imaging is done at intermediate times, the enhancement reflects a combination of both intravascular and interstitial components.

Because of its high tissue contrast and noninvasiveness, magnetic resonance (MR) imaging is accepted as the most sensitive method for diagnosing diseases of the CNS.[3,4] MR imaging enables accurate recognition and determination of the dimensions of CNS pathologies and their surrounding tissue. This requires a high CNS-to-lesion contrast, which both depends on the signal intensity of the lesion relative to that of the surrounding normal tissue and the best description of the physiologic tissue and vasculature not affected. Furthermore, detailed information on the internal morphology of the lesion is essential for differential diagnosis, grading, and for the selection and planning of therapy.

Although MR imaging using standard nonenhanced T1-weighted and T2-weighted sequences has proven to be very sensitive in the detection of pathologic lesions, for most CNS diseases and for many of the currently available functional MR imaging methods, the use of MR contrast media is mandatory. The standard dose used for MR imaging of the CNS is 0.1 mmol/kg body weight, although numerous studies have shown that lesion detection may be improved with the use of higher doses and dedicated sequences.[5,6] A higher dosage also allows for the combination of a number of advanced, mostly contrast-enhanced MR imaging techniques that have been developed that provide new insights into the pathophysiology of CNS diseases, as well as to better describe the angioarchitecture using contrast-enhanced MR angiography (CE-MRA). One of these techniques, perfusion MR imaging, is now recognized as an important new means for assessing tumor grading and follow-up of various treatment strategies or to better assess cerebrovascular diseases. Another of these techniques, dynamic contrast-enhanced MR imaging, is also gaining acceptance for the same purposes. In this article, the reader is provided with the fundamental features of the contrast mechanisms in MR imaging neuroimaging, the basic methodologies and the first clinical experience with the contrast-enhanced functional imaging tools, and some of the classical indications for contrast media. The different properties of the currently available contrast media and the dosage and field dependencies have been discussed in the article by Dr. Kanal, elsewhere in this issue.

In neuroimaging, pathologic enhancement can occur in several regions:

1. Abnormal enhancement within vessels without breakdown of the blood-brain-barrier (BBB), which reflects neovascularity, macrovasodilatation or microvasodilatation (aneurysm), and shortened transit time or shunting, including arteriovenous malformations (**Fig. 1**).
2. Extra-axial lesions with no BBB, such as meningioma, acoustic schwannoma, or granulomatous disease.
3. Breakdown of BBB with leakage of contrast, including neoplastic disease, infection, infarction, inflammation with demyelinating disease, and trauma.

LISTING AND DEFINITION OF CONTRAST MEDIA INDICATIONS
Mechanism of Contrast Enhancement in CNS

Owing to the presence of the BBB, the currently available contrast media do not leak into the brain tissue.[7,8] Only vascular structures and areas of the brain that have no BBB (choroid plexus, pineal and anterior lobe of pituitary gland) physiologically enhance after contrast injection. The BBB consists of a complex of capillary endothelial cells, pericytes, and astroglial and perivascular macrophages and serves as an effective physical barrier to the entry of lipophobic substances into the brain.[7] The BBB blocks all molecules except those that cross cell membranes by means of lipid solubility (such as oxygen, carbon dioxide, ethanol, and steroid hormones) and those that are allowed in by specific transport systems (such as sugars and some amino acids). Substances with a molecular weight higher than 180 Da, which include all available imaging contrast media, generally cannot cross the BBB.[9]

The integrity of the BBB can be altered by a variety of pathologic and physiologic circumstances that increase the permeability, both for contrast media

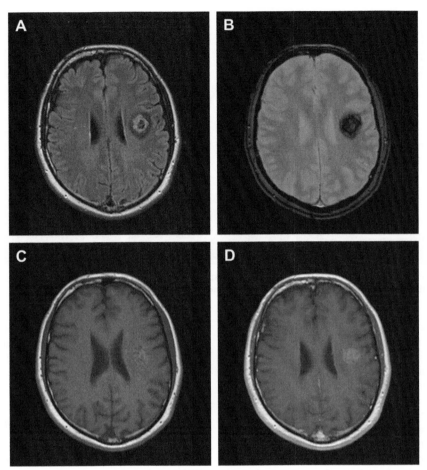

Fig. 1. Fluid attenuated inversion recovery (FLAIR) (*A*), gradient-echo T2 (*B*), T1 spin echo (SE) (*C*), and contrast-enhanced T1 SE (*D*) in a patient with cerebral arteriovenous malformations. The malformation presents on FLAIR and T2 a signal drop, which is partially related to flow-void and partially attributable to microbleedings. The high signal on unenhanced T1 is attributable to blood, the marked contrast enhancement represents vascularization in the center of the malformation.

and drug delivery. A disruption of the BBB may be caused by osmotic means (eg, steroids), biochemically by the use of vasoactive substances, such as bradykinin, or even by localized exposure to focused ultrasound.[10–13] In addition, the permeability of the BBB can be increased by inflammation (either infectious or noninfectious), hypertension, or cerebral ischemia.[2,14] Moreover, common physiologic processes such as hyperemia (of primary or secondary cause) and neovascularity usually have increased blood volume and blood flow. Abnormal hyperenhancement is usually a result of a combination of increased blood volume/flow and capillary permeability.

Mechanisms of Extra-axial Contrast Enhancement

In extra-axial benign or malignant processes, enhancement occurs because extracerebral vessels (located within the dura mater) do not have a BBB. A leakage of contrast agent is therefore possible in the interstitial compartment and a slightly dural enhancement is seen on MR imaging. After neurosurgery or sometimes lumbar puncture, a diffuse, thick linear dural enhancement may occur and is probably attributable to postintervention inflammatory changes and intracranial hypotension.[15,16] The pressure exercised on the veins in the subarachnoid space drops when the cerebrospinal fluid pressure is low, enabling vasodilatation and edema.[17] Furthermore, patients having intracranial hypotension are predisposed to subdural hemorrhage after minor trauma as a result of "stretching" of the dural veins.

The most frequent primary extra-axial tumor is the meningioma (**Fig. 2**): a tumor of meningiothelial cells arising from the arachnoid. This neoplasm is rarely malignant and enhances strongly after contrast medium injection because of the lack of BBB. A thickening of the neighbored dura at the

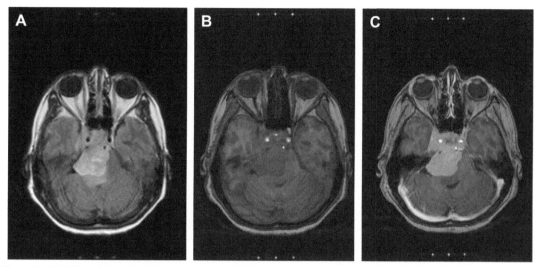

Fig. 2. FLAIR (*A*), T1 (*B*), and contrast-enhanced T1 fast spin echo (FSE) (*C*) in a patient with skull base meningeoma representing a strong and homogeneous enhancement in an extra-axial tumor without a BBB.

edge of the menigioma is often seen; this is the "dura tail" reflecting edema and congestion of the dura.[18–20]

Extra-axial malignant tumors show a contrast enhancement because of the lack of BBB and the presence of angiogenesis (see the following section, Mechanisms of Contrast Enhancement in Intra-axial Brain Tumors). The most common extra-axial malignant neoplasm is the metastatic disease carcinomatous meningitis (**Fig. 3**), usually arising from breast carcinoma in women and prostate cancer in men.

Granulomatous diseases, including sarcoid, tuberculosis, Wegener granulomatous, and rheumatoid nodules, may produce enhancing meningeal nodules without presence of neo-angiogenesis. The mechanisms of enhancement in infectious meningitis are more complex and involve additionally the release of inflammatory mediators facilitating the disruption of the BBB and sometimes leakage of contrast agent in the cerebrospinal fluid.[21]

Mechanisms of Contrast Enhancement in Intra-axial Brain Tumors

In intra-axial primary tumors, mainly gliomas, the BBB can be compromised by neovascularization and direct tumorous damage. Because non-neoplastic astrocytes are required to induce BBB features of cerebral endothelial cells, it is conceivable that malignant astrocytes have lost this ability owing to dedifferentiation. Alternatively, glioma cells might actively degrade previously intact

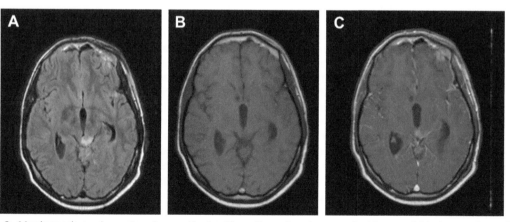

Fig. 3. Meningeosis carcinomatosa in a patient with malignant melanoma. Besides a solid lesion on FLAIR (*A*) with solid enhancing center (*C*), a meningeal enhancement is present in both hemispheres. The unenhanced SE sequences (*B*) did not visualize the meningeal involvement.

BBB tight junctions.[22,23] Although the integrity of the barrier is often compromised within the tumor, this alteration in permeability is variable and dependent on the tumor type and size. Moreover, it is extremely heterogeneous in a given lesion (**Fig. 4**).[24] Although the BBB is frequently leaky in the center of malignant brain tumors, the well-vascularized actively proliferating edge of the tumor, in the brain adjacent to tumor area, has been shown to have variable and complex barrier integrity. In secondary, metastatic intra-axial tumors, the vessels are different from normal cerebral vasculature and have no or strongly disturbed BBB.[25,26] The enhancement pattern is therefore more homogeneous than in primary tumor.

As brain edema is also thought to be attributable to breakdown of the BBB, one can expect a correlation between the degree of enhancement and the volume of the peritumoral edema. Holodny and colleagues[27–29] studied this correlation in malignant gliomas as a representative of primary intra-axial tumors and meningeomas as representative of an extra-axial tumor. In their study, no correlation was found for meningeomas, which proved that the meningeoma vessels have no BBB or no effect on the BBB in the surrounding brain tissue. For malignant gliomas, a strong correlation was found, which offers evidence that the defect of the BBB is directly both related to the degree of lesion enhancement and amount of edema and both should interfere between each other. The interference may influence both the conventional contrast-enhanced imaging as well as some of the flow-dependent functional imaging MR techniques. The contrast-enhancement patterns change substantially after corticosteroid treatment, as first presented by the group of Sheffield.[30]

However, the concept of permeability across a disrupted or disturbed BBB in patients with brain tumor has recently gained further interest in monitoring modern treatment strategies. First, changes in permeability may serve as a surrogate marker for other important physiologic processes in brain tumors, such as angiogenesis. Second, an understanding of permeability can elucidate the mechanisms by which therapeutic agents enter brain parenchyma. Third, an understanding of methods for increasing permeability can help in the development of methods to selectively alter the BBB to enhance drug delivery.

Modern MR-neuroimaging strategies, such as dynamic contrast-enhanced MR imaging, focus on the visualization and quantification of the BBB breakdown, which is described in detail in the article on dynamic MR imaging, elsewhere in this issue.

Mechanisms of Contrast Enhancement in Cerebral Infection

Encephalitis

Viral encephalitis usually occurs either as a direct effect of an acute infection, or as one of the sequelae of a latent infection. Sometimes, a serpentine contrast enhancement along gyri can be observed in the subacute phase. In the particular case of herpes virus encephalitis, the contrast enhancement is usually located in the superficial gray matter, often in the medial temporal lobes and in the cingulated gyrus of the medial frontal and parietal lobes.[31–34] Pathologic specimens reveal spots of petechial hemorrhage and inflammation in almost every case. The slight contrast enhancement is attributable to the inflammatory

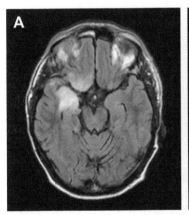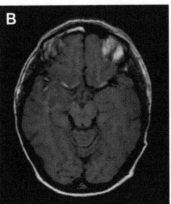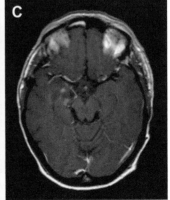

Fig. 4. FLAIR (A), T1 SE (B), and contrast-enhanced T1 SE (C) in a patient with suspected low-grade astrocytoma. The lesion appears to be homogeneous on the unenhanced sequences. The small central enhancement is suspicious for an anaplastic transformation, which was confirmed in the histologic examination.

reaction with altered permeability of the native vessels.

Abscess

Contiguous spread of severe sinus or mastoid infection through the dura is the main cause of pyogenic infections of the brain. Less frequently, cerebral abscesses are attributable to hematogenous septic emboli or occur after trauma.[35] After an initial unorganized, poor demarcated inflammation, the immune system will circumscribe the infection in an abscess, forming a membrane made with granulation tissue and collagen layer, which is surrounded by a layer of astrogliosis.[36,37] Perifocal edema is always present. The well-defined ring enhancement of the wall is attributable to the increased permeability of the capillaries in the granulation tissue (**Fig. 5**). In addition, the vascularity is augmented within the abscess wall. Typically, pyogenic abscesses demonstrate restricted

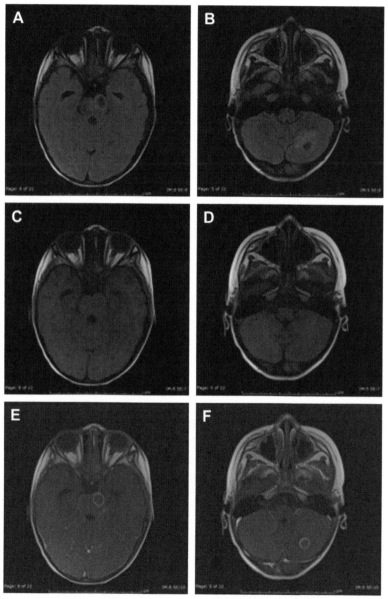

Fig. 5. A 2-year-old male patient with cerebral tuberculosis. The patient presented with hyponatremia of unknown etiology, slightly hypertensive, and with pneumonia The MR imaging with T2 FLAIR (*A, B*), T1 FSE unenhanced (*C, D*), and T1 FSE contrast enhanced (*E, F*) shows 2 abscess typical dominant peripherally enhancing centrally isodense to brain parenchyma lesions within the left pons and left cerebellum. Additionally, there is a small circumference of the edema around these lesions.

diffusion on diffusion-weighted imaging (DWI), owing to the high viscosity of pus, and there is usually a decreased perfusion within the central portion and in the region of surrounding edema. The perfusion is increased only in the contrast-enhanced wall (or in the very closeness of it). Intracranial fungal infection may have findings similar to bacterial infection, and if a patient is immunocompromised, fungal infection should be considered.

Mechanism of Contrast Enhancement in Multiple Sclerosis

The enhancement of multiple sclerosis (MS) plaques is usually seen during the "active phase," and this enhancement lasts for 2 to 6 weeks and rarely longer. The pathophysiological cause of enhancement in the MS demyelination lesions is attributable to inflammation only. That is why the enhancement of MS plaques is usually faint, because the inflammation is limited to the perivenular/perivascular area, and is not accompanied by angiogenesis or relevant permeability changes of the BBB. This is also the reason why there is usually no perilesional vasogenic edema.

The enhancing rim may be thin and sometimes incomplete with an appearance of an "open ring" sign.[38,39] This appearance strongly suggests demyelination process and is usually to be distinguished from those of an abscess (which typically has a surrounding edema) and necrotic neoplasm (which has a thick rim). An "incomplete ring" may be seen in active demyelination, both in MS and in tumefactive demyelination.[40] If MS is suspected, MR imaging of the spinal cord may demonstrate additional lesions to help support the diagnosis; however, although imaging may help, the diagnosis of MS remains a clinical diagnosis.

Use of Contrast Media in Stroke Assessment

In the event of suspected acute stroke assessment, a conventional noncontrast brain CT is usually performed before starting any therapy to detect intracerebral hemorrhage that is contraindicated for thrombolytic treatment and also to exclude tumors, vascular malformations, or subdural/extradural hematomas that can imitate the clinical symptoms of stroke. The early signs of acute ischemic stroke can be very subtle, however (hyperdense middle cerebral artery sign, hypoattenuation in basal ganglia, edema in insular cortex, disappearance of gray-white matter discrimination, and midline shift because of edema). Noncontrast CT has limited sensitivity for the diagnosis of ischemic stroke in the initial hours. Improved accuracy of stroke diagnosis, such as perfusion or diffusion-

weighted MR imaging is therefore mandatory.[41,42] Although CT or MRA helps in identification of vascular occlusion and collateral blood supplies, perfusion imaging provides additional information about the extension and hemodynamic status of ischemic tissue.[43]

Use of Contrast Media for Functional Imaging Techniques

Today there are several indications for cerebral perfusion imaging. The major indications in which perfusion MR imaging is routinely used in increasing numbers of imaging centers include cerebrovascular disease, tumor imaging, infectious diseases, epilepsy, and, most recently, psychiatric disorders such as Alzheimer disease and schizophrenia. Because of the radiation dose, perfusion CT is performed mainly in cerebrovascular disease or tumor imaging.

CT AND MR PERFUSION IN STROKE

The acquisition procedure consists of rapid, repetitive, or continuous scanning through a defined volume of interest immediately before and during the injection of a bolus of contrast agent. In CT, the changes in attenuation, expressed in Hounsfield units, are measured during the contrast injection and reflect the changes in contrast agent concentration. Even with large multidetector CT, perfusion CT does not allow for whole-brain perfusion assessment. But a modern CT scanner with 64-row or 128-row multidetector CT allows for volumetric coverage of 3 to 4 cm in length and the acquisition is usually done at the basal ganglia level.

In MR, very fast sequences allow for whole brain evaluation over a period of usually 30 to 60 seconds at a temporal resolution of 1 image every 1 to 2 seconds. During the perfusion scan, the passage of a bolus of contrast agent is recorded through the vasculature of the brain. After the acquisition is completed, data are analyzed through dedicated postprocessing and is mathematically transformed into quantitative parameters using a kinetic model of cerebral perfusion.[44] The parameters obtained are the cerebral blood flow (CBF), cerebral blood volume (CBV), mean transit time (MTT), and time to peak (TTP). The MTT can be calculated through the division of CBV/CBF and reflects the time between the arterial inflow and the venous outflow. TTP refers to the time taken by the contrast medium to achieve maximum enhancement in the selected region of interest. CBV is the volume of blood available per unit of brain tissue.

In stroke imaging, MR DWI can identify the regions of the brain that have already succumbed to ischemia The cytotoxic edema seen on MR diffusion reflects the volume of dead brain tissue and has an important prognostic value.[45] However, perfusion imaging has the potential to assess the volume of potentially salvageable brain tissue and the extension and severity of the ischemia. Therefore, perfusion imaging has increased relevance in the therapeutic management of the patient.

In an ischemic stroke, the decrease of the blood flow to a particular area of the brain is compensated to some extent by collateral supply from normal surrounding vessels and from leptomeningeal vessels. The peripheral region where the compensation occurs is called the penumbra and is potentially salvageable by thrombolytic therapy.[46]

In CBF decrease, owing to any cause, the cerebral autoregulation ensures adequate CBV by vasodilatation (increase in MTT and CBV). When CBF reaches a critical level (20%–30% of its normal value), the mechanisms of blood supply compensation are exceeded and the CBV and CBF decrease. The brain compensates the diminution of CBF by increasing the extraction of oxygen from the blood. If both CBF and CBV fall below 30% or 40% of the normal value, the oxygen metabolism is disrupted, causing cellular dysfunction and eventually irreversible damages for CBF values below 10 mL/100 g/min.[47]

PERFUSION IN BRAIN TUMOR

Perfusion imaging in brain tumors has benefits for 3 major fields: differential diagnosis, biopsy planning, and treatment monitoring. Together with other imaging methods, such as DWI and spectroscopic, perfusion imaging has the ability to provide quantitative cellular, hemodynamic, and metabolic information about brain tumor biology.

Brain tumors are a heterogeneous group of neoplasms with a correspondingly wide variation in histology and a variety of imaging features. Accurate diagnosis and grading of brain tumors, however, is critical to determine prognosis and therapy schemes that base on the 3 main columns: surgery, radiotherapy, and chemotherapy. MR imaging is the modality of choice for depiction and delineation of intracerebral neoplasms. However, tumor specification is limited and sometimes conventional MR imaging cannot discriminate glioblastomas from solitary metastases, CNS lymphomas, or other glioma grades. Because their management and prognosis are different, early differentiation is important. The results of the available studies in literature, all with relatively limited patient numbers, indicate that dynamic susceptibility contrast (DSC) MR imaging is useful in the preoperative diagnosis of gliomas, CNS lymphomas, and solitary metastases, as well as in the differentiation of these neoplastic lesions from infections and tumorlike manifestations of demyelinating disease.[48–51] For these issues, it delivers higher predicting values than conventional MR imaging.

Our experience on brain tumor differentiation is that perfusion-weighted imaging (PWI) has superior diagnostic performance in predicting glioma grade (Fig. 6) and in differentiating glioblastoma from other tumor entities (metastases, meningiomas, and CNS lymphomas) when compared with spectroscopic imaging and dynamic contrast-enhanced (DCE) MR imaging.[51] Because of the shorter acquisition time and the better predictive values in differential diagnosis, we would favor the use of perfusion over spectroscopic imaging and DCE MR imaging on a 1.5-T MR unit. This may be the case in patients with reduced physical condition and compliance, often encountered in patients with brain tumor, which results in a limited imaging time.

Because of a significantly higher tumor perfusion in glioblastomas compared with CNS lymphomas, a threshold value of 1.4 for relative CBV provided sensitivity, specificity, positive predictive value (PPV), and negative predicting value (NPV) of 100%, 50%, 90%, and 100%.[51] Although conventional MR imaging characteristics of solitary metastases and primary high-grade gliomas may sometimes be similar, MR perfusion and spectroscopic imaging enable distinction between the two.[51,52] Although both intratumoral metabolite ratios, rCBV or rrCBF values did not allow for discrimination between the 2 entities, analyzing the peritumoral T2-weighted hyperintense region enables the discrimination between high-grade gliomas and metastases, as CBV was significantly higher in peritumoral nonenhancing T2-hyperintense regions of glioblastomas compared with metastases. Thus, elevated perfusion in the peritumoral region of the lesion represents with high specificity glioma in differentiation of glioma from metastasis or grade 1 meningioma.[51,52] Hence, PWI allows us to readily appreciate tumor extension past obvious gross anatomic boundaries on conventional MR imaging.

Correct grading of gliomas has significant clinical impact, because adjuvant therapy after surgery is usually administered to high-grade but not low-grade gliomas. Histopathology as gold standard based on biopsy samples is limited owing to the inherent sampling error in these heterogeneous tumors.[53] Several studies reported that high-grade gliomas had higher relative regional CBV[51,52] and CBF[51,54,55] than low-grade gliomas,

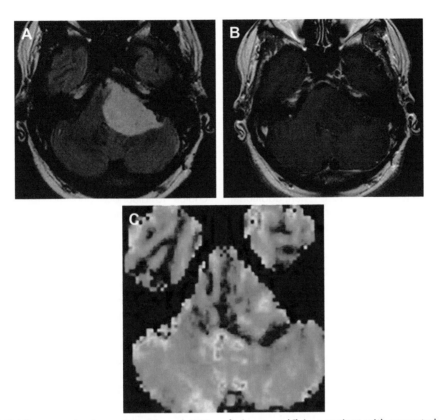

Fig. 6. FLAIR (*A*), contrast-enhanced T1 (*B*), and CBV perfusion map (*C*) in a patient with suspected low-grade astrocytoma. The low-grade tumor was suspected because of the homogeneous signal changes on FLAIR and T2 and the missing contrast enhancement. The perfusion CBV map presented a highly perfused area in the center of the lesion, which was used as a target for stereotactic biopsy and revealed an anaplastic transformation of the tumor.

and glioblastomas have the highest tumor perfusion among all other glioma grades (see **Fig. 5**). However, there is a significant overlap of tumor perfusion between high-grade and low-grade gliomas, which may be explained by the inherent glioma heterogeneity and the sampling error of biopsy samples. This overlap leads to a low specificity, especially when differentiating grade 3 from grade 2 gliomas. Thus, PWI has limited utility for an individual patient in making a specific diagnosis, but they may be of great clinical value for biopsy guidance because of the potential glioma heterogeneity with high-grade components that might be interspersed among low-grade components. Nevertheless, PWI increases the sensitivity, specificity, PPV, and NPV compared with conventional MR imaging, which is only 73%, 65%, 86%, and 44%, for discriminating high-grade from low-grade gliomas. Future work has to focus on the optimum threshold values to be used in a clinical setting to evaluate tumors preoperatively for histologic grade.

Although PWI has a better diagnostic performance than conventional MR imaging techniques in distinguishing different tumor entities, PWI cannot eliminate the need for a biopsy and histologic confirmation because modern treatment regimens also take genetic mutations of tumor cells into account.

Because histopathology as gold standard based on biopsy samples is limited owing to the inherent sampling error in these heterogeneous tumors, biopsy guidance by functional MR imaging methods, especially in the homogeneous-appearing low-grade gliomas, is crucial. PWI is suitable for determining tumor areas of increased microcirculation that very well correspond to anaplastic areas of active tumor growth. These areas should be the target of stereotactic biopsy. Several recent studies report that by using PWI it may become possible to reduce potential errors attributable to sampling bias from a stereotactic biopsy.[48,51,56]

It is very important is to evaluate for tumor status during therapy to assess for therapeutic response and treatment-related complications (eg, the differentiation between recurrent tumor and treatment-related complications). Studies on PWI for these issues show that it helps in better assessing the tumor response to therapy, residual tumor after therapy, and possible treatment failure and therapy-related complications, such as radiation necrosis. In case of the latter, new enhancing lesions might appear years after radiotherapy that are indistinguishable from tumor recurrence with conventional MR imaging. In this issue, an enhancing lesion with relative regional CBV ratios of higher than 2.6 suggests tumor recurrence, whereas ratios lower than 0.6 suggest therapy-related non-neoplastic contrast enhancement.[57] Problematic is contrast-enhancing tissue with a CBV ratio between 0.6 and 2.6. Then, additional nuclear medicine or spectroscopic imaging approaches must be performed.

PWI has tremendous impact on treatment monitoring of low-grade gliomas, besides the advantages in biopsy planning. Because of the intact BBB, valid quantification of perfusion is possible in these entities. In case of a disrupted BBB, leakage of contrast agents from tumor vessels causes underestimation of tumor CBV in PWI. In low-grade gliomas, determination of relative regional CBV measurements can be used to predict clinical response. In a recent study, low-grade gliomas that had progressed more rapidly (mean time to progression of 245 days) had significantly higher CBV than those with stable tumor volumes at follow-up (mean time to progression of 4620 days). The investigators proposed a threshold value of relative regional CBV (>1.75) to indicate a propensity for malignant transformation.[58] The reason for this finding is presumably, as in biopsy planning, that PWI depicts focal anaplastic areas in low-grade gliomas that have not yet led to a disruption of the BBB and therefore to a contrast-enhancement on conventional MR imaging. The same applies for low-grade gliomas after radiotherapy. PWI also detects a subset of patients with higher tumor CBV and shorter progression-free survival.[59] Thus, PWI enables a better prediction of prognosis after radiotherapy than conventional MR imaging. But also after anti-angiogenic chemotherapy of gliomas, PWI has shown its potential to better predict treatment outcome than tumor volume determined on conventional MR imaging.[60] For other intra-axial lesions, such as brain metastases,[61,62] PWI has also shown its potential to better predict treatment outcome than tumor volume. In this context, a reduction of CBV was highly predictive of treatment response, whereas an increase in CBV was a hint for nonresponse. In extra-axial lesions, such as meningiomas, DCE MR imaging might be a good alternative to DSC MR imaging for treatment monitoring[63,64] (see also the following section), because the technique is not as susceptible to

susceptibility artifacts arising from bone and air as DSC MR imaging.

In summary, PWI delivers higher predicting values than conventional MR imaging by providing maps of the regional variations in cerebral microvasculature of normal and diseased brains. PWI can easily be incorporated as part of the routine clinical evaluation of intracranial mass lesions owing to the relatively short imaging and data-processing times and the use of a standard dose of contrast agent. Thus, PWI together with conventional MR imaging should be regarded as the test of choice to diagnose and monitor brain tumors before, during, and after therapy.

DCE MR PERFUSION

DCE magnetic resonance perfusion (DCE-MRP) is the acquisition of serial images before, during and after the administration of extracellular low-molecular weighted MR contrast media. The resulting signal intensity measurements of the tumor reflect a composite of tumor perfusion, vessel permeability, and the extravascular-extracellular space.[65,66]

DCE-MR imaging has been investigated for a range of clinical oncologic applications, including cancer detection, diagnosis, staging, and assessment of treatment response.[67–70] DCE-MR imaging parameters measures permeability and its aberrations, whereas microvascular density (MVD) measures only the histopathological partial picture of the tissue microvasculature. Furthermore, MVD is also a heterogeneous property of tumors and is limited by histopathologic sampling and are generally hotspot values. Tumor microvascular measurements by DCE-MR imaging have been found to correlate with prognostic factors, such as tumor grade, microvessel density (MVD), and vascular endothelial growth factor expression (VEGF) and with recurrence and survival outcomes.[71,72]

In addition, changes of DCE-MR imaging in follow-up studies during therapeutic intervention have been shown to correlate with outcome, suggesting a role for DCE-MR imaging as a predictive marker.[68–70]

In contrast to conventional (static postcontrast T1-weighted) enhanced MR imaging, which simply presents a snapshot of enhancement at one time point, DCE-MR imaging permits a fuller depiction of the wash-in and wash-out contrast kinetics within tumors, and this provides insight into the nature of the bulk tissue properties on its microvascular level. Such data are readily to 2-compartment pharmacokinetic modeling from which parameters based on the rates of exchange between the compartments can be generated.

This modeling condenses the 4-dimensional information (3-dimensional contrast media delivery over time) via parametric mapping into a 3-dimensional image data set. These color codes aid the visual assessment of tumor microvascular environment.

CONTRAST MEDIA DOSAGE

As described, the use of gadolinium (Gd) contrast media is standard for the assessment of different CNS diseases. Whereas in the beginning of MR imaging only one contrast medium (Gd-DTPA, Magnevist, Bayer Healthcare, Wayne, NJ) was available, there are several Gd-based contrast agents available today and use up to a dosage of 0.3 mmol/kg of body weight.

This topic is ongoing in MR imaging and will be continuing with further improvement of the hardware technology and changes in sequence design and more advanced CM application strategies. By looking only at gadopentetate dimeglumine, the pioneer being used now worldwide in more than 45 million applications,[73] we find the same dosage recommendations in the package inserts for the minimum dose by looking at France, Germany, Italy, Japan, the United Kingdom, and the United States, but different results if the maximal dose is considered. The maximum dose of 0.3 mmol/kg body weight did not gain approval in Japan or in the United States.[73] It has been shown, however, that a higher dose of gadolinium chelate–based contrast agents may help reveal more subtle disease states of the BBB.[74,75]

Several studies exist both for detection and characterization of focal CNS lesions. Initial investigations by Yuh and colleagues[75] have demonstrated that a dosage of 0.2 mmol/kg and up to 0.3 mmol/kg allow detection of additional brain metastases in about 20% of patients. Although they detected highly significant differences in small lesions, there was no difference in the detection rate for lesions larger than 10 mm. The application of a triple dose was also superior compared with delayed imaging. In-between the highest dose group, the detection rate did not correlate with the application scheme. For screening of metastases, Sze and colleagues[76] compared single-dose and triple-dose contrast-enhanced MR imaging quantifying lesion load at single and triple dose in patients with risk of cerebral metastases and those who could benefit from the possible increased sensitivity in lesion detection. In their series in all 70 negative single-dose studies, the triple-dose studies depicted no additional metastases in terms of the standard of reference. No statistically significant difference was seen between the results of the single-dose and triple-

dose studies. For 10 equivocal single-dose studies, the triple-dose study helped clarify the presence or absence of metastases in 50% of the cases. In 12 patients with a solitary metastasis seen on the single-dose study, the triple-dose study depicted additional metastases in 25% of the cases. In the results of 1 of the 2 blinded readers, use of triple-dose contrast led to a statistical difference by decreasing the number of equivocal readings but at the expense of increasing the number of false-positive readings. The authors therefore conclude that routine triple-dose contrast administration in all cases of suspected brain metastasis is not helpful.

The effect of higher dosage on lesion size in metastatic brain tumors was assessed in a study from.[77] The contrast of brain metastases after cumulative doses of gadolinium chelate was quantified and compared to assess the clinical utility of high dosage in a series of 39 patients with metastatic brain tumors. The post-Gd MR imaging contrast doubled with dose escalation from 0.1 to 0.3 mmol/kg and also increased with lesion size, by a factor of 2.5 between metastases of 3 and 16 mm diameter. At 0.2 and 0.3 mmol/kg, the respective numbers of visible metastases increased by 15% and 43% compared with 0.1 mmol/kg ($P<.0001$). Image contrast figures differed significantly between doses ($P = .018$). Both the number of metastases and the image contrast are significantly higher when dose escalation is performed. It is indicated that the number of detected metastases will increase further at Gd doses beyond 0.3 mmol/kg. Post-Gd MR imaging contrast increases with lesion size, to an extent that cannot be attributed to partial volume attenuation.

Regarding the effect of field strength, no differences were described. In a study comparing 3.0-T and 1.5-T, cumulative triple-dose images of both field strengths were superior to standard field strengths. However, administration of a better contrast medium, such as gadodiamide contrast agent, produces higher contrast between tumor and normal brain on 3.0 T than on 1.5 T, resulting in better detection of brain metastases and leptomeningeal involvement.[78]

Besides the better detection, the high dose may also allow a better characterization of gliomas. In suspected low-grade tumors, a mild enhancement pattern might be better visualized, and a tumor recurrence may be better visualized, as has been shown by Erickson and colleagues.[5]

In a prospective study protocol, Erickson and colleagues[5] evaluated if there is a subset of brain tumors that demonstrate contrast enhancement with triple dose and magnetization transfer saturation (MTS) that do not enhance with standard imaging and standard contrast dose. In 15 patients with either newly diagnosed primary brain tumor or brain tumor that had been followed for more than 2 years, T1-weighted MTS images without IV contrast, with 0.1 mmol/kg without MTS (single-dose images), and with additional 0.2 mmol/kg Gd and MTS ("TD/MTS") were obtained. None of the patients had enhancement on single-dose imaging whereas 6 patients had areas of enhancement on triple-dose MTS images. So far, it might be possible that those small areas of enhancement seen only with triple-dose MTS might represent areas of higher-grade tumor, which may benefit form a more intensive initial tumor therapy.

MR CONTRAST AGENTS USED AT DIFFERENT FIELD STRENGTH

Over the past decade, most clinical experience in the field of cerebral MR imaging has been with 1.5-T systems with a dose of 0.1 mmol/kg body weight of the conventional Gd chelates, as this combination seems to be an acceptable compromise between imaging expense and diagnostic sensitivity.[79,80] The number of 3.0-T systems in clinical settings has been increasing over the past few years, and systems operating at even higher field strengths are being used in clinical trials already.[81]

One of the main features of MR imaging at 3.0 T is the general gain in signal-to-noise ratio (SNR) compared with that at lower field strengths. Therefore, one may anticipate that the increased SNR associated with a higher magnetic field will translate, at least to a certain degree, into a higher contrast-to-noise ratio (CNR) between enhancing and nonenhancing tissues. The increased CNR should improve the delineationof contrast agent–induced changes and, thus, could increase the sensitivity of detection of such signal-intensity changes (**Fig. 7**).

In addition, the effectiveness of the T1-shortening effect of a Gd-based contrast agent depends on the baseline T1 relaxation time of local tissue. With the longer baseline, T1 relaxation times brought about by a higher magnetic field strength, the T1-shortening effect of Gd-based contrast agents will be greater, as the relaxivity of such contrast agents changes only marginally between 1.5-T MR imaging and 3.0-T MR imaging.[82,83] Accordingly, the signal intensity changes caused by contrast enhancement observable in T1-weighted images should generally be stronger at 3.0 T than they are at 1.5 T.

Giesel and colleagues[84] described that contrast media with affinity for serum human serum albumin, eg, weak protein binding Gd-chelates a decrease in T1 relaxation rate with higher field strength.

A study comparing 1.5-T and 3.0-T imaging[85] showed that the CNR increased more than twofold with respect to 1.5-T imaging, with a median relative CNR (ratio of change of CNR with full dose) of 2.8. Moreover, even with the reduced contrast agent dose, CNR at 3.0 T was significantly higher (ratio of change of CNR with half dose; median, 1.3-fold) compared with the same patient's examination at 1.5 T with the full dose of contrast agent (*P*<.01). Trattnig and colleagues[86] found that the cumulative triple-dose at 3.0 T still showed the best results in the detection of brain metastases but that CM dose for dynamic susceptibility–weighted CE perfusion MR imaging can be reduced to 0.1 mmol compared with 0.2 mmol at 1.5 T.

There are 2 different clinical strategies to exploit this CNR increase. First, the higher CNR can be invested to improve the visualization of subtle disruptions of the BBB, thus possibly improving the sensitivity for depiction of small metastases or early inflammatory changes. Second, the higher CNR could, in principle, be traded to reduce the dose of contrast agent for contrast-enhanced brain imaging at 3.0 T.

With regard to the first approach, that of a possible improvement in sensitivity, this may be said. In standard clinical settings, a dose of 0.10 mmol/kg gadolinium chelate is generally considered sufficient for contrast-enhanced MR imaging of the brain at 1.5 T,[79,80,87] as this dose delivers acceptable diagnostic sensitivity at a reasonable cost. Imaging for certain indications, however, has been shown to benefit from double or triple the dose of contrast agent. Typically, these indications include clinical situations in which the detection of even subtle disruptions in the BBB has an effect on patient treatment.[88–90] Yuh and colleagues[74,75] found that studies at 1.5 T with triple the dose of contrast agent were more effective in the detection of metastatic brain lesions than were studies with the full dose of gadolinium chelate.

With regard to the second approach, that of a reduction in the dose of contrast agent, this may be said. By using the reduced contrast agent dose at 3.0-T MR imaging, CNR was still higher compared with that at 1.5-T imaging with the full dose of contrast agent. This suggests that even with half the contrast agent dose, the diagnostic sensitivity in the depiction of disruptions of the BBB should be maintained at 3.0 T compared

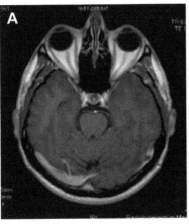
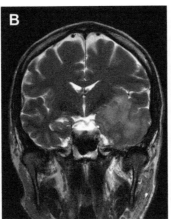
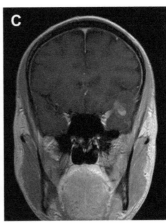

Fig. 7. Patient with a suspected low-grade astrocytoma referred from an outpatient 1.5-T MR imaging center without an enhancement on the MR imaging (A). For treatment planning, MR imaging was performed on a 3-T MR imaging scanner using the same dose of contrast media. In this exam, an oval-shaped contrast enhancement in the center of the homogeneous T2 changes (B) became obvious on the postcontrast T1 FSE sequences (C).

with the 1.5-T standard setting. In fact, all lesions depicted at 1.5 T with the full dose of contrast agent were also diagnosed prospectively and independently at 3.0 T with half the dose of contrast agent; lesion conspicuity was rated to be equivalent.

Haba and colleagues[91] showed that dose can be reduced by using MTS by 50% without loss of contrast enhancement in investigation of meningiomas. No matter which dose is used, MTS can also be helpful to further improve detection of small areas of enhancement.[5]

SUMMARY

Since their introduction, Gd-based contrast media are routinely used in most CNS MR imaging indications, including assessment of CNS tumors, vascular pathologies, infections, degenerative diseases, and posttreatment imaging. Contrast media are applied to improve the sensitivity and specificity of CNS diseases and to allow a better treatment decision, planning, and follow-up.

The standard dose used is 0.1 mmol/kg of body weight with some exceptions that allow injection of up to a triple dose.

More recently, contrast media have also been used to allow the measurement of tissue perfusion and to follow the time course of enhancement in dynamic contrast-enhanced imaging or dynamic MRA studies.

With the presence of the BBB, contrast media does not leak into the tissue. Only vascular structures and areas of the brain that have no BBB (choroid plexus, pineal and anterior lobe of pituitary gland) physiologically enhance after contrast

injection. The mechanisms of tissue enhancement in the brain are related to a higher vascularity of the pathology or a disruption of the BBB.

Tissue enhancement is, besides the degree of BBB disruption, further dependent on the applied magnetic field strength, with higher field providing a better enhancement and the applied dose of contrast media.

REFERENCES

1. McMicken DB. Emergency CT head scans in traumatic and atraumatic conditions. Ann Emerg Med 1986;15(3):274–9.
2. Smirniotopoulos JG, Murphy FM, Rushing EJ, et al. Patterns of contrast enhancement in the brain and meninges. Radiographics 2007;27(2):525–51.
3. Brant-Zawadzki M, Norman D, Newton TH, et al. Magnetic resonance of the brain: the optimal screening technique. Radiology 1984;152(1):71–7.
4. Muroff LR, Runge VM. The use of MR contrast in neoplastic disease of the brain. Top Magn Reson Imaging 1995;7(3):137–57.
5. Erickson BJ, Campeau NG, Schreiner SA, et al. Triple-dose contrast/magnetization transfer suppressed imaging of 'non-enhancing' brain gliomas. J Neurooncol 2002;60(1):25–9.
6. Schneider G, Kirchin MA, Pirovano G, et al. Gadobenate dimeglumine-enhanced magnetic resonance imaging of intracranial metastases: effect of dose on lesion detection and delineation. J Magn Reson Imaging 2001;14(5):525–39.
7. Bart J, Groen HJ, Hendrikse NH, et al. The blood-brain barrier and oncology: new insights into function and modulation. Cancer Treat Rev 2000;26(6): 449–62.

8. Neuwelt EA. Mechanisms of disease: the blood-brain barrier. Neurosurgery 2004;54(1):131–40.

9. Gururangan S, Friedman HS. Innovations in design and delivery of chemotherapy for brain tumors. Neuroimaging Clin N Am 2002;12(4):583–97.

10. Demeule M, Regina A, Jodoin J, et al. Drug transport to the brain: key roles for the efflux pump P-glycoprotein in the blood-brain barrier. Vascul Pharmacol 2002;38(6):339–48.

11. Kemper EM, Boogerd W, Thuis I, et al. Modulation of the blood-brain barrier in oncology: therapeutic opportunities for the treatment of brain tumours? Cancer Treat Rev 2004;30(5):415–23.

12. Rautioa J, Chikhale PJ. Drug delivery systems for brain tumor therapy. Curr Pharm Des 2004;10(12):1341–53.

13. Kroll RA, Neuwelt EA. Outwitting the blood-brain barrier for therapeutic purposes: osmotic opening and other means. Neurosurgery 1998;42(5):1083–99.

14. Sage MR, Wilson AJ, Scroop R. Contrast media and the brain: the basis of CT and MR imaging enhancement. Neuroimaging Clin N Am 1998;8:695–707.

15. Meltzer CC, Fukui MB, Kanal E, et al. MR imaging of the meninges. I. Normal anatomic features and non-neoplastic disease. Radiology 1996;201:297–308.

16. Burke JW, Podrasky AE, Bradley WG Jr. Meninges: benign postoperative enhancement on MR images. Radiology 1990;174:99–102.

17. Paldino M, Mogilner AY, Tenner MS. Intracranial hypotension syndrome: a comprehensive review. Neurosurg Focus 2003;15:1–8.

18. Buetow MP, Buetow PC, Smirniotopoulos JG. Typical, atypical, and misleading features in meningioma. Radiographics 1991;11:1087–106.

19. Gupta S, Gupta RK, Banerjee D, et al. Problems with the dural tail sign. Neuroradiology 1993;35:541–2.

20. Nagele T, Petersen D, Klose U, et al. The dural tail adjacent to meningiomas studied by dynamic contrast-enhanced MRI: a comparison with histopathology. Neuroradiology 1994;36:303–7.

21. Van Sorge NM, Doran KS. Defense at the border: the blood-brain barrier versus bacterial foreigners. Future Microbiol 2012;7(3):383–94.

22. Kido G, Wright JL, Merchant RE. Acute effects of human recombinant tumor necrosis factor-alpha on the cerebral vasculature of the rat in both normal brain and in an experimental glioma model. J Neurooncol 1991;10(2):95–109.

23. Schneider SW, Ludwig T, Tatenhorst L, et al. Glioblastoma cells release factors that disrupt blood-brain barrier features. Acta Neuropathol 2004;107(3):272–6.

24. Earnest F, Kelly PJ, Scheithauer BW, et al. Cerebral astrocytomas: histopathologic correlation of MR and CT contrast enhancement with stereotactic biopsy. Radiology 1988;166(3):823–7.

25. Fidler IJ, Yano S, Zhang RD, et al. The seed and soil hypothesis: vascularisation and brain metastases. Lancet Oncol 2002;3(1):53–7.

26. Groothuis DR. The blood-brain and blood-tumor barriers: a review of strategies for increasing drug delivery. Neuro Oncol 2000;2(1):45–59.

27. Holodny AI, Nusbaum AO, Festa S, et al. Correlation between the degree of contrast enhancement and the volume of peritumoral edema in meningiomas and malignant gliomas. Neuroradiology 1999;41(11):820–5.

28. Pronin IN, Holodny AI, Petraikin AV. MRI of high-grade glial tumors: correlation between the degree of contrast enhancement and the volume of surrounding edema. Neuroradiology 1997;39(5):348–50.

29. Runge VM. A review of contrast media research in 1999–2000. Invest Radiol 2001;36(2):123–30.

30. Wilkinson ID, Jellineck DA, Levy D, et al. Dexamethasone and enhancing solitary cerebral mass lesions: alterations in perfusion and blood-tumor barrier kinetics shown by magnetic resonance imaging. Neurosurgery 2006;58(4):640–6.

31. Burke JW, Mathews VP, Elster AD, et al. Contrast-enhanced magnetization transfer saturation imaging improves MR detection of herpes simplex encephalitis. AJNR Am J Neuroradiol 1996;17:773–6.

32. Davis JM, Davis KR, Kleinman GM, et al. Computed tomography of herpes simplex encephalitis, with clinicopathological correlation. Radiology 1978;129:409–17.

33. Zimmerman RD, Russell EJ, Leeds NE, et al. CT in the early diagnosis of herpes simplex encephalitis. AJR Am J Roentgenol 1980;134:61–6.

34. Enzmann DR, Ranson B, Norman D, et al. Computed tomography of herpes simplex encephalitis. Radiology 1978;129:419–25.

35. Mullins ME. Emergent neuroimaging of intracranial infection/inflammation. Radiol Clin North Am 2011;49(1):47–62.

36. Brant-Zawadzki M, Enzmann DR, Placone RC Jr, et al. NMR imaging of experimental brain abscess: comparison with CT. AJNR Am J Neuroradiol 1983;4:250–3.

37. Britt RH, Enzmann DR, Placone RC Jr, et al. Experimental anaerobic brain abscess. J Neurosurg 1984;60:1148–59.

38. Masdeu JC, Moreira J, Trasi S, et al. The open ring: a new imaging sign in demyelinating disease. J Neuroimaging 1996;6:104–7.

39. Masdeu JC, Quinto C, Olivera C, et al. Open-ring imaging sign: highly specific for atypical brain demyelination. Neurology 2000;54:1427–33.

40. Bot JC, Barkhof F, Nijeholt G, et al. Differentiation of multiple sclerosis from other inflammatory disorders and cerebrovascular disease: value of spinal MR imaging. Radiology 2002;223:46–56.

41. Von Kummer V, Meyding-Lamade U, Forsting M, et al. Sensitivity and prognostic value of early CT in occlusion of middle cerebral artery trunk. AJNR Am J Neuroradiol 1994;15:9–15.

42. Moulin T, Cattin F, Crepin-Leblond T, et al. Early CT signs in acute middle cerebral artery infarction: predictive value for subsequent infarct locations and outcome. Neurology 1996;47:366–75.

43. Koenig M, Kraus M, Theek C, et al. Quantitative assessment of the ischemic brain by means of perfusion related parameters derived from perfusion CT. Stroke 2001;32:431–7.

44. Tomandl BF, Klotz E, Handsch u R, et al. Comprehensive imaging of ischemic stroke with multisection CT. Radiographics 2003;23:565–92.

45. Srinivasan A, Goyal M, Al Azri F, et al. State-of-the-art imaging of acute stroke. Radiographics 2006; 26(Suppl 1):S75–95.

46. Karonen JO, Vanninen RL, Liu Y, et al. Combined diffusion and perfusion MRI with correlation to single-photon emission CT in acute ischemic stroke. Ischemic penumbra predicts infarct growth. Stroke 1999;30:1583–90.

47. Furlan M, Marchal G, Viader F, et al. Spontaneous neurological recovery after stroke and the fate of the ischemic penumbra. Ann Neurol 1996;40:216–26.

48. Cha S, Knopp EA, Johnson G, et al. Intracranial mass lesions: dynamic contrast-enhanced susceptibility-weighted echo-planar perfusion MR imaging. Radiology 2002;223(1):11–29.

49. Hartmann M, Heiland S, Harting I, et al. Distinguishing of primary cerebral lymphoma from high-grade glioma with perfusion-weighted magnetic resonance imaging. Neurosci Lett 2003;338(2):119–22.

50. Law M, Yang S, Wang H, et al. Glioma grading: sensitivity, specificity, and predictive values of perfusion MR imaging and proton MR spectroscopic imaging compared with conventional MR imaging. AJNR Am J Neuroradiol 2003;24(10):1989–98.

51. Weber MA, Zoubaa S, Schlieter M, et al. Diagnostic performance of spectroscopic and perfusion MRI for distinction of brain tumors. Neurology 2006;66(12): 1899–906.

52. Law M, Cha S, Knopp EA, et al. High-grade gliomas and solitary metastases: differentiation by using perfusion and proton spectroscopic MR imaging. Radiology 2002;222(3):715–21.

53. Law M. MR spectroscopy of brain tumors. Top Magn Reson Imaging 2004;15(5):291–313.

54. Shin JH, Lee HK, Kwun BD, et al. Using relative cerebral blood flow and volume to evaluate the histopathologic grade of cerebral gliomas: preliminary results. AJR Am J Roentgenol 2002;179(3): 783–9.

55. Warmuth C, Gunther M, Zimmer C. Quantification of blood flow in brain tumors: comparison of arterial spin labeling and dynamic susceptibility-weighted contrast-enhanced MR imaging. Radiology 2003; 228(2):523–32.

56. Lev A, Barzilay E. Synchronized intermittent mandatory insufflation of the endotracheal tube cuff. Intensive Care Med 1983;9(5):291–3.

57. Sugahara T, Korogi Y, Tomiguchi S, et al. Post therapeutic intraaxial brain tumor: the value of perfusion-sensitive contrast-enhanced MR imaging for differentiating tumor recurrence from nonneoplastic contrast-enhancing tissue. AJNR Am J Neuroradiol 2000;21(5):901–9.

58. Uematsu H, Maeda M. Double-echo perfusion-weighted MR imaging: basic concepts and application in brain tumors for the assessment of tumor blood volume and vascular permeability. Eur Radiol 2006;16(1):180–6.

59. Law M, Oh S, Babb JS, et al. Low-grade gliomas: dynamic susceptibility-weighted contrast-enhanced perfusion MR imaging—prediction of patient clinical response. Radiology 2006;238(2):658–67.

60. Cha S, Knopp EA, Johnson G, et al. Dynamic contrast-enhanced T2-weighted MR imaging of recurrent malignant gliomas treated with thalidomide and carboplatin. AJNR Am J Neuroradiol 2000;21(5):881–90.

61. Essig M, Waschkies M, Wenz F, et al. Assessment of brain metastases with dynamic susceptibility-weighted contrast-enhanced MR imaging: initial results. Radiology 2003;228(1):193–9.

62. Weber MA, Thilmann C, Lichy MP, et al. Assessment of irradiated brain metastases by means of arterial spin-labeling and dynamic susceptibility-weighted contrast-enhanced perfusion MRI: initial results. Invest Radiol 2004;39(5):277–87.

63. Hawighorst H, Engenhart R, Knopp MV, et al. Intracranial meningeomas: time- and dose-dependent effects of irradiation on tumor microcirculation monitored by dynamic MR imaging. Magn Reson Imaging 1997;15(4):423–32.

64. Hawighorst H, Knopp MV, Debus J, et al. Pharmacokinetic MRI for assessment of malignant glioma response to stereotactic radiotherapy: initial results. J Magn Reson Imaging 1998;8(4):783–8.

65. Brix G, Semmler W, Port R, et al. Pharmacokinetic parameters in CNS Gd-DTPA enhanced MR imaging. J Comput Assist Tomogr 1991;15(4):621–8.

66. Tofts PS, Kermode AG. Measurement of the blood-brain barrier permeability and leakage space using dynamic MR imaging. 1. Fundamental concepts. Magn Reson Med 1991;17(2):357–67.

67. Padhani AR, Husband JE. Dynamic contrast-enhanced MRI studies in oncology with an emphasis on quantification, validation and human studies. Clin Radiol 2001;56(8):607–20.

68. Giesel FL, Bischoff H, von Tengg-Kobligk H, et al. Dynamic contrast-enhanced MRI of malignant pleural mesothelioma: a feasibility study of

noninvasive assessment, therapeutic follow-up, and possible predictor of improved outcome. Chest 2006;129(6):1570–6.

69. Martincich L, Montemurro F, De Rosa G, et al. Monitoring response to primary chemotherapy in breast cancer using dynamic contrast-enhanced magnetic resonance imaging. Breast Cancer Res Treat 2004; 83(1):67–76.

70. Hawighorst H, Bock M, Knopp MV, et al. Magnetically labeled water perfusion imaging of the uterine arteries and of normal and malignant cervical tissue: initial experiences. Magn Reson Imaging 1998; 16(3):225–34.

71. de Lussanet QG, Langereis S, Beets-Tan RG, et al. Dynamic contrast-enhanced MR imaging kinetic parameters and molecular weight of dendritic contrast agents in tumor angiogenesis in mice. Radiology 2005;235(1):65–72.

72. Tuncbilek N, Karakas HM, Altaner S. Dynamic MRI in indirect estimation of microvessel density, histologic grade, and prognosis in colorectal adenocarcinomas. Abdom Imaging 2004;29(2):166–72.

73. Knopp MV, Balzer T, Esser M, et al. Assessment of utilization and pharmacovigilance based on spontaneous adverse event reporting of gadopentetate dimeglumine as a magnetic resonance contrast agent after 45 million administrations and 15 years of clinical use. Invest Radiol 2006;41(6):491–9.

74. Yuh WT, Nguyen HD, Tali ET, et al. Delineation of gliomas with various doses of MR contrast material. AJNR Am J Neuroradiol 1994;15(5):983–9.

75. Yuh WT, Tali ET, Nguyen HD, et al. The effect of contrast dose, imaging time, and lesion size in the MR detection of intracerebral metastasis. AJNR Am J Neuroradiol 1995;16(2):373–80.

76. Sze G, Johnson C, Kawamura Y, et al. Comparison of single- and triple-dose contrast material in the MR screening of brain metastases. AJNR Am J Neuroradiol 1998;19(5):821–8.

77. Van DP, Sijens PE, Schmitz PI, et al. Gd-enhanced MR imaging of brain metastases: contrast as a function of dose and lesion size. Magn Reson Imaging 1997;15(5):535–41.

78. Ba-Ssalamah A, Nobauer-Huhmann IM, Pinker K, et al. Effect of contrast dose and field strength in the magnetic resonance detection of brain metastases. Invest Radiol 2003;38(7):415–22.

79. Haustein J, Laniado M, Niendorf HP, et al. Administration of gadopentetate dimeglumine in MR imaging of

intracranial tumors: dosage and field strength. AJNR Am J Neuroradiol 1992;13(4):1199–206.

80. Schubeus P, Schorner W, Haustein J, et al. Optimization of gadolinium-DTPA dose: an inter-individual study of patients with intracranial tumors. Rofo 1990;153(1):29–35 [in German].

81. Yang M, Christoforidis GA, Figueredo T, et al. Dosage determination of ultrasmall particles of iron oxide for the delineation of microvasculature in the Wistar rat brain. Invest Radiol 2005;40(10): 655–60.

82. Elster AD. How much contrast is enough? Dependence of enhancement on field strength and MR pulse sequence. Eur Radiol 1997;5(Suppl 7): 276–80.

83. Chang KH, Ra DG, Han MH, et al. Contrast enhancement of brain tumors at different MR field strengths: comparison of 0.5 T and 2.0 T. AJNR Am J Neuroradiol 1994;15(8):1413–9.

84. Giesel FL, von Tengg-Kobligk H, Griffiths PD, et al. Effects of field strength and protein content on R1 and R2 of different contrast agents. RSNA; 2005. SSG 20–07.

85. Krautmacher C, Willinek WA, Tschampa HJ, et al. Brain tumors: full- and half-dose contrast-enhanced MR imaging at 3.0 T compared with 1.5 T—initial experience. Radiology 2005;237(3):1014–9.

86. Trattnig S, Pinker K, Ba-Ssalamah A, et al. The optimal use of contrast agents at high field MRI. Eur Radiol 2006;16(6):1280–7.

87. Brekenfeld C, Foert E, Hundt W, et al. Enhancement of cerebral diseases: how much contrast agent is enough? Comparison of 0.1, 0.2, and 0.3 mmol/kg gadoteridol at 0.2 T with 0.1 mmol/kg gadoteridol at 1.5 T. Invest Radiol 2001;36(5):266–75.

88. Runge VM, Gelblum DY, Pacetti ML, et al. Gd-HP-DO3A in clinical MR imaging of the brain. Radiology 1990;177(2):393–400.

89. Haustein J, Laniado M, Niendorf HP, et al. Triple-dose versus standard-dose gadopentetate dimeglumine: a randomized study in 199 patients. Radiology 1993;186(3):855–60.

90. Runge VM, Kirsch JE, Burke VJ, et al. High-dose gadoteridol in MR imaging of intracranial neoplasms. J Magn Reson Imaging 1992;2(1):9–18.

91. Haba D, Pasco PA, Tanguy JY, et al. Use of half-dose gadolinium-enhanced MRI and magnetization transfer saturation in brain tumors. Eur Radiol 2001;11(1):117–22.

Contrast-Enhanced MR Imaging in Neuroimaging

Bum-soo Kim, MD[a], Juan E. Gutierrez, MD[b],*

KEYWORDS

- Gadolinium-based contrast agents (GBCAs) • Contrast-enhanced MR imaging (CE MR imaging)
- Microcyclic agent • Lineal agent • Susceptibility-weighted imaging (SWI)
- Diffusion-weighted imaging (DWI) • MR spectroscopy (MRS) • Perfusion MR imaging (pMR imaging)

KEY POINTS

- Combined MR imaging without and with gadolinium-based contrast agents (GBCAs) is an important imaging tool for defining normal anatomy and characteristics of lesions.
- GBCAs have been used in contrast-enhanced (CE) MR imaging in defining and characterizing both cranial and spinal lesions of the central nervous system (CNS) for more than 20 years.
- Normally, the blood-brain barrier (BBB) prevents GBCAs from crossing from the blood to the brain.
- The combination of unenhanced and GBCA-enhanced MR imaging is the clinical gold standard for the noninvasive detection and delineation of most intracranial and spinal lesions.
- MR imaging has a high predictive value that reliably rules out neoplasm and most inflammatory and demyelinating processes of the CNS.

INTRODUCTION

MR imaging is a proved and well-established imaging modality in the evaluation and assessment of normal and abnormal conditions of the brain with superior accuracy compared with other imaging modalities.[1–4] With intravenous administration of GBCAs, conventional CE MR imaging has been a valuable method for visualization of lesions with breakdown of the BBB, with improved sensitivity and specificity. At present, there are 7 GBCAs approved in the United States or the European Union for use in the CNS (**Table 1**).[5–7] Most available GBCAs that shorten the T1 relaxation time to enhance MR images are low-molecular-weight polyaminocarboxylate compounds.[8] All these GBCAs share low rates of qualitatively similar adverse drug reaction in surveillance studies.[9–12] The standard dose of GBCA for most MR imaging applications is 0.1 mmol/kg body weight; although it is proved that higher doses can improve lesion detection.[13,14]

GBCAs can be classified on the basis of ionicity (ionic vs nonionic), biochemical structures (macrocyclic vs linear), or binding to serum albumin (see **Table 1**).

EFFECT OF GBCAS ON MR SEQUENCES ON NEUROIMAGING

In clinical practice, CE MR imaging is performed with either spin-echo or gradient-echo (GRE) T1-weighted (T1W) MR imaging sequences, and there has been controversy regarding which sequence is better for use for CE MR imaging in neuroimaging. Spin-echo images have been the preferred sequence due to better contrast enhancement of the brain lesions.[15] GRE sequences, alternatively,

[a] Department of Radiology, Seoul St. Mary's Hospital, The Catholic University of Korea, #505 Banpo-dong, Seocho-gu, Seoul 137-701, Korea; [b] Department of Radiology, University of Texas Health Science Center, San Antonio, TX, USA
* Corresponding author.
E-mail address: gutierrezje@uthscsa.edu

Magn Reson Imaging Clin N Am 20 (2012) 649–685
http://dx.doi.org/10.1016/j.mric.2012.07.003
1064-9689/12/$ – see front matter © 2012 Elsevier Inc. All rights reserved.

Table 1
Gadolinium-based contrast agents approved for CNS use in the US and/or the European Union

Generic Name	Product/ Trade Name	Manufacturer	Formulation	Concentration (mol/L)	Serum Albumen Binding
Gadopentetate dimeglumine	Magnevist	Bayer Healthcare	Ionic linear	0.5	No
Gadoterate meglumine	Dotarem	Guerbet	Macrocyclic	0.5	No
Gadodiamide	Omniscan	GE Healthcare	Nonionic linear	0.5	No
Gadoteridol	ProHance	Bracco Diagnostics	Macrocyclic	0.5	No
Gadobutrol	Gadovist	Bayer Healthcare	Macrocyclic	1	No
Gadoversetamide	Optimark	Mallinckrodt	Nonionic linear	0.5	No
Gadobenate disodium	MultiHance	Bracco Diagnostics	Ionic linear	0.5	Weak

Data from Refs.[5–7]

provide improved spatial resolution in reduced imaging time and reduced motion artifact; thus, small neoplastic lesions may be better visualized in thin-slice 3-D GRE images.[15–19] When it comes to 3-T MR, in which the T1 relaxation times of gray and white matter tend to become longer, T1 contrast of the brain on sequences without contrast administration is reduced, and specific absorption rate limitation matters. Therefore, opportunity to use the GRE sequence may be increased in clinical examination at 3 T. Although there have been several reports that GRE cannot surpass SE imaging for detecting brain lesions because of inherently weaker enhancement,[20,21] GRE at 3 T with administration of high relaxavity GBCAs, high doses of gadolinium, and suitable scanning delay time improves diagnostic accuracy of brain tumor.[20,22,23] Recent studies that used 3-D T1 turbo spin-echo sequence with variable flip angle echo train in reasonable imaging duration and specific absorption rate limit showed higher enhancement brain metastasis than 3-D GRE.[24–26]

Contrast enhancement is also seen on fluid-attenuated inversion recovery (FLAIR) brain MR imaging after intravenous injection of GBCA. Contrast enhancement on FLAIR imaging is the result of a mild T1 effect, produced by the long inversion time used to nullify the signal intensity of water. As in CE T1W imaging, choroid plexus, pituitary stalk, pineal gland, and dural sinuses show normal enhancement on CE FLAIR MR imaging.[27] Degree of contrast enhancement in normal intracranial

structures on CE FLAIR is less intense than that on CE T1W imaging, because of a mild T1 effect on the FLAIR sequence. Alternatively, most blood vessels do not enhance on CE FLAIR, probably due to a T2 effect of the FLAIR sequence. Thus, CE FLAIR is useful in depicting the superficial abnormalities, such as leptomeningeal inflammation or carcinomatosis, cranial nerve lesion, and inner ear abnormalities (**Fig. 1**).[28–37] CE FLAIR is also suggested as having a complementary role for detecting intracranial tumors and demyelinating disease.[38–47] In stroke imaging, vascular hyperintensity on CE FLAIR in patients with acute ischemic stroke, intracranial stenosis, moyamoya disease, and transient ischemic attack represents disordered blood flow from collaterals distal to the arterial occlusion or stenosis (not an indicator of infarction but rather of tissue at risk for infarction).[48–50]

Susceptibility-weighted imaging (SWI) is sensitive sequence for parenchymal bleed and calcifications, allows noninvasive visualization of small veins in the brain, and can be used to depict venous architecture in normal and pathologic tissues.[51–53] In SWI images, veins appear hypointense due to the presence of deoxyhemoblobin and the arteries are hyperintense due to time-of-flight effects and lack of T2* effects, giving natural separation of arteries and veins.[51,54] SWI can be performed after gadolinium has been injected, without loss or signal change in the parenchyma (**Fig. 2**).[55,56] CE SWI is useful in the evaluation of arteriovenous shunt in patients with brain vascular

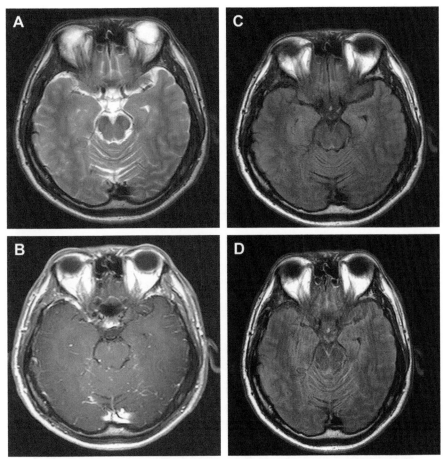

Fig. 1. A 31-year-old male patient with viral meningitis with lymphocyte-dominant leukocytosis in CSF. T2W (*A*) and FLAIR (*B*) images show no abnormal signal intensity. CE T1W image (*C*) shows subtle increase in leptomeningeal contrast enhancement on the surface of midbrain and cerebellum. Contrast enhancement is more prominently seen on CE FLAIR image (*D*). (*Courtesy of* S. Park, Department of Radiology, Boramae Medical Center, College of Medicine, Seoul National University, Seoul, Korea.)

malformation, in which presence of high signal intensity within the venous structure is an accurate indicator of arteriovenous shunt.[57] CE SWI can also visualize the architecture of brain neoplasm, demonstrating the leakage of contrast material due to breakdown of the BBB.[58]

Diffusion-weighted imaging (DWI) has become a powerful tool in the evaluation of brain lesions and mainly used in assessment of acute stroke, but it has become widely used in the assessment of tumor, infection, inflammation, and trauma.[59–63] DWI after administration of contrast agent may be necessary in circumstances with motion of the head, especially in acute stroke. DWI can be obtained after contrast administration of GBCA without causing a significant change in visual evaluation of normal and infarcted brain.[64–66] Apparent diffusion coefficient (ADC) values decrease, however, after contrast agent injection on early CE DWI in normal brain tissue (1%) and brain lesions (3%–6%). Thus, if ADC measurements are planned, DWI must be performed after an acceptable delay after contrast medium injection of at least 6 to 10 minutes.[66]

Magnetic resonance spectroscopy (MRS) is increasingly used in neuroimaging, including evaluation of brain tumor. Magnetic resonance spectra of brain tumors show elevated levels of Cho peak and decreased levels of N-acetyl aspartate (NAA) peak relative to normal brain, reflecting increased cellularity.[67,68] MRS is helpful in differentiation of brain tumors and characterization of metabolic changes associated with tumor progression, degree of malignancy, and response to treatment.[69] In some cases, need for MRS may not be determined until after contrast agent had been administered, and the placement of region of interest at the enhancing part of the tumor may be more valuable than that of remaining nonenhancing part. Sijens and colleagues[70] reported

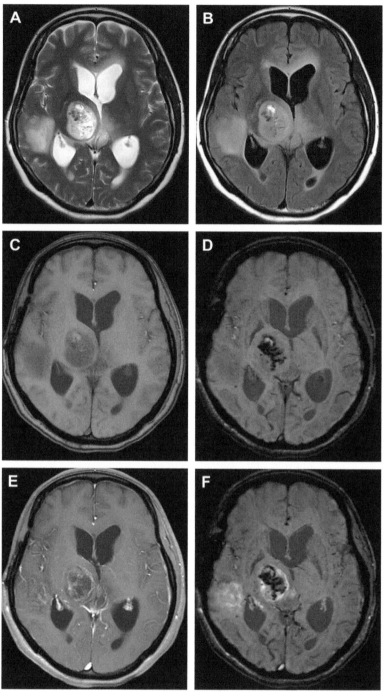

Fig. 2. A 23-year-old female patient with a recurrent glioma. T2W (*A*), FLAIR (*B*), and T1W (*C*) images and SWI (*D*) show well-marginated mass with internal hemorrhage and necrotic change involving the right thalamus and another smoothly marginated mass in right temporal lobe. CE T1W (*E*) image shows irregular marginal contrast enhancement in and around the right thalamic mass and faintly in right temporal mass lesion. CE SWI (*F*) shows more prominent contrast enhancement of the masses.

a decrease in the Cho peak after administration of gadolinium contrast that lasted for nearly 5 minutes, and with little further change with time. The presence of contrast material, however, after 5 to 10 minutes of administration does not alter the diagnostic quality of MRS in brain tumors.[70–72] Manual reshimming the gradients immediately before obtaining the postcontrast spectra might further decrease any effect of magnetic field changes by gadolinium.[72]

CONTRAST ENHANCEMENT IN NORMAL CE MR IMAGING

Most of brain is not enhanced with administration of contrast agent because the BBB prevents the contrast from reaching the cerebral extravascular space. The pituitary gland and stalk, choroid plexus, and intracavernous portions of cranial nerves III–VI, which have an incomplete BBB, enhance greatly (**Fig. 3**).[73] Enhancement in these structures persists for 1 hour but is usually maximal or nearly maximal at 3 minutes. Also, the mucosal surfaces of the nasopharynx and sinuses, slowly flowing blood, and the retinal choroid all show prominent contrast enhancement after administration of a magnetic resonance contrast agent. The dura mater, which usually shows enhancement of the falx and tentorium on CE CT images, does not routinely demonstrate similar enhancement on MR images. Although normal dura mater does not have a BBB,

it lacks sufficient water to show the T1 shortening required for enhancement on MR images.[74,75] Meningeal enhancement, alternatively, has been seen in the pathologic conditions, including leptomeningeal metastases, bacterial and granulomatous meningitis, and after intracranial surgery.[75–78] Also visualized is the enhancement of normal superficial venous structures, although this may be both variable and asymmetric. Normally, there is little or no enhancement of gray matter, white matter, cerebrospinal fluid (CSF), muscle, fat, and cortical bone.

CLINICAL APPLICATION

MR imaging has been accepted as the most sensitive method, and diagnosing brain lesions and has been the first step in classifying a lesion according to location, contrast enhancement, perilesional edema, mass effect, necrosis, and hemorrhage.[79,80] Contrast enhancement in brain lesion could be a sign of BBB breakdown by the abnormal structure of tumor vessels (extravascular) or of increased vascularity (intravascular).[74] Interstitial enhancement is related to alterations in the permeability of the BBB, whereas intravascular enhancement is proportional to increases in blood flow or blood volume. Conventional CE MR imaging improves the capability to identify lesions not visible on unenhanced MR imaging and to provide additional information on lesion morphology, delineation, physiology, and biology.[81–83] In the

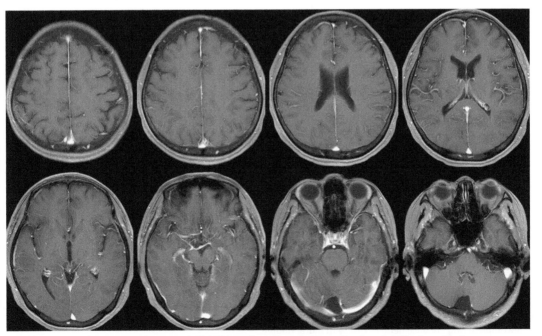

Fig. 3. Contrast enhancement in normal CE MR imaging. The pituitary gland and stalk, choroid plexus, cavernous sinus, cortical veins, and dural sinuses show contrast enhancement.

imaging of neoplastic brain lesion, however, conventional CE MR imaging has the limitation in the evaluation of early response after treatment and differential diagnosis of recurrent tumor, pseudo-progression, and radiation necrosis.[80,84–87] Use of functional MR imaging techniques, such as DWI, MRS, and perfusion MR imaging, can improve the diagnostic accuracy and provide more reliable differentiation of brain tumors.[69,80,88–95] Use of GBCAs in perfusion MR imaging, including dynamic susceptibility contrast and dynamic CE MR imaging, are discussed by Law elsewhere in this issue.

Knowledge of the patterns and mechanisms of contrast enhancement facilitates radiologic differential diagnosis, and understanding the classic patterns of lesion enhancement can improve image assessment and differential diagnosis of brain lesions. Smirniotopoulos and colleagues[74] summarized patterns of contrast enhancement in the brain and meninges (**Table 2**). Extra-axial enhancing lesions include primary neoplasms (meningioma), granulomatous disease (sarcoid), and metastases. Linear pachymeningeal (dura-arachnoid) enhancement occurs after surgery and with spontaneous intracranial hypotension. Leptomeningeal (pia-arachnoid) enhancement is present in meningitis and meningoencephalitis. Superficial gyral enhancement is seen after reperfusion in cerebral ischemia, during the healing phase of cerebral infarction, and with encephalitis. Nodular subcortical lesions are typical for hematogenous dissemination and may be neoplastic (metastases) or infectious (septic emboli). Deeper lesions may form rings or affect the ventricular margins. Ring enhancement that is smooth and thin is typical of an organizing abscess, whereas thick irregular rings suggest a necrotic neoplasm. Some low-grade neoplasms are fluid secreting,

Table 2
Patterns of contrast enhancement in the brain and meninges

	Location	Enhancement Pattern	Lesions
Extra-axial	Pachymeningeal	• Thin, linear, discontinuous, • Mass with dural attachment and dural tail • Basilar meningeal	• Postoperative change, intracranial hypotension • Meningioma, metastasis, secondary CNS lymphoma, • Granulomatous disease
	Leptomeningeal	• Gyriform/serpentine • Thick, lumpy, nodular • Along the cranial nerve	• Meningitis, meningoencephalitis • Fungal meningitis, carcinomatous meningitis • Viral meningitis, schwannoma
Intra-axial	Superficial gyral	• Serpentine	• Reperfusion in cerebral ischemia, subacute infarction, PRES, meningitis, encephalitis, postictal
	Cortical/subcortical Deep gray/white matter	• Nodular • Deep gray matter • Deep ring enhancement • Incomple ring enhancement[a]	• Hematogenous metastasis • Metabolic disease, leukoencephalopathy, yoxoplasmosis and primary CNS lymphoma in immunocompromised patients • Malignant glioma, metastasis, abscess, demyelinating disease • Pilocystic astrocytoma, hemangioblastoma
	Periventricular	• Nodular • Linear along the ventricle	• Primary CNS lymphoma, glioma, • Infectious ependymitis

Abbreviations: PRES, posterior reversible encephalopathy syndrome.
[a] Incomplete ring enhancement → cyst with mural nodule.
Data from Smirniotopoulos JG, Murphy FM, Rushing EJ, et al. Patterns of contrast enhancement in the brain and meninges. Radiographics 2007;27(2):525–51.

and they may form heterogeneously enhancing lesions with an incomplete ring sign as well as the classic cyst-with-nodule morphology. Demyelinating lesions, including both classic multiple sclerosis and tumefactive demyelination, may also create an open ring or incomplete ring sign. Thick and irregular periventricular enhancement is typical for primary CNS lymphoma. Thin enhancement of the ventricular margin occurs with infectious ependymitis (see **Table 2**).

NEOPLASTIC DISEASE

The goals of tumor imaging are multiplex according to the stage of management for initial diagnosis, during the treatment, and on follow-up immediately and longer after therapy.[81] During the initial diagnosis of brain tumor, neuroimaging has essential roles: (1) to differentiate it from nontumorous condition, (2) to precisely define the location and extent of the lesion, (3) to make a diagnosis and a differential diagnosis, (4) to estimate the grade of tumor, (5) to evaluate possible complication made by the tumor (hemorrhage, herniation, hydrocephalus, and so forth.).[79,96–98] During the therapeutic planning and surgical/radiosurgical treatment, neuroimaging is an essential part of the decision-making process for therapy and provides valuable anatomic information to guide biopsy, resection, and radiosurgical therapy.[99–102] For therapeutic follow-up, neuroimaging is also mandatory to monitor disease progression and therapeutic response, including the differentiation of recurrent tumor from radiation necrosis and possible side effects.[84,86,103]

Evolution of applications and protocols for MR imaging and GBCA prompts a continued reassessment of the optimal use of these technique and agents. From the consensus discussion of small group of experts in neuroradiology, neuro-oncology, neurosurgery and radio-oncology, Essig and colleagues[81] have recently proposed recommendations on practical application of MR imaging of neoplastic CNS lesions as follows. (1) MR imaging is the technique of choice for the differential diagnosis, tumor grading, and treatment planning of neoplastic CNS lesions, and advanced MR imaging techniques provide physiologic data relevant to diagnosis and grading that may assist conventional MR imaging. (2) MR imaging is an important reference point for monitoring treatment response and recurrence, but the McDonald criteria have limitations. New criteria for assessing enhancing/nonenhancing lesions[104] offer amended guidance for response assessment. Advanced MR imaging techniques may help assess the post-therapeutic brain when

contrast enhancement is nonspecific. (3) As optimization of the protocol sequence enhances CNS lesion characterization, a standardized protocol sequence for conventional MR imaging includes T1W precontrast, T2-weighted (T2W) DWI, and T1W contrast imaging. Additional advanced MR imaging techniques can be selected according to the clinical scenario. Higher field strengths (eg, 3 T vs 1.5 T) provide superior image quality, if available. Image acquisition at up to 20 minutes post–contrast injection offers improved lesion detection; (4) a single dose (0.1 mmol/kg of body weight) of GBCA is recommended for suspected primary lesions, with a second administration in cases of diagnostic doubt. In patients with a glomerular filtration rate below 30 mL/min/1.73 m^2, a single dose only is recommended. With a glomerular filtration rate of 30 mL/min/1.73 m^2 to 60 mL/min/1.73 m^2, a single dose or double dose may be used; and (5) contrast media with a macrocyclic structure (eg, gadobutrol, gadoterate dimeglumine, and gadoteridol) have a higher chelate stability than linear agents. Contrast agents with high gadolinium concentration and higher relaxivity are preferred for superior enhancement. Gadobutrol offers the highest gadolinium concentration (1 mol/L) and high relaxivity to provide the highest T1 shortening effect among currently available agents.

Tumors of Neuroepithelial Tissue

Astrocytic tumors

Glioma is a tumor arising in the supportive parenchymal cells or glial cells of the brain, which are made up of astrocytes, oligodendrocytes, ependymal cells, and microglial cells. Primary brain tumors account for two-thirds of all brain tumors, and gliomas are approximately 45% to 50% of primary brain tumors. They occur most commonly in the cerebrum and occur most frequently between the ages of 40 and 70 years. Grading of tumors can be difficult both by diagnostic imaging and from surgical biopsy, because gliomas may be heterogeneous in terms of tumor grade.

In glioma, contrast enhancement on CE MR imaging is determined by the degree of intratumoral angiogenesis and BBB breakdown (see **Fig. 2**). Contrast enhancement is generally correlated with grade of malignancy for diffuse astrocytomas (low-grade astrocytoma, anaplastic astrocytoma, and gliblastoma multiforme)[105]; however, it is not usually for circumscribed astrocytomas (pilocytic astrocytoma, subependymal giant cell astrocytoma, and pleomorphic xanthoastrocytoma).[106,107] It is frequent that a single astrocytoma has both low-grade and high-grade histologic components.

If there is focal area of contrast enhancement within the low-grade astrocytoma, it may have high chance of localized malignant transformation (**Fig. 4**).[108]

Low-grade astrocytoma consists of well-differentiated fibrillary astrocyte and subtle increase in cell density and cellular atypia but has no other finding of anaplasia. Low-grade glioma may eventually progress to high-grade glioma. Because low-grade astrocytoma has low cellular density, it shows T1 low, T2 bright signal intensity, and, rarely, contrast enhancement because BBB is

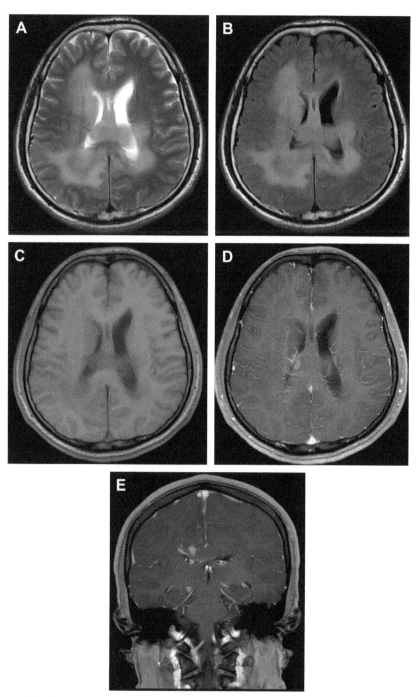

Fig. 4. A 43-year-old male patient with gliomatosis cerebri. T2W (*A*), FLAIR (*B*), and T1W (*C*) images show ill-defined, diffusely infiltrating mass lesion in cerebral white matters of both cerebral hemispheres, including corpus callosum. Axial (*D*) and coronal (*E*) CE T1W images show focal contrast enhancement near the corpus callosum.

generally intact.[109,110] The absence of contrast enhancement is also consistent with the absence of any histologic vascular changes.

Anaplastic astrocytoma is a lesion of intermediate aggression, between simple astrocytoma (World Health Organization grade 2) and glioblastoma multiforme (World Health Organization grade 4). Anaplastic astrocytomas show variable enhancement characteristics.[111–113] They may present as a nonenhancing, homogeneous region of abnormal signal intensity and/or expanded brain. In some cases, there may be patchy contrast enhancement (**Fig. 5**). Because there is no necrosis by pathologic definition, heterogeneous ring-like enhancement does not occur.[112,114]

Glioblastoma multiforme is the most malignant of the glial neoplasm and comprises more than half of all adult glial tumors.[115] The magnetic resonance appearance of glioblastoma multiforme includes a mass lesion with irregular ring-like enhancement, prominent surrounding vasogenic edema, and heterogeneity of signal. These tumors may exhibit cystic and solid components and hemorrhage is common. The central necrosis does not enhance and is surrounded by living tumor, which shows prominent ring-like, irregular enhancement of variable thickness (**Fig. 6**). Because the tumor vessels sprout from pre-existing normal vasculature, the enhancing rim may be thicker on the cortical or outer surface compared with the thinner, deep or white matter margin.[74,116] Contrast enhancement is important in patient management. CE MR imaging can be particularly helpful in planning of surgical biopsy, because enhancement correlates with tumor viability.[117,118]

Pilocystic astrocytoma is one of the most benign of all primary CNS tumors and is the most common posterior fossa tumor in childhood. It is often cystic or partially cystic, usually encapsulated, and grows slowly. It can be totally cured by surgical removal with the best prognosis of all astrocytomas. On MR imaging, pilocytic astrocytomas may appear as a well-circumscribed cystic mass with prominent contrast-enhancing nodule in posterior fossa (cyst with nodule). This nodular portion usually demonstrates contrast enhancement,[106,119] and variable degree of wall enhancement may also occur (**Fig. 7**). In addition to pilocytic astrocytoma, supratentorial brain tumor having cyst with contrast-enhancing nodule may also include pleomorphic xanthoastrocytoma, gangliogioma, and hemangioblastoma.

Pleomorphic xanthoastrocytoma originates from subpial astrocytes and occurs superficially in the brain.[107,120] Although the histology may appear malignant, most pleomorphic xanthoastrocytoma have a benign clinical course. It occurs mainly in childhood and adolescence. The most common tumor location is the temporal lobe followed by parietal frontal and occipital lobes. The tumors are mostly superficially located with common involvement of the cortex. They appear as cystic, mixed cystic-solid, or solid lesions. The mural nodules of the mixed cystic-solid tumors are closed to the leptomeningeal surface (**Fig. 8**). Multiple minute cysts are also noted in the solid tumors. The solid components of tumors, including the mural nodules or thick cystic walls, show marked enhancement with contrast media.[107,120,121]

Subependymal giant cell astrocytoma is a clinically benign tumor arising from the wall of the lateral ventricle near the foramen of Monro. It is associated with tuberous sclerosis and is believed to originate from subependymal tuberous sclerosis nodules. On MR imaging, subependymal giant cell astrocytoma typically shows a well-circumscribed mass at the foramen of Monro, which frequently exhibits partial calcification or cyst formation. Enhancement after contrast administration is strong but inhomogeneous.[122–124]

Oligodendroglial tumors
Oligodendroglioma is a well-differentiated, diffusely infiltrating tumor of adults that is typically located in the cerebral hemispheres. The tumors are derived from supportive cells and may also present as oligoastrocytoma with mixed histology. They are most commonly located in the frontal

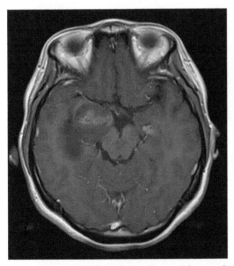

Fig. 5. A 26-year-old female patient with anaplastic astrocytoma. CE T1W image shows mass involving the medial aspect of right temporal lobe, with focal area of patchy contrast enhancement.

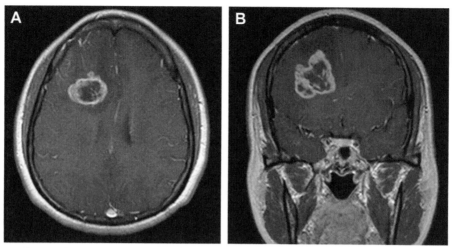

Fig. 6. A 45-year-old female patient with glioblastoma multiforme. Axial (*A*) and coronal (*B*) contrast enhanced T1W images show mass with ring-like, irregular enhancement of variable thickness. Enhancing rim is thicker on the cortical (outer) surface.

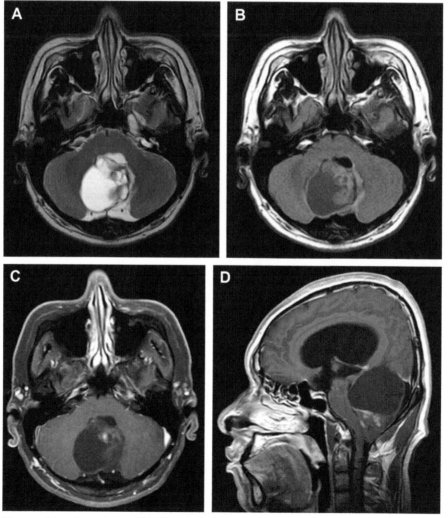

Fig. 7. A 39-year-old male patient with pilocytic astrocytoma. T2W (*A*) and FLAIR (*B*) images show a well-circumscribed cystic mass with solid nodule in posterior fossa (cyst with nodule). Axial (*C*) and sagittal (*D*) CE T1W images show contrast enhancement in the nodular portion.

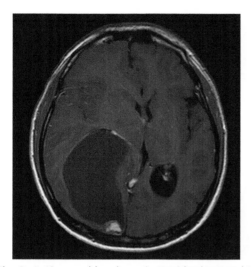

Fig. 8. A 43-year-old male patient with pleomorphic xanthoastrocytoma. CE T1W image shows mixed cystic and solid mass involving the right occipital lobe, with contrast-enhancing mural nodule on the leptomeningeal (outer) surface.

lobes. They tend to grow toward the cortex rather than infiltrating into the centrally located corpus callosum. They are slowly growing and often heterogeneous. Because of the slow-growing manner, the lesions may be large at the time of presentation; 90% of oligodendrogliomas show histologic calcification (**Fig. 9**). Oligodendrogliomas have been reported to show frequent postcontrast enhancement on MR imaging. Contrast enhancement is suggested as proportional to tumor vascularity.[125] Contrast enhancement as well as perilesional edema is associated with high-grade oligodendroglioma.[125–128]

Ependymal tumors

Ependymomas are rare tumors of neuroectodermal origin, arising from the epithelium lining the ventricles. They are classified as myxopapillary ependymoma and subependymoma (grade I), ependymoma (grade II), and anaplastic ependymoma (grade III). Ependymoma is generally a tumor of childhood and located in the fourth ventricle region, although in adults they can be seen in the lateral and third ventricles. Lesions appear as soft plastic masses that squeeze out fourth ventricle foramina into cerebellopontine angle or cisterna magna, pushing against the walls of the ventricle without invasion. Myxopapillary ependymomas are typically and almost exclusively located in the conus–cauda equina–filum terminale region. Subependymomas are typically located in the fourth and lateral ventricles.[129,130] On CE MR imaging, ependymoma is well

vascularized and enhances intensely with gadolinium.[131–133] On the contrary, subependymoma shows different MR imaging features depending on anatomic location; calcification and heterogeneous contrast enhancement are common features of fourth ventricular subependymomas, whereas lack of calcification and minimal or no contrast enhancement in the lateral ventricular lesions (**Fig. 10**).[130]

Choroid plexus tumors

Choroid plexus tumors arise from choroid plexus, and there are 2 primary types: the well-differentiated and benign choroid plexus papilloma and the malignant less-differentiated choroid plexus carcinoma. They are most common in the first decade of life. Choroid plexus tumors are almost invariably intraventricular masses, usually seen in lateral ventricle in children, not infrequently in fourth ventricle in adults. On CE MR imaging, choroid plexus papilloma typically shows densely contrast-enhancing intraventricular mass (**Fig. 11**).[134,135] Choroid plexus papilloma usually has limited focal parenchymal invasion; thus, presence of extensive subependymal invasion should raise the suspicion of choroid plexus carcinoma.[136]

Neuronal and mixed neuroglial tumors

Dysembrioplastic neuroepithelial tumor (DNT) is mixed neuroglial tumor, usually associated with chronic epilepsy in adolescents and young adults. It is most commonly located in the temporal lobe as intracortical lesion and causes no neurologic deficit.[137] Multicystic appearance on MR images is a characteristic feature of DNT and corresponds to its myxoid matrix and multinodular architecture. The cystic, in most cases even multicystic, appearance on MR images is a typical feature of DNT despite the absence of true cysts intraoperatively or on microscopic examination.[138,139] On CE MR imaging, multifocal faintly nodular or ring enhancement is seen in one-third of cases (**Fig. 12**).

Gangliogliomas are slow-growing neoplasms composed of 2 types of cells: neoplastic glial cells and neoplastic ganglion cells. They most commonly occur in children and young adults. The most common location in the brain is the temporal lobe, followed by frontal lobe.[140] On MR imaging, they are typically well-circumscribed masses, often with partially cystic change and with no or little edema. Contrast enhancement is reported in approximately one-half of tumors (**Fig. 13**).[140–142]

Central neurocytoma occurs in adults and typically in the lateral ventricle or in the subependymal region. The imaging appearance of central neurocytoma is characteristic and consists of an entirely

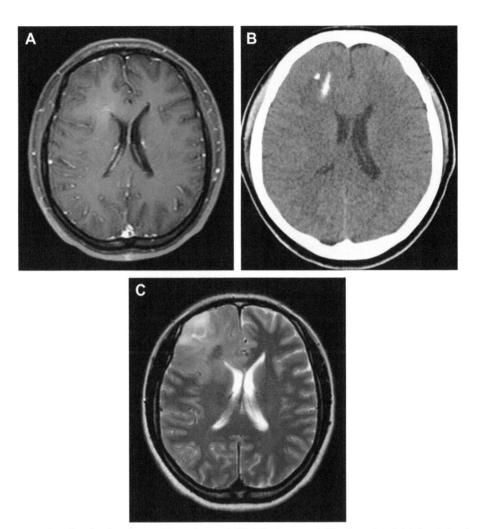

Fig. 9. Low-grade oligodendroglioma. Nonenhanced CT (*A*) shows calcifications in right frontal subcortical region. T2W image (*B*) shows cortical to subcortical involvement of the mass in right frontal lobe. CE T1W image (*C*) shows no contrast enhancement.

intraventricular mass near the foramen of Monro, showing well-circumscribed tumor lesion with iso-intense to hyperintense signal on most MR sequences. Contrast enhancement is variable in degree and pattern, from slight to heterogeneously intense contrast enhancement (**Fig. 14**).[143,144]

Tumors of the pineal region
Pineocytoma and more malignant pineoblastoma are rare and have been estimated as less than 15% of all pineal region tumors.[145,146] On MR imaging, pineocytomas on T1W images show rounded, sometimes or slightly lobulated low signal intensity masses with strong and homogeneous contrast enhancement. Their margin is clear, without invasion of adjacent structures. The pineoblastomas, however, show multilobulated tumor with heterogeneous contrast enhancement and poorly defined margin with adjacent structures, including posterior thalamus or corpus callosum by more invasive nature.[145]

Embryonal tumors
Medulloblastomas (most common type of Primitive neuroectodermal tumors [PNETs]) comprise a heterogeneous group of undifferentiated malignant tumors of brain. PNETs of the cerebellum are historically referred to as medulloblastomas, whereas supratentorial PNETs have been called cerebral medulloblastoma, cerebral neuroblastomas or ganglioneuroblastoma, ependymoblastoma, and undifferentiated small cell neoplasms of the brain.[147–149] They are highly malignant due to locally aggressive behavior and subarachnoid dissemination, for which contrast enhancement is helpful to delineate extent. Most of the lesions

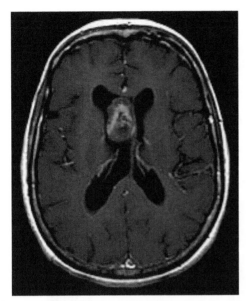

Fig. 10. Subependymoma. CE T1W image shows intra-ventricular mass in right lateral ventricle, with mild focal contrast enhancement.

show variable contrast enhancement from mild to intense degree.[147,150,151]

Tumors of Cranial and Paraspinal Nerves

Schwannoma is the second most common intra-cranial extra-axial neoplasm in adults, and 90% of them arise from the acoustic nerve, followed by trigeminal and facial nerves. Vestibular schwannoma is the most common solid mass involving the cer-ebellopontine angle and internal auditory canal. It is mostly a solitary lesion but may be multiple in patients with neurofibromatosis type 2. On CE MR imaging, it generally shows strong contrast enhancement, which is sometimes heterogeneous with cystic changes (**Fig. 15**).[152,153] Contrast enhancement pattern may be similar to cerebello-pontine angle meningioma, but menigioma usually has broad base to the adjacent dura and dural tail, and schwannomas often cause flaring of the porus acousticus with extension into the internal auditory canal.

Tumors of the Meninges

Tumors of meningothelial cells
Meningiomas account for 15% to 18% of all intra-cranial neoplasms and are the most common primary nonglial lesions. They are most common in middle-aged and elderly adults, twice as common in women as in men. Typical locations include the parasagittal region of the anterior, middle, and posterior segments of the sagittal sinus, cerebral falx, convexity, olfactory groove,

tuberculum sellae, medial and lateral sphenoid wings, Meckel cave, tentorium, cerebellopontine angle, clivus, and craniocervical junction. The great majority of meningioma is benign and well differentiated and has low proliferative capacity. Meningiomas are classified histologically as grade I tumors (benign tumors without atypia or mitosis) for approximately 90% of cases, grade II tumors (rare mitosis and some cellular atypia) for 5% of cases, and grade III tumors (abundant vasculariza-tion, numerous mitoses, and presence of cell aty-pia) for 3% to 5% of cases. MR imaging demonstrates imaging features that vary accord-ing to the presence of histologic atypia, cysts, calcification, and grade of vascularization. Usually, meningiomas are isointense to gray matter and show homogeneous dense contrast enhancement in more than 95% of cases. The extent of dura mater involvement is demarcated by the dural tail sign of meningioma (**Fig. 16**).[154]

Other neoplasms related to the meninges
Hemangioblastoma is benign vascular neoplasm of unknown origin and generally presents as a well-circumscribed mass. Approximately 10% to 20% of patients with hemangioblastoma are associated with von Hippel-Lindau disease, and approximately 45% of patients with von Hippel-Lindau disease have hemangioblastoma.[155] It is usually located in the cerebellar hemisphere, vermis, or medullar near the area postrema. It is seen as cyst with nodule in 60% of cases (**Fig. 17**) and as solid mass in remaining 40%. The typical cerebellar he-mangioblastoma is a well-circumscribed lesion with an enhancing nodule in superficial and subpial location and shows intratumoral vascular signal void on MR imaging.[156,157]

Lymphomas and Hematopoietic Neoplasms

Primary CNS lymphomas are rare, although they have increased in incidence in immunocompro-mised patients. They are generally non-Hodgkin lymphoma of B-cell type. They have a distinct affinity for perivascular extension. Although gran-ular nodules may be seen at gross pathologic inspection, diffuse microscopic spread is always present, which accounts for the ability of this tumor to produce distant disease and local recurrences. The dense cellularity of the tumor and its predilec-tion for the periventricular region also explains its typical hyperattenuated appearance on unen-hanced CT and hypointensity on T2W MR images. Virtually all lesions enhance with contrast material (**Fig. 18**).[158] Lymphoma also can be seen in immu-nosuppressed patients, and imaging findings are variable in appearance. Contrast enhancement may be ring-shaped and irregular.[83,159]

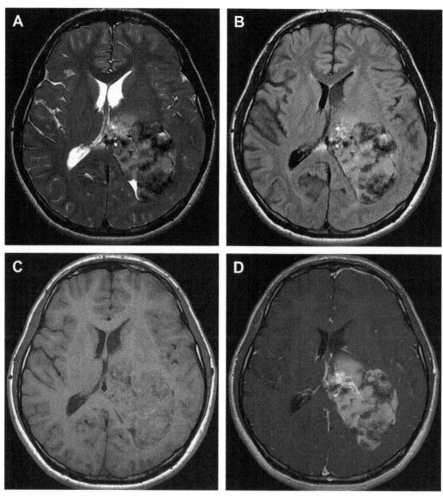

Fig. 11. Choroid plexus papilloma. T2W (A), FLAIR (B), and T1W (C) images show intraventricular mass involving the left lateral ventricle. CE T1W image (D) shows dense contrast enhancement.

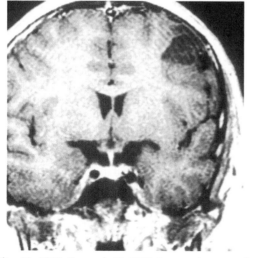

Fig. 12. DNT. Coronal CE T1W image shows well-circumscribed cystic cortical lesion involving the left frontal lobe, with little contrast enhancement.

Germ Cell Tumors

Germ cell tumors are classified into 6 histologic types: germinoma, embryonal carcinoma, yolk-sac tumor, choriocarcinoma, teratoma (mature, immature, and teratoma with malignant transformation), and mixed germ cell tumor.[160,161] Germ cell tumors in the pineal region and basal ganglia have a predominantly male preponderance, whereas neurohypophyseal germ cell tumors have a slight female preponderance.[161,162] On MR imaging, the solid portion of the tumor is isointense to the gray matter on T2W image. Cystic change is seen in approximately 50% of germinomas and in most of nongerminomatous germ cell tumors. CE MR imaging shows contrast enhancement of solid portion in more than half of the germinoma and most of nongerminomatous tumors.[157,161,163,164] Contrast enhancement is also helpful in depicting CSF spread of these tumors (Fig. 19).[83]

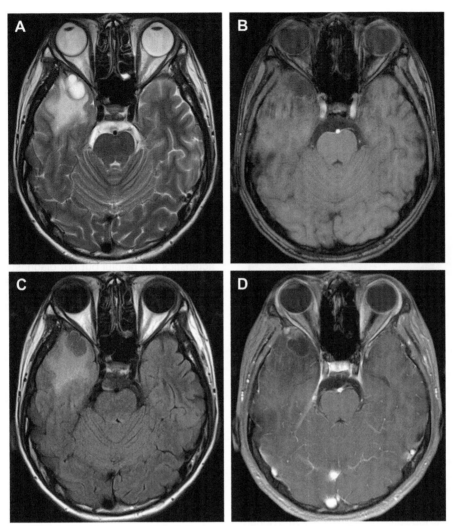

Fig. 13. Ganglioglioma. T2W (*A*), T1W (*B*) and FLAIR (*C*) images show well-defined mass with cystic change involving the right anterior temporal cortical region. CE T1W image (*D*) shows marginal contrast enhancement on the wall of cystic change and nodular contrast enhancement on anterior surface of the lesion.

Tumors of the Sella Region

Pituitary adenoma is a slowly growing benign tumor arising from adenohypophysis and is approximately 10% to 15% of total brain tumor. Approximately 25% of lesions are nonfunctional and remaining 75% are functioning tumor with variable symptoms according to the hypersecreting hormone. Microadenoma is less than 10 mm in diameter. On MR imaging, microadenomas usually show delayed contrast enhancement compared with normal pituitary gland. Sakamoto and colleagues[165] reported gradual contrast enhancement pattern of normal pituitary gland and adenoma. The earliest contrast material enhancement of normal structures is in the infundibulum and posterior lobe of the pituitary gland at 20 seconds, followed by gradual contrast

material enhancement of the anterior lobe of the pituitary gland from the junction of the infundibulum to the peripheral portion of the anterior lobe of the pituitary gland within 80 seconds after gadolinium injection. The peak enhancement of pituitary adenomas occurred at 60 to 200 seconds, usually after the most marked enhancement of the normal pituitary gland. Microadenomas are best visualized at earlier phases of dynamic CE MR imaging, with signal intensity lower than that seen on images of normal pituitary glands (**Fig. 20**).[165,166] Evaluation of cavernous sinus invasion from the macroadenoma may be difficult to determine with certainty but can be suspected when the lesion encircles the internal carotid artery and asymmetric tentorial enhancement is associated.[167]

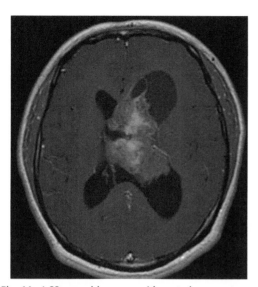

Fig. 14. A 33-year-old woman with central neurocytoma. CE T1W image shows intraventricular mass near the foramen of Monro, with slightly heterogeneous and patch CE in the isointense solid portion of the mass.

Craniopharyngioma is an intracranial epithelial neoplasm occurring in an intrasellar and/or supra-sellar location.[168–170] It is the most common supra-sellar mass in children and has bimodal peak in incidence, the larger first peak in children and second peak in early sixth decade. In children, lesions are commonly adamantinomatous type, which frequently shows cystic change and calcifi-cation with poor prognosis. The adamantinoma-tous craniopharyngioma is mixed solid-cystic or mainly cystic lobulated mass, typically with nonen-hancing hyperintense cysts on T1W image. In adults, the squamous-papillary type is more common and has less cystic change and better prognosis. The squamous-papillary craniophar-yngioma is a predominantly solid or mixed solid-cystic suparsellar tumor, appearing as a hy-pointense cyst on noncontrast T1W images.[170] Lesions show well-defined heterogeneous mass with cystic changes on MR imaging. Contrast enhancement does not play a role in tumor detec-tion, although enhancement can best define the extent of the lesion and its relationship to normal adjacent structures.[83]

Metastatic Tumors

Hematogeneous spread of primary neoplasm can result in CNS disease burdening various anatomi-cally distinct regions: intraparenchymal, leptome-ningeal, pachymeningeal, and calvarial.[171–173]

Parenchymal metastasis accounts for up to 50% of all brain tumors and 10% to 50% of patients with systemic malignancy develop brain metastases during the course of their disease, and metastases account for more than half of all brain tumors in adults. In adults, the primary tumors most likely to metastasize to the brain are located, in decreasing order, in the lung, breast, skin, colon-rectum, and kidney, but in general any malignant tumor is able to metastasize to the brain.[172,173] There are no pathognomonic features on MR imaging that distinguish brain metastases from primary brain tumors (more commonly malig-nant gliomas and lymphomas) or non-neoplastic conditions (abscesses, infections, demyelinating diseases, and vascular lesions). A peripheral loca-tion, spherical shape, ring enhancement with prominent peritumoral edema, and multiple lesions all suggest metastatic disease: these char-acteristics are helpful but not diagnostic, even in patients with a positive history of cancer. CE MR imaging is the preferred imaging modality for the evaluation of cerebral metastasis.[171,174,175] Paren-chymal metastases are generally well-defined cir-cumscribed nodular or ring-enhancing lesion of variable size, located at corticomedullary junction (**Figs. 21** and **22**).

Leptomeningeal carcinomatosis may be either from primary CNS malignancy (medulloblastoma, ependymoma, glioblastoma, and oligodendroglioma) or extracranial primary malignancy (lung, stom-ach, breast, ovary, melanoma, lymphoma, and leukemia).[74] Leptomeningeal metastases may produce thin or thick linear, nodular, or miliary thickening with contrast enhancement on CE MR imaging. CE MR imaging is complementary to CSF examinations and can be invaluable, detect-ing up to 50% of false-negative lumbar punctures. MR findings range from diffuse linear lepto-meningeal enhancement to multiple enhancing extra-axial nodules and obstructive communi-cating and noncommunicating hydrocephalus (**Fig. 23**).[171,176] Recently, CE FLAIR sequence has been found effective in the detection of lepto-meningeal carcinomatosis.[32,43] Because of the suppression of CSF signal intensity, there is marked delineation of meningeal lesion abutting the border of the CSF. In addition, slow-flowing blood is not usually hyperintense on postcontrast FLAIR images but frequently hyperintense on post-contrast T1W images, partly accounting for the clearer distinction of enhancing meninges and enhancing cortical veins with FLAIR imaging.[28,43]

Pachymeningeal carcinomatosis or dural metastases may be from direct invasion of calvari-al malignancy or from primary malignancy of breast, prostate, systemic lymphoma, and lung.[74,171] Bone metastases extending intracrani-ally and primary dural metastases show the

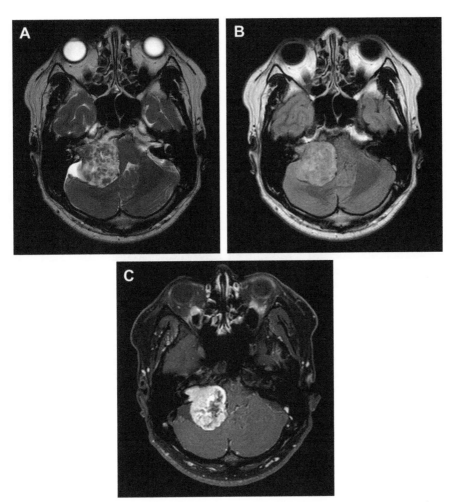

Fig. 15. A 31-year-old male patient with vestibular schwannoma. T2W (*A*) and FLAIR (*B*) images show solid mass with cystic changes involving the right cerebellopontine angle and internal auditory canal with flaring of the porus acousticus. CE T1W image (*C*) shows strong and heterogeneous contrast enhancement.

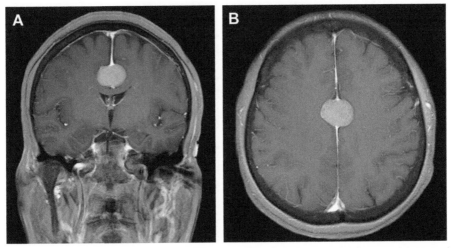

Fig. 16. A 57-year-old female patient with meningioma. Axial (*A*) and coronal (*B*) CE T1W images show well-defined, extra-axial mass with strong and homogeneous contrast enhancement, involving the cerebral falx. There is associated dural thickening (dural tail).

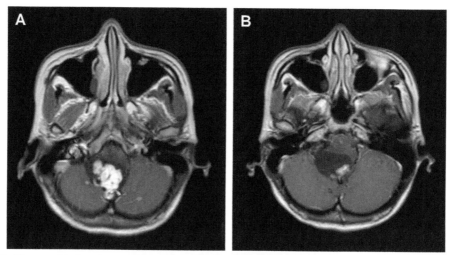

Fig. 17. A 22-year-old female patient with hemangioblastoma. Axial CE T1W images (*A*, *B*) show well-circumscribed, mixed solid and cystic mass with strong nodular contrast enhancement in cerebellum.

characteristic biconvex shape, usually associated with brain displacement away from the inner table. Although CT is better in detecting skull base erosion, MR is more sensitive and provides more detailed information about dural involvement.[176] CE MR imaging may show multiple nodules, diffuse dural thickening, or combination.[171,177]

NON-NEOPLASTIC DISEASE
Infection and Inflammatory Disease

Leptomeningeal/pachymeningeal inflammation
Meningitis is inflammation of subarachnoid space and surrounding meninges and can be classified as acute pyogenic meningitis, acute viral lymphocytic meningitis, and chronic tuberculous or mycobacterial meningitis. Diagnosis of meningitis is made by clinical history, physical examination findings, and laboratory results. Imaging findings are usually nonspecific, varying according to the temporal evolution of the disease, degree of inflammation, and etiologic agents. Thus, the role of imaging is mostly delineating the complication, such as hydrocephalus, subdural empyema, ventriculitis, or abscess.[178]

Acute pyogenic meningitis is mostly from hematogenous spread of inflammation, although direct extension of mastoiditis or paranasal sinusitis may

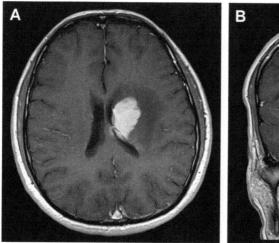
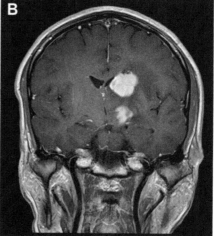

Fig. 18. A 51-year-old male patient with primary CNS lymphoma. Axial (*A*) and coronal (*B*) CE T1W images show 2 masses with homogeneous and strong contrast enhancement, involving the left frontal periventricular and thalamic regions.

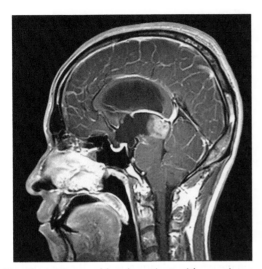

Fig. 19. A 26-year-old male patient with germinoma. Sagittal CE T1W image shows contrast-enhancing mass with cystic change involving the pineal region, with cystic changes. There are associated linear contrast enhancement on the surface of the brain, suggesting CSF spread, and hydrocephalus.

not infrequently result in meningitis. CE MR imaging is the preferred imaging modality in the evaluation of lesional localization and extent of meningitis and associated complication, such as hydrocephalus, ventriculitis, subdural effusion, emphyema,

cerebritis, and abscess. In the early phase of uncomplicated pyogenic meningitis, CE MR imaging shows normal findings or mild hydrocephalus. As disease progresses, effacement of sulci, leptomeningeal contrast enhancement, and hydrocephalus is seen. Mechanism of contrast enhancement is either from leakage of gadolinium from abnormal vasculatures or from vascular contrast enhancement in the granulation tissues.[179] CE FLAIR may also have an important role in the early screening for infectious meningitis, with increased sensitivity of leptomeningeal contrast enhancement compared with CE T1W image.[31]

Tuberculous meningitis arises from hematogeneous spread and usually develops gelatinous exudate in suprasellar cistern, sylvian fissure, and ambient cistern. Hydrocephalus is more frequent than pyogenic meningitis. Diagnosis may be made from a combination of clinical symptoms and laboratory and imaging findings. Laboratory findings include increased protein, lymphocytosis, decreased glucose in CSF, and, not infrequently, acid-fast bacteria smear and culture that may show negative findings. Imaging findings are effacement of basal cisterns, leptomeningeal enhancement at basal cistern, and communicating hydrocephalus. CE MR imaging shows irregular and thick leptomeningeal contrast enhancement.[180] Tuberculous granuloma may develop with tuberculous meningitis or independently.

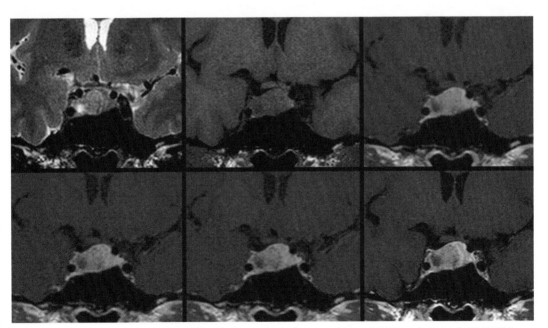

Fig. 20. A 32-year-old female patient with pituitary microadenoma. Coronal T2W and dynamic CE T1W images show mass involving the right lateral aspect of the sella, with decreased contrast enhancement compared with densely contrast-enhancing pituitary gland.

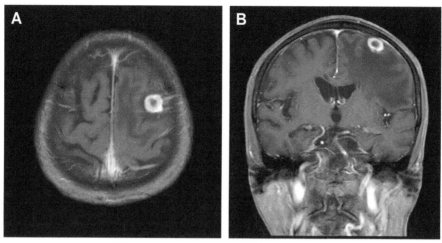

Fig. 21. A 70-year-old male patient with solitary brain metastasis from lung cancer. Axial (*A*) and coronal (*B*) CE T1W images show well-defined, ring-enhancing lesion involving the left frontal cortical region. There is extensive white matter compared with small size of contrast-enhancing lesion.

Granuloma shows signal intensities similar to the brain on nonenhanced MR imaging; thus, is it often difficult to find granuloma without contrast enhancement. Small granulomas (<1 cm) usually show solid, homogeneous contrast enhancement, and larger granulomas may show ring enhancement with caseation necrosis.[181]

Cerebritis and brain abscess
Brain abscess starts as localized cerebritis and develops central liquefaction necrosis in a short period and focal parenchymal inflammation surrounded by fibrocollageneous capsule. Brain abscess mostly arises from pyogenic bacteria but can also arise from mycobacteria, actinomyces,

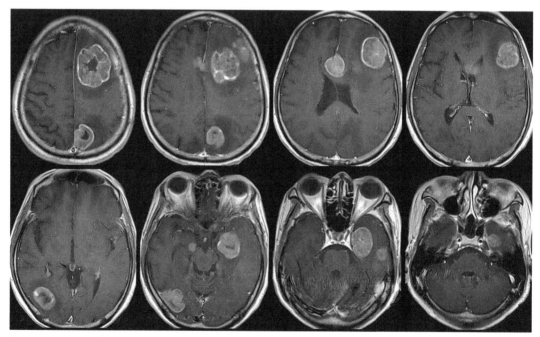

Fig. 22. A 65-year-old male patient with multiple brain metastasis from lung cancer. CE T1W images show multiple nodular contrast-enhancing masses scattered in cortical and subcortical regions of both cerebral hemispheres, with variable degree of peritumoral edema.

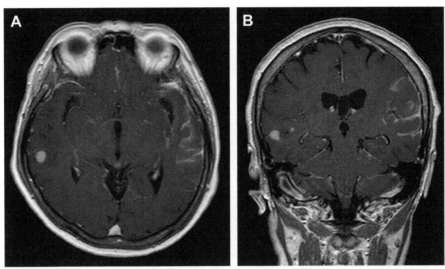

Fig. 23. A 63-year-old female patient with leptomeningeal metastasis from lung cancer. Axial (*A*) and coronal (*B*) CE T1W images shows diffuse and linear leptomeningeal contrast enhancement in left temporal lobe and cerebellum and nodular contrast enhancement in leptomeningeal surface of right temporal lobe.

fungi, and parasites. Cerebritis usually develops from hematogeneous spread or direct extension of mastoiditis and paranasal sinusitis. Imaging findings of brain abscess correlate with pathologic changes related to stage of disease progression.[182,183] In acute cerebritis stage (1 to approximately 5 days), there are focal infiltration of inflammatory cells, edema, and necrosis, and imaging findings show lesions with irregularly marginated contrast enhancement, mass effect, and ill-defined edema. In late cerebritis stage (5 to approximately 14 days), central necrotic areas conglomerates, and CE MR imaging shows irregular and thick ring enhancement (**Fig. 24**). In mature capsular stage (later than 14 days), capsule is made of 3 layers: (1) inner granulation tissue and macrophage, (2) intermediate collagen layer, and (3) outer gliosis. Central necrotic portion liquefies and produce pus. Capsule is isointense to slightly hyperintense on T1WI, and hypointense to isointense on T2W imaging on MR imaging, and contrast-enhancing wall becomes smooth and thinner than the cerebritis stage.[183] There can be a stellate abscess around the main abscess cavity at this stage. Ring enhancement can last several weeks after disappearance of active inflammation.

Viral CNS infection
Acute viral encephalitis widely describes CNS involvement of viral infection, and it more frequently involves the meninges, resulting in aseptic meningitis or mild meningoencephalitis

rather than pure encephalitis. Viral meningitis usually shows better prognosis and does not induce serious complication. Laboratory findings, including increased protein, normal glucose level, and lymphocyte proliferation in CSF, lead to diagnosis of viral meningitis. CE MR imaging shows normal or mild leptomeningeal contrast enhancement (see **Fig. 1**).[184]

Herpes simplex encephalitis occurs as 2 distinct entities. Type 1 herpes simplex encephalitis occurs in children older than 3 months and in adults and is typically localized to the temporal and frontal lobes, whereas type 2 occurs in neonates, is acquired at the time of delivery, and shows generalized involvement of the brain. Type 1 herpes simplex encephalitis is acute fulminating necrotizing encephalitis and shows high mortality. It involves typical sites, including inferomedial aspect of temporal lobe, orbital side of frontal lobe, insula, and cingulate gyrus. CE MR imaging rarely shows contrast enhancement in early phase; however, a patchy parenchymal or gyral contrast enhancement may develop slightly later after the T2 signal changes within 1 to 2 weeks (**Fig. 25**).[185]

Fungal CNS infection
Cryptococcal infection occurs in patients with lymphoma, leukemia, organ transplantation, steroid administration, and HIV infection. It hematogeneously spreads from lung, and the most commonly involved site is the CNS. It may present as meningitis, meningoencephalitis, or

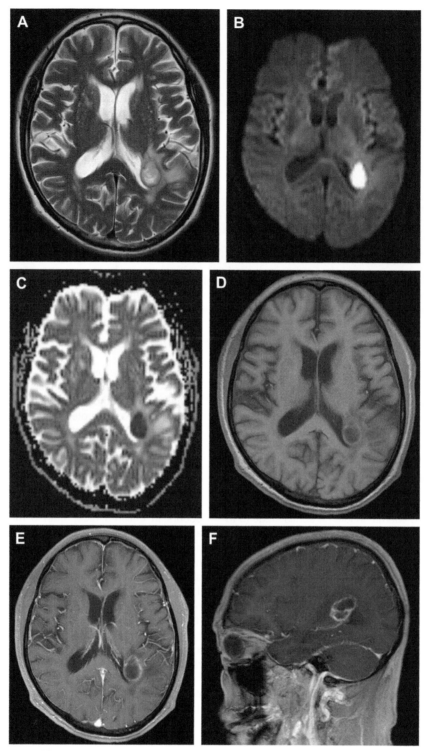

Fig. 24. A 71-year-old male patient with brain abscess. T2W image (*A*) shows lesion with isointense to hypointense capsule and internal bright signal intensity. DWI (*B*) and ADC map (*C*) show decreased ADC of internal content due to thick pus. Capsule is hyperintense on T1W image (*D*) and shows ring-like contrast enhancement on axial (*E*) and sagittal (*F*) CE T1W images.

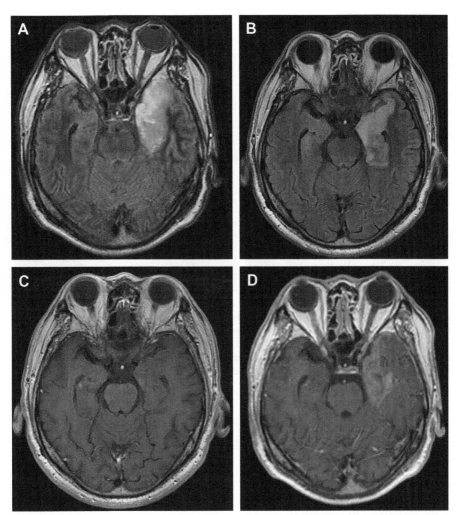

Fig. 25. A 72-year-old male patient with herpes encephalitis. FLAIR (*A & B*) images show gyral swelling with bright signal intensity involving the medial aspect of temporal lobe. CE T1W image (*C*) shows no contrast enhancement at this early phase. Follow-up CE T1W image (*D*), 2 weeks later, shows patchy gyral contrast enhancement.

cryptococooma in the brain. Imaging findings frequently show normal findings. Cryptococci may spread along the Virchow-Robin space from basal cistern, forming gelatinous pseudocyst filled with yeast mostly involving the basal ganglia, thalamus, or cerebral cortex. It generally shows little contrast enhancement on CE MR imaging, especially in immunocompromised patients, but may show nodular or ring-like contrast enhancement, or multiple enhancing nodules in brain parenchyma or leptomeninges.[186,187] It rarely shows basal or leptomeningeal contrast enhancement.

Aspergillosis and mucormycosis may occur by hematogeneous spread from lung or direct invasion from paranasal sinus and orbit, predominantly in immunosuppressed patients. They present as meningitis, multiple abscess, granuloma, or craniofacial lesion with dural involvement. Vascular invasion or thrombosis frequently results in multiple hemorrhagic mycetoma, mycotic aneurysm, and subcortical hemorrhagic infarction. CE MR imaging shows little or no contrast enhancement in severely immunosuppressed patients; however, lesions with ring or nodular enhancement are typically seen with the development of an abscess or granuloma in immunocompetent and in some immunosuppressed patients (**Fig. 26**).[188,189]

Vascular Disease

Cerebral infarction

The role of imaging in patients with acute stroke includes exclusion of hemorrhage, differentiation

A   **B**

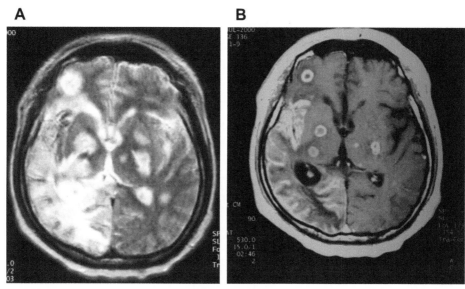

Fig. 26. A 44-year-old male patient with acute myelogneous leukemia with left hemiplegia and altered mentality. T2W image (A) shows large high signal intensity in the right temporo-occipital region. Multiple nodular high signal lesions are scattered in both cerebral hemispheres with central intermediate or low signal intensity. CE T1W image (B) shows diffuse gyral enhancement of the right temporo-occipital lobe, suggesting either fungal meningitis or associated subacute infarction and multiple ring enhancing nodules in both cerebral hemispheres. Stereotaxic biopsy from ring-enhancing lesion revealed aspergillosis.

between irreversibly infarcted brain tissue and reversibly impaired tissue (penumbra), and identification of stenosis or occlusion of major arteries. GRE MR sequence and SWI can be helpful for detecting a hemorrhage. DWI is most sensitive sequence for acute cerebral infarction, and combining the perfusion MR imaging to demonstrate mismatch can give valuable information to predict the presence of a penumbra. The status of extracranial and intracranial arteries can be evaluated with MR angiography. Conventional MR imaging is more sensitive and more specific than CT for the detection of acute cerebral ischemia within the first few hours after the onset of stroke. Typical MR imaging findings in patients with hyperacute cerebral infarction include hyperintense signal in white matter on T2W images and FLAIR images, with a resultant loss of gray matter–white matter differentiation, sulcal effacement, and mass effect; loss of the arterial flow voids seen on T2W images; and stasis of contrast material within vessels in the affected territories.[190–192]

CE MR imaging in patients with cerebral infarction shows different location and pattern of enhancement according to the location of occluded artery and stage of cerebral infarction.[193] In transient ischemic attack patients, enhanced lesions on MR imaging may be associated with a cardiac emboli or arterial disease.[194] In patients with cerebral infarction, CE MR imaging usually shows arterial enhancement followed by parenchymal enhancement. Intravascular enhancement can be early (largely within 1–2 days) and is due to slow blood flow in arteries surrounding the ischemic tissue (Fig. 27). Vascular hyperintensity on CE FLAIR may also represent disordered blood flow from collaterals distal to the arterial occlusion or stenosis (not an indicator of infarction but rather of penumbra).[48–50] Parenchymal enhancement at the infarcted lesion is generally considered to result from breakdown of the BBB,[193] which is also believed a precursor to hemorrhagic transformation and poor outcome (Fig. 28). Early parenchymal contrast enhancement after thrombolytic therapy may also predict hemorrhagic transformation.[195–197] CE FLAIR can also demonstrate early opening of BBB after cerebral infarction, seen as contrast enhancement in the CSF, and in the sulci or ventricle (hyperintense acute reperfusion marker).[198] Although this sign reflects disruption of BBB, it usually becomes apparent on delayed MR imaging.

Vascular malformation
Brain arteriovenous malformation is a vascular malformation with tangled cluster of vessels and abnormal direct connection between the arteries and veins without intervening capillary. It is a

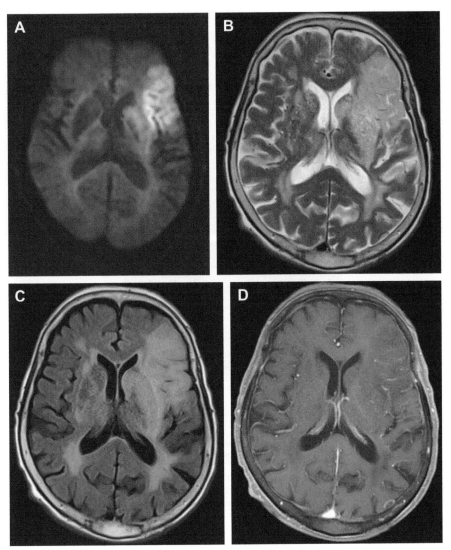

Fig. 27. A 99-year-old female patient with dysarthria and right hemiplegia. DWI (*A*) obtained at 3 hours after onset of symptom shows bright signal intensity of hyperacute infarction involving left frontal lobe and insula. T2W (*B*) and FLAIR (*C*) images, 2 days later, shows swelling of the infarcted region with effaced sulci. CE T1W image (*D*) shows intravascular contrast enhancement on the surface of affected region.

common cause of intracranial hemorrhage among the brain vascular malformations. Brain MR imaging is the preferred imaging modality, allowing detailed evaluation of relationship between the nidus and surrounding brain structures. On MR imaging, brain arteriovenous malformation is identified as a cluster of serpentine signal voids on T1W/T2W images. CE MR imaging, including postenhanced T1W images and SWI (CE SWI), are useful in the evaluation of brain arteriovenous malformation, in which presence of high signal intensity within the venous structure is an indicator of arteriovenous shunt (**Fig. 29**).[57]

Cavernous malformation (CM) is a malformation of the capillaries with widened sinusoidal spaces. There is variable amount of thrombosis and surrounding hemorrhage at different stage in and around the CM. It can cause hemorrhage, seizure, and headache or be asymptomatic. CM appears as punctuate dark lesion on T2W image, GRE, and SWI. On CE MR imaging, approximately half of CMs show contrast enhancement in variable degree of contrast enhancement (**Fig. 30**). The low flow vascular architecture within CMs seems to be the main factor contributing to the degree of contrast enhancement.[199]

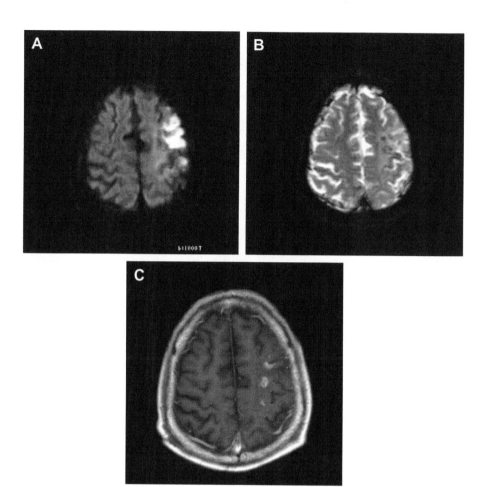

Fig. 28. An 82-year-old male patient with acute cerebral infarction and early focal hemorrhage. DWI (*A*) shows acute cerebral infarction involving the left frontal lobe. Echo-planar GRE image (*B*) shows small focal dark signal intensities of early hemorrhagic transformation, where patchy and nodular contrast enhancement is seen on CE T1W image (*C*).

Capillary telangiectasia is a lesion with abnormally dilated capillaries within normal brain tissue. It most commonly occurs in the pons but can also involve anywhere in the brain and spinal cord. MR imaging shows characteristic finding. On CE MR imaging, capillary telangiectasia has mild contrast material enhancement but is otherwise undetectable on conventional MR images,[200] with lack of hemosiderin rim on T2W image, which is characteristic finding of CM.

Developmental venous anomaly is a congenital variation with dilated venous channels and the most common CNS vascular malformation. Developmental venous anomalies are usually found incidentally and rarely cause symptoms. They can be associated with CM in 10% to 20%. CE MR imaging usually shows contrast-enhancing small medullary veins draining into dilated main transcerebral vein (**Fig. 31**).[201]

White Matter Disease

Multiple sclerosis

MR imaging has an important role in the diagnosis and management of multiple sclerosis (**Fig. 32**). MR imaging shows high sensitivity for depicting focal white matter abnormalities and clinically silent lesions in the initial evaluation of a patient suspected of multiple sclerosis, and it is also used as a tool to estimate prognosis at initial diagnosis and to evaluate outcome during and after treatment.[202] The use of gadolinium contrast agents increases both the reliability and sensitivity of detecting active lesions in multiple sclerosis. On CE MR imaging, enhancing lesions may vary in size, shape, or pattern of enhancement. This considerable variability may be associated with the different severity of inflammation and extent of BBB breakdown. Homogeneous nodular

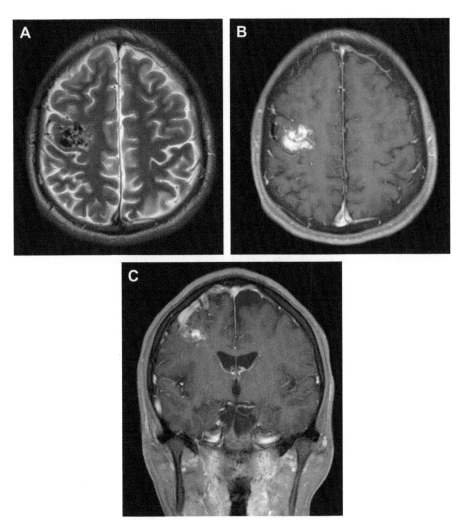

Fig. 29. A 29-year-old male patient with brain arteriovenous malformation. T2W image (*A*) shows cluster of serpentine signal voids involving the right frontal lobe. Axial (*B*) and coronal (*C*) CE T1W images show strong contrast enhancement in the nidus and dilated cortical draining vein.

enhancement is the predominant enhancement pattern (68%) for new multiple sclerosis lesions, followed by ring-like enhancement (23%) and other enhancement patterns (9%).[203] The temporal course of enhancement is usually shorter than 6 months. The enhancement corresponds to areas of transient impairment of BBB associated with inflammatory infiltration. Although contrast enhancement can be increased during clinical relapses, most enhancing lesions are clinically silent.[204] Corticosteroid administration significantly reduces the number of enhancing lesions and suppresses their appearance. Administration of increased dose of GBCA with delayed MR imaging, combining the MRS, diffusion MR imaging and DTI, perfusion MR imaging, and

imaging at higher field strength, enhance the sensitivity to active lesions.[205–209]

SUMMARY

It is well known that combined MR imaging without and with GBCA is the one of the best imaging methods to define normal anatomy and characteristics of lesions (location, size, number, border delineation, degree of edema, contrast enhancement, and so forth).

GBCAs have been used in CE MR imaging in defining and characterizing both cranial and spinal lesions of the CNS for more than 20 years.[3,13,83,109,210,211] Normally, the BBB prevents GBCAs from crossing from the blood to the brain.

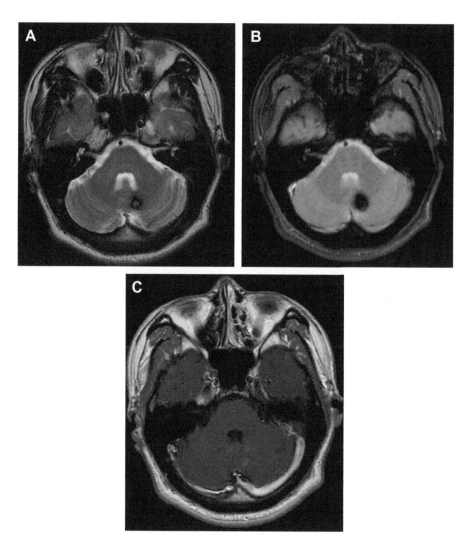

Fig. 30. CM. T2W image (*A*) shows marginal dark signal intensity involving the cerebellum. GRE (*B*) image shows dark blooming of the lesion, which is larger than that on T2W image. CE T1W image (*C*) shows subtle contrast enhancement in the lesion.

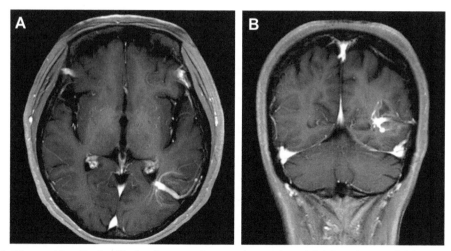

Fig. 31. A 75-year-old patient with developmental venous anomaly. Axial (*A*) and coronal (*B*) CE T1W images show contrast-enhancing small medullary veins draining into dilated transcerebral vein involving the left temporal lobe.

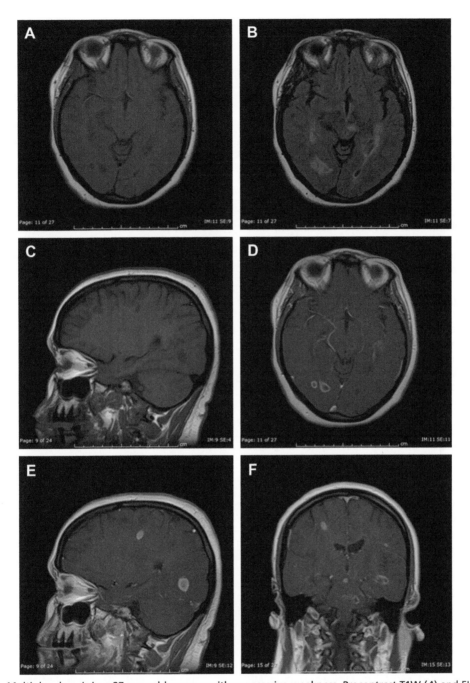

Fig. 32. Multiple sclerosis in a 27-year-old woman with progressive weakness. Precontrast T1W (*A*) and FLAIR (*B*) axial, T1W sagittal (*C*), and CE T1W axial (*D*), sagittal (*E*) and coronal (*F*) images showing multiple areas of high FLAIR and low T1 signal throughout the subcortical and periventricular white matter of cerebral lobes, corpus callosum, midbrain, and pons as well as in cerebellar peduncle and cerebellum, which demonstrate postcontrast enhancement. Findings are compatible with active, enhancing multiple sclerosis plaques.

Some pathologic conditions, however, such as primary or metastatic brain tumor lesions, cause local disruption to the BBB, allowing GBCAs to diffuse into the lesions and increasing their visual impact on CE MR sequences. As such, the combination of unenhanced and GBCA-enhanced MR imaging is the clinical gold standard for the noninvasive detection and delineation of most intracranial and spinal lesions.[212]

MR imaging has a high predictive value that reliably rules out neoplasm and most inflammatory and demyelinating processes of the CNS. Also, CE MR imaging is the primary method for neurodiagnostic work-up, especially due to its established role in the detection, localization, and depiction of the intrinsic properties of a CNS lesion, and can provide important information for both therapy planning and prognosis of patients.

REFERENCES

1. Kidwell CS, Chalela JA, Saver JL, et al. Comparison of MRI and CT for detection of acute intracerebral hemorrhage. JAMA 2004;292(15):1823–30.
2. Kondziolka D, Dempsey PK, Lunsford LD, et al. A comparison between magnetic resonance imaging and computed tomography for stereotactic coordinate determination. Neurosurgery 1992;30(3):402–6 [discussion: 406–7].
3. Schellinger PD, Meinck HM, Thron A. Diagnostic accuracy of MRI compared to CCT in patients with brain metastases. J Neurooncol 1999;44(3):275–81.
4. Brant-Zawadzki M, Norman D, Newton TH, et al. Magnetic resonance of the brain: the optimal screening technique. Radiology 1984;152(1):71–7.
5. Sherry AD, Caravan P, Lenkinski RE. Primer on gadolinium chemistry. J Magn Reson Imaging 2009; 30(6):1240–8.
6. de Haen C, Cabrini M, Akhnana L, et al. Gadobenate dimeglumine 0.5 M solution for injection (Multi-Hance) pharmaceutical formulation and physicochemical properties of a new magnetic resonance imaging contrast medium. J Comput Assist Tomogr 1999;23(Suppl 1):S161–8.
7. Tombach B, Benner T, Reimer P, et al. Do highly concentrated gadolinium chelates improve MR brain perfusion imaging? intraindividually controlled randomized crossover concentration comparison study of 0.5 versus 1.0 mol/L gadobutrol. Radiology 2003;226(3):880–8.
8. Strijkers GJ, Mulder WJ, van Tilborg GA, et al. MRI contrast agents: current status and future perspectives. Anticancer Agents Med Chem 2007;7(3): 291–305.
9. Forsting M, Palkowitsch P. Prevalence of acute adverse reactions to gadobutrol—a highly concentrated macrocyclic gadolinium chelate: review of 14,299 patients from observational trials. Eur J Radiol 2010;74(3):e186–92.
10. Nelson KL, Gifford LM, Lauber-Huber C, et al. Clinical safety of gadopentetate dimeglumine. Radiology 1995;196(2):439–43.
11. Shellock FG, Parker JR, Venetianer C, et al. Safety of gadobenate dimeglumine (MultiHance): summary of findings from clinical studies and postmarketing surveillance. Invest Radiol 2006;41(6): 500–9.
12. Oudkerk M, Sijens PE, Van Beek EJ, et al. Safety and efficacy of dotarem (Gd-DOTA) versus magnevist (Gd-DTPA) in magnetic resonance imaging of the central nervous system. Invest Radiol 1995; 30(2):75–8.
13. Knauth M, Forsting M, Hartmann M, et al. MR enhancement of brain lesions: increased contrast dose compared with magnetization transfer. AJNR Am J Neuroradiol 1996;17(10):1853–9.
14. Kramer H, Runge VM, Naul LG, et al. Brain MRI with single-dose (0.1 mmol/kg) Gadobutrol at 1.5 T and 3 T: comparison with 0.15 mmol/kg Gadoterate meglumine. AJR Am J Roentgenol 2010;194(5): 1337–42.
15. Cherryman G, Golfieri R. Comparison of spin echo T1-weighted and FLASH 90 degrees gadolinium-enhanced magnetic resonance imaging in the detection of cerebral metastases. Br J Radiol 1990;63(753):712–5.
16. Mirowitz SA. Intracranial lesion enhancement with gadolinium: T1-weighted spin-echo versus three-dimensional Fourier transform gradient-echo MR imaging. Radiology 1992;185(2):529–34.
17. Mugler JP 3rd, Brookeman JR. Theoretical analysis of gadopentetate dimeglumine enhancement in T1-weighted imaging of the brain: comparison of two-dimensional spin-echo and three-dimensional gradient-echo sequences. J Magn Reson Imaging 1993;3(5):761–9.
18. Pui MH, Fok EC. MR imaging of the brain: comparison of gradient-echo and spin-echo pulse sequences. AJR Am J Roentgenol 1995;165(4):959–62.
19. Li D, Haacke EM, Tarr RW, et al. Magnetic resonance imaging of the brain with gadopentetate dimeglumine-DTPA: comparison of T1-weighted spin-echo and 3D gradient-echo sequences. J Magn Reson Imaging 1996;6(3):415–24.
20. Furutani K, Harada M, Mawlan M, et al. Difference in enhancement between spin echo and 3-dimensional fast spoiled gradient recalled acquisition in steady state magnetic resonance imaging of brain metastasis at 3-T magnetic resonance imaging. J Comput Assist Tomogr 2008;32(2):313–9.
21. Rand S, Maravilla KR. Uses and limitations of spoiled gradient-refocused imaging in the evaluation of suspected intracranial tumors. Top Magn Reson Imaging 1992;4(4):7–16.

22. Wintersperger BJ, Runge VM, Biswas J, et al. Brain tumor enhancement in MR imaging at 3 Tesla: comparison of SNR and CNR gain using TSE and GRE techniques. Invest Radiol 2007;42(8):558–63.

23. Kakeda S, Korogi Y, Hiai Y, et al. Detection of brain metastasis at 3T: comparison among SE, IR-FSE and 3D-GRE sequences. Eur Radiol 2007;17(9): 2345–51.

24. Kato Y, Higano S, Tamura H, et al. Usefulness of contrast-enhanced T1-weighted sampling perfection with application-optimized contrasts by using different flip angle evolutions in detection of small brain metastasis at 3T MR imaging: comparison with magnetization-prepared rapid acquisition of gradient echo imaging. AJNR Am J Neuroradiol 2009;30(5):923–9.

25. Komada T, Naganawa S, Ogawa H, et al. Contrast-enhanced MR imaging of metastatic brain tumor at 3 tesla: utility of T(1)-weighted SPACE compared with 2D spin echo and 3D gradient echo sequence. Magn Reson Med Sci 2008;7(1):13–21.

26. Park J, Kim J, Yoo E, et al. Detection of small metastatic brain tumors: comparison of 3D contrast-enhanced whole-brain black-blood imaging and MP-RAGE imaging. Invest Radiol 2012;47(2): 136–41.

27. Goo HW, Choi CG. Post-contrast FLAIR MR imaging of the brain in children: normal and abnormal intracranial enhancement. Pediatr Radiol 2003;33(12): 843–9.

28. Mathews VP, Caldemeyer KS, Lowe MJ, et al. Brain: gadolinium-enhanced fast fluid-attenuated inversion-recovery MR imaging. Radiology 1999; 211(1):257–63.

29. Tsuchiya K, Katase S, Yoshino A, et al. FLAIR MR imaging for diagnosing intracranial meningeal carcinomatosis. AJR Am J Roentgenol 2001; 176(6):1585–8.

30. Griffiths PD, Coley SC, Romanowski CA, et al. Contrast-enhanced fluid-attenuated inversion recovery imaging for leptomeningeal disease in children. AJNR Am J Neuroradiol 2003;24(4):719–23.

31. Splendiani A, Puglielli E, De Amicis R, et al. Contrast-enhanced FLAIR in the early diagnosis of infectious meningitis. Neuroradiology 2005; 47(8):591–8.

32. Fukuoka H, Hirai T, Okuda T, et al. Comparison of the added value of contrast-enhanced 3D fluid-attenuated inversion recovery and magnetization-prepared rapid acquisition of gradient echo sequences in relation to conventional postcontrast T1-weighted images for the evaluation of leptomeningeal diseases at 3T. AJNR Am J Neuroradiol 2010;31(5):868–73.

33. Alkan O, Kizilkilic O, Yildirim T, et al. Comparison of contrast-enhanced T1-weighted FLAIR with BLADE, and spin-echo T1-weighted sequences in intracranial MRI. Diagn Interv Radiol 2009;15(2): 75–80.

34. Yamazaki M, Naganawa S, Kawai H, et al. Signal alteration of the cochlear perilymph on 3 different sequences after intratympanic Gd-DTPA administration at 3 tesla: comparison of 3D-FLAIR, 3D-T1-weighted imaging, and 3D-CISS. Magn Reson Med Sci 2010;9(2):65–71.

35. Naganawa S, Kawai H, Sone M, et al. Increased sensitivity to low concentration gadolinium contrast by optimized heavily T2-weighted 3D-FLAIR to visualize endolymphatic space. Magn Reson Med Sci 2010;9(2):73–80.

36. Yamazaki M, Naganawa S, Kawai H, et al. Increased signal intensity of the cochlea on pre- and post-contrast enhanced 3D-FLAIR in patients with vestibular schwannoma. Neuroradiology 2009;51(12):855–63.

37. Galassi W, Phuttharak W, Hesselink JR, et al. Intracranial meningeal disease: comparison of contrast-enhanced MR imaging with fluid-attenuated inversion recovery and fat-suppressed T1-weighted sequences. AJNR Am J Neuroradiol 2005;26(3): 553–9.

38. Bagheri MH, Meshksar A, Nabavizadeh SA, et al. Diagnostic value of contrast-enhanced fluid-attenuated inversion-recovery and delayed contrast-enhanced brain MRI in multiple sclerosis. Acad Radiol 2008;15(1):15–23.

39. Tomura N, Narita K, Takahashi S, et al. Contrast-enhanced multi-shot echo-planar FLAIR in the depiction of metastatic tumors of the brain: comparison with contrast-enhanced spin-echo T1-weighted imaging. Acta Radiol 2007;48(9):1032–7.

40. Terae S, Yoshida D, Kudo K, et al. Contrast-enhanced FLAIR imaging in combination with pre- and postcontrast magnetization transfer T1-weighted imaging: usefulness in the evaluation of brain metastases. J Magn Reson Imaging 2007; 25(3):479–87.

41. Zhou ZR, Shen TZ, Chen XR, et al. Diagnostic value of contrast-enhanced fluid-attenuated inversion-recovery MRI for intracranial tumors in comparison with post-contrast T1W spin-echo MRI. Chin Med J (Engl) 2006;119(6):467–73.

42. Sasiadek M, Wojtek P, Sokolowska D, et al. Evaluation of contrast-enhanced FLAIR sequence in MR assessment of intracranial tumours. Med Sci Monit 2004;10(Suppl 3):94–100.

43. Ercan N, Gultekin S, Celik H, et al. Diagnostic value of contrast-enhanced fluid-attenuated inversion recovery MR imaging of intracranial metastases. AJNR Am J Neuroradiol 2004;25(5):761–5.

44. Essig M, Schoenberg SO, Debus J, et al. Disappearance of tumor contrast on contrast-enhanced FLAIR imaging of cerebral gliomas. Magn Reson Imaging 2000;18(5):513–8.

45. Kataoka H, Taoka T, Ueno S. Early contrast-enhanced magnetic resonance imaging with fluid-attenuated inversion recovery in multiple sclerosis. J Neuroimaging 2009;19(3):246–9.

46. Kubota T, Yamada K, Kizu O, et al. Relationship between contrast enhancement on fluid-attenuated inversion recovery MR sequences and signal intensity on T2-weighted MR images: visual evaluation of brain tumors. J Magn Reson Imaging 2005;21(6):694–700.

47. Naganawa S, Satake H, Iwano S, et al. Contrast-enhanced MR imaging of the brain using T1-weighted FLAIR with BLADE compared with a conventional spin-echo sequence. Eur Radiol 2008;18(2):337–42.

48. Sanossian N, Saver JL, Alger JR, et al. Angiography reveals that fluid-attenuated inversion recovery vascular hyperintensities are due to slow flow, not thrombus. AJNR Am J Neuroradiol 2009;30(3):564–8.

49. Lee KY, Latour LL, Luby M, et al. Distal hyperintense vessels on FLAIR: an MRI marker for collateral circulation in acute stroke? Neurology 2009;72(13):1134–9.

50. Azizyan A, Sanossian N, Mogensen MA, et al. Fluid-attenuated inversion recovery vascular hyperintensities: an important imaging marker for cerebrovascular disease. AJNR Am J Neuroradiol 2011;32(10):1771–5.

51. Haacke EM, Mittal S, Wu Z, et al. Susceptibility-weighted imaging: technical aspects and clinical applications, part 1. AJNR Am J Neuroradiol 2009;30(1):19–30.

52. Mittal S, Wu Z, Neelavalli J, et al. Susceptibility-weighted imaging: technical aspects and clinical applications, part 2. AJNR Am J Neuroradiol 2009;30(2):232–52.

53. Sehgal V, Delproposto Z, Haacke EM, et al. Clinical applications of neuroimaging with susceptibility-weighted imaging. J Magn Reson Imaging 2005; 22(4):439–50.

54. Barnes SR, Haacke EM. Susceptibility-weighted imaging: clinical angiographic applications. Magn Reson Imaging Clin N Am 2009;17(1):47–61.

55. El-Koussy M, Schenk P, Kiefer C, et al. Susceptibility-weighted imaging of the brain: does gadolinium administration matter? Eur J Radiol 2012; 81(2):272–6.

56. Noebauer-Huhmann IM, Pinker K, Barth M, et al. Contrast-enhanced, high-resolution, susceptibility-weighted magnetic resonance imaging of the brain: dose-dependent optimization at 3 tesla and 1.5 tesla in healthy volunteers. Invest Radiol 2006;41(3):249–55.

57. Jagadeesan BD, Delgado Almandoz JE, Benzinger TL, et al. Postcontrast susceptibility-weighted imaging: a novel technique for the detection of arteriovenous shunting in vascular malformations of the brain. Stroke 2011;42(11):3127–31.

58. Hori M, Ishigame K, Kabasawa H, et al. Precontrast and postcontrast susceptibility-weighted imaging in the assessment of intracranial brain neoplasms at 1.5 T. Jpn J Radiol 2010;28(4): 299–304.

59. Le Bihan D, Breton E, Lallemand D, et al. MR imaging of intravoxel incoherent motions: application to diffusion and perfusion in neurologic disorders. Radiology 1986;161(2):401–7.

60. Kealey SM, Kim Y, Whiting WL, et al. Determination of multiple sclerosis plaque size with diffusion-tensor MR imaging: comparison study with healthy volunteers. Radiology 2005;236(2):615–20.

61. Maier SE, Mamata H, Mulkern RV. Characterization of normal brain and brain tumor pathology by chisquares parameter maps of diffusion-weighted image data. Eur J Radiol 2003;45(3):199–207.

62. Schaefer PW, Huisman TA, Sorensen AG, et al. Diffusion-weighted MR imaging in closed head injury: high correlation with initial glasgow coma scale score and score on modified rankin scale at discharge. Radiology 2004;233(1):58–66.

63. Sener RN. Diffusion MRI in Rasmussen's encephalitis, herpes simplex encephalitis, and bacterial meningoencephalitis. Comput Med Imaging Graph 2002;26(5):327–32.

64. Yamada K, Kubota H, Kizu O, et al. Effect of intravenous gadolinium-DTPA on diffusion-weighted images: evaluation of normal brain and infarcts. Stroke 2002;33(7):1799–802.

65. Fitzek C, Mentzel HJ, Fitzek S, et al. Echoplanar diffusion-weighted MRI with intravenous gadolinium-DTPA. Neuroradiology 2003;45(9):592–7.

66. Firat AK, Sanli B, Karakas HM, et al. The effect of intravenous gadolinium-DTPA on diffusion-weighted imaging. Neuroradiology 2006;48(7):465–70.

67. Miller BL, Chang L, Booth R, et al. In vivo 1H MRS choline: correlation with in vitro chemistry/histology. Life Sci 1996;58(22):1929–35.

68. Usenius JP, Vainio P, Hernesniemi J, et al. Choline-containing compounds in human astrocytomas studied by 1H NMR spectroscopy in vivo and in vitro. J Neurochem 1994;63(4):1538–43.

69. Bulakbasi N, Kocaoglu M, Ors F, et al. Combination of single-voxel proton MR spectroscopy and apparent diffusion coefficient calculation in the evaluation of common brain tumors. AJNR Am J Neuroradiol 2003;24(2):225–33.

70. Sijens PE, Oudkerk M, van Dijk P, et al. 1H MR spectroscopy monitoring of changes in choline peak area and line shape after Gd-contrast administration. Magn Reson Imaging 1998;16(10): 1273–80.

71. Alkan A, Burulday V, Oztanir N, et al. Effects of contrast material on the metabolite ratios in single-voxel MR spectroscopy of intraaxial brain tumors. Med Hypotheses 2012;79(2):129–31.

72. Smith JK, Kwock L, Castillo M. Effects of contrast material on single-volume proton MR spectroscopy. AJNR Am J Neuroradiol 2000;21(6):1084–9.

73. Kilgore DP, Breger RK, Daniels DL, et al. Cranial tissues: normal MR appearance after intravenous injection of Gd-DTPA. Radiology 1986;160(3):757–61.

74. Smirniotopoulos JG, Murphy FM, Rushing EJ, et al. Patterns of contrast enhancement in the brain and meninges. Radiographics 2007;27(2):525–51.

75. Burke JW, Podrasky AE, Bradley WG Jr. Meninges: benign postoperative enhancement on MR images. Radiology 1990;174(1):99–102.

76. Davis PC, Friedman NC, Fry SM, et al. Leptomeningeal metastasis: MR imaging. Radiology 1987; 163(2):449–54.

77. Mathews VP, Kuharik MA, Edwards MK, et al. Dyke award. Gd-DTPA-enhanced MR imaging of experimental bacterial meningitis: evaluation and comparison with CT. AJR Am J Roentgenol 1989; 152(1):131–6.

78. Krol G, Sze G, Malkin M, et al. MR of cranial and spinal meningeal carcinomatosis: comparison with CT and myelography. AJR Am J Roentgenol 1988;151(3):583–8.

79. Asari S, Makabe T, Katayama S, et al. Evaluation of MRI score in the differentiation between glioblastoma multiforme and metastatic adenocarcinoma of the brain. Acta Neurochir (Wien) 1993;122(1–2): 54–9.

80. Faehndrich J, Weidauer S, Pilatus U, et al. Neuroradiological viewpoint on the diagnostics of space-occupying brain lesions. Clin Neuroradiol 2011; 21(3):123–39.

81. Essig M, Anzalone N, Combs SE, et al. MR imaging of neoplastic central nervous system lesions: review and recommendations for current practice. AJNR Am J Neuroradiol 2012;33(5):803–17.

82. Runge VM, Muroff LR, Wells JW. Principles of contrast enhancement in the evaluation of brain diseases: an overview. J Magn Reson Imaging 1997;7(1):5–13.

83. Runge VM, Muroff LR, Jinkins JR. Central nervous system: review of clinical use of contrast media. Top Magn Reson Imaging 2001;12(4):231–63.

84. Kumar AJ, Leeds NE, Fuller GN, et al. Malignant gliomas: MR imaging spectrum of radiation therapy- and chemotherapy-induced necrosis of the brain after treatment. Radiology 2000;217(2): 377–84.

85. Brandsma D, Stalpers L, Taal W, et al. Clinical features, mechanisms, and management of pseudoprogression in malignant gliomas. Lancet Oncol 2008;9(5):453–61.

86. Mullins ME, Barest GD, Schaefer PW, et al. Radiation necrosis versus glioma recurrence: conventional MR imaging clues to diagnosis. AJNR Am J Neuroradiol 2005;26(8):1967–72.

87. Rachinger W, Goetz C, Popperl G, et al. Positron emission tomography with O-(2-[18F]fluoroethyl)-l-tyrosine versus magnetic resonance imaging in the diagnosis of recurrent gliomas. Neurosurgery 2005;57(3):505–11 [discussion: 505–11].

88. Al-Okaili RN, Krejza J, Woo JH, et al. Intraaxial brain masses: MR imaging-based diagnostic strategy–initial experience. Radiology 2007; 243(2):539–50.

89. Maeda M, Itoh S, Kimura H, et al. Tumor vascularity in the brain: evaluation with dynamic susceptibility-contrast MR imaging. Radiology 1993;189(1):233–8.

90. Ott D, Hennig J, Ernst T. Human brain tumors: assessment with in vivo proton MR spectroscopy. Radiology 1993;186(3):745–52.

91. Bitzer M, Klose U, Nagele T, et al. Echo planar perfusion imaging with high spatial and temporal resolution: methodology and clinical aspects. Eur Radiol 1999;9(2):221–9.

92. Mills SJ, Soh C, O'Connor JP, et al. Enhancing fraction in glioma and its relationship to the tumoral vascular microenvironment: a dynamic contrast-enhanced MR imaging study. AJNR Am J Neuroradiol 2010;31(4):726–31.

93. Pauliah M, Saxena V, Haris M, et al. Improved T(1)-weighted dynamic contrast-enhanced MRI to probe microvascularity and heterogeneity of human glioma. Magn Reson Imaging 2007;25(9): 1292–9.

94. Lam WW, Chan KW, Wong WL, et al. Pre-operative grading of intracranial glioma. Acta Radiol 2001; 42(6):548–54.

95. Essig M, Weber MA, von Tengg-Kobligk H, et al. Contrast-enhanced magnetic resonance imaging of central nervous system tumors: agents, mechanisms, and applications. Top Magn Reson Imaging 2006;17(2):89–106.

96. Vaghi MA, Strada L, Visciani A, et al. Magnetic resonance imaging in intracranial gliomas. Comparison with computed tomography and serial stereotactic biopsy. Acta Radiol Suppl 1986;369:151–3.

97. Mut M, Turba UC, Botella AC, et al. Neuroimaging characteristics in subgroup of GBMs with p53 overexpression. J Neuroimaging 2007;17(2): 168–74.

98. Schumacher DJ, Tien RD, Friedman H. Gadolinium enhancement of the leptomeninges caused by hydrocephalus: a potential mimic of leptomeningeal metastasis. AJNR Am J Neuroradiol 1994; 15(4):639–41.

99. Schad LR, Boesecke R, Schlegel W, et al. Three dimensional image correlation of CT, MR, and PET studies in radiotherapy treatment planning of brain tumors. J Comput Assist Tomogr 1987; 11(6):948–54.

100. Shuman WP, Griffin BR, Haynor DR, et al. The utility of MR in planning the radiation therapy of

oligodendroglioma. AJR Am J Roentgenol 1987; 148(3):595–600.

101. Krol G, Galicich J, Arbit E, et al. Preoperative localization of intracranial lesions on MR. AJNR Am J Neuroradiol 1988;9(3):513–6.

102. Zamorano L, Dujovny M, Chavantes C, et al. Image-guided stereotactic centered craniotomy and laser resection of solid intracranial lesions. Stereotact Funct Neurosurg 1990;54-55:398–403.

103. Dequesada IM, Quisling RG, Yachnis A, et al. Can standard magnetic resonance imaging reliably distinguish recurrent tumor from radiation necrosis after radiosurgery for brain metastases? A radiographic-pathological study. Neurosurgery 2008;63(5):898–903 [discussion: 904].

104. Wen PY, Macdonald DR, Reardon DA, et al. Updated response assessment criteria for high-grade gliomas: response assessment in neuro-oncology working group. J Clin Oncol 2010; 28(11):1963–72.

105. Dean BL, Drayer BP, Bird CR, et al. Gliomas: classification with MR imaging. Radiology 1990;174(2): 411–5.

106. Fulham MJ, Melisi JW, Nishimiya J, et al. Neuroimaging of juvenile pilocytic astrocytomas: an enigma. Radiology 1993;189(1):221–5.

107. Tien RD, Cardenas CA, Rajagopalan S. Pleomorphic xanthoastrocytoma of the brain: MR findings in six patients. AJR Am J Roentgenol 1992; 159(6):1287–90.

108. Pallud J, Capelle L, Taillandier L, et al. Prognostic significance of imaging contrast enhancement for WHO grade II gliomas. Neuro Oncol 2009;11(2): 176–82.

109. Stack JP, Antoun NM, Jenkins JP, et al. Gadolinium-DTPA as a contrast agent in magnetic resonance imaging of the brain. Neuroradiology 1988;30(2): 145–54.

110. Kelly PJ, Daumas-Duport C, Scheithauer BW, et al. Stereotactic histologic correlations of computed tomography- and magnetic resonance imaging-defined abnormalities in patients with glial neoplasms. Mayo Clin Proc 1987;62(6):450–9.

111. Kondziolka D, Lunsford LD, Martinez AJ. Unreliability of contemporary neurodiagnostic imaging in evaluating suspected adult supratentorial (low-grade) astrocytoma. J Neurosurg 1993;79(4): 533–6.

112. Ginsberg LE, Fuller GN, Hashmi M, et al. The significance of lack of MR contrast enhancement of supratentorial brain tumors in adults: histopathological evaluation of a series. Surg Neurol 1998; 49(4):436–40.

113. Scott JN, Brasher PM, Sevick RJ, et al. How often are nonenhancing supratentorial gliomas malignant? A population study. Neurology 2002;59(6): 947–9.

114. Asari S, Makabe T, Katayama S, et al. Assessment of the pathological grade of astrocytic gliomas using an MRI score. Neuroradiology 1994;36(4): 308–10.

115. Bruner JM. Neuropathology of malignant gliomas. Semin Oncol 1994;21(2):126–38.

116. Rees JH, Smirniotopoulos JG, Jones RV, et al. Glioblastoma multiforme: radiologic-pathologic correlation. Radiographics 1996;16(6):1413–38 [quiz: 1462–3].

117. Kelly PJ. Volumetric stereotactic surgical resection of intra-axial brain mass lesions. Mayo Clin Proc 1988;63(12):1186–98.

118. Kelly PJ. Stereotactic imaging, surgical planning and computer-assisted resection of intracranial lesions: methods and results. Adv Tech Stand Neurosurg 1990;17:77–118.

119. Strong JA, Hatten HP Jr, Brown MT, et al. Pilocytic astrocytoma: correlation between the initial imaging features and clinical aggressiveness. AJR Am J Roentgenol 1993;161(2):369–72.

120. Yu S, He L, Zhuang X, et al. Pleomorphic xanthoastrocytoma: MR imaging findings in 19 patients. Acta Radiol 2011;52(2):223–8.

121. Crespo-Rodriguez AM, Smirniotopoulos JG, Rushing EJ. MR and CT imaging of 24 pleomorphic xanthoastrocytomas (PXA) and a review of the literature. Neuroradiology 2007;49(4):307–15.

122. Kashiwagi N, Yoshihara W, Shimada N, et al. Solitary subependymal giant cell astrocytoma: case report. Eur J Radiol 2000;33(1):55–8.

123. Nishio S, Morioka T, Suzuki S, et al. Subependymal giant cell astrocytoma: clinical and neuroimaging features of four cases. J Clin Neurosci 2001;8(1): 31–4.

124. Pascual-Castroviejo I, Pascual-Pascual SI, Velazquez-Fragua R, et al. Subependymal giant cell astrocytoma in tuberous sclerosis complex. A presentation of eight paediatric patients. Neurologia 2010;25(5):314–21 [in Spanish].

125. Quon H, Hasbini A, Cougnard J, et al. Assessment of tumor angiogenesis as a prognostic factor of survival in patients with oligodendroglioma. J Neurooncol 2010;96(2):277–85.

126. Reiche W, Grunwald I, Hermann K, et al. Oligodendrogliomas. Acta Radiol 2002;43(5):474–82.

127. Daumas-Duport C, Tucker ML, Kolles H, et al. Oligodendrogliomas. Part II: a new grading system based on morphological and imaging criteria. J Neurooncol 1997;34(1):61–78.

128. Khalid L, Carone M, Dumrongpisutikul N, et al. Imaging characteristics of oligodendrogliomas that predict grade. AJNR Am J Neuroradiol 2012; 33(5):852–7.

129. Brown DF, Rushing EJ. Subependymomas: clinicopathologic study of 14 tumors. Arch Pathol Lab Med 1999;123(10):873.

130. Chiechi MV, Smirniotopoulos JG, Jones RV. Intracranial subependymomas: CT and MR imaging features in 24 cases. AJR Am J Roentgenol 1995; 165(5):1245–50.

131. Jelinek J, Smirniotopoulos JG, Parisi JE, et al. Lateral ventricular neoplasms of the brain: differential diagnosis based on clinical, CT, and MR findings. AJNR Am J Neuroradiol 1990;11(3):567–74.

132. Spoto GP, Press GA, Hesselink JR, et al. Intracranial ependymoma and subependymoma: MR manifestations. AJR Am J Roentgenol 1990; 154(4):837–45.

133. Furie DM, Provenzale JM. Supratentorial ependymomas and subependymomas: CT and MR appearance. J Comput Assist Tomogr 1995;19(4): 518–26.

134. Coates TL, Hinshaw DB Jr, Peckman N, et al. Pediatric choroid plexus neoplasms: MR, CT, and pathologic correlation. Radiology 1989;173(1):81–8.

135. Girardot C, Boukobza M, Lamoureux JP, et al. Choroid plexus papillomas of the posterior fossa in adults: MR imaging and gadolinium enhancement. Report of four cases and review of the literature. J Neuroradiol 1990;17(4):303–18.

136. Meyers SP, Khademian ZP, Chuang SH, et al. Choroid plexus carcinomas in children: MRI features and patient outcomes. Neuroradiology 2004;46(9):770–80.

137. Daumas-Duport C, Scheithauer BW, Chodkiewicz JP, et al. Dysembryoplastic neuroepithelial tumor: a surgically curable tumor of young patients with intractable partial seizures. Report of thirty-nine cases. Neurosurgery 1988;23(5):545–56.

138. Ostertun B, Wolf HK, Campos MG, et al. Dysembryoplastic neuroepithelial tumors: MR and CT evaluation. AJNR Am J Neuroradiol 1996;17(3): 419–30.

139. Kuroiwa T, Bergey GK, Rothman MI, et al. Radiologic appearance of the dysembryoplastic neuroepithelial tumor. Radiology 1995;197(1):233–8.

140. Zentner J, Wolf HK, Ostertun B, et al. Gangliogliomas: clinical, radiological, and histopathological findings in 51 patients. J Neurol Neurosurg Psychiatry 1994;57(12):1497–502.

141. Castillo M, Davis PC, Takei Y, et al. Intracranial ganglioglioma: MR, CT, and clinical findings in 18 patients. AJR Am J Roentgenol 1990;154(3):607–12.

142. Provenzale JM, Ali U, Barboriak DP, et al. Comparison of patient age with MR imaging features of gangliogliomas. AJR Am J Roentgenol 2000; 174(3):859–62.

143. Chang KH, Han MH, Kim DG, et al. MR appearance of central neurocytoma. Acta Radiol 1993; 34(5):520–6.

144. Zhang B, Luo B, Zhang Z, et al. Central neurocytoma: a clinicopathological and neuroradiological study. Neuroradiology 2004;46(11):888–95.

145. Nakamura M, Saeki N, Iwadate Y, et al. Neuroradiological characteristics of pineocytoma and pineoblastoma. Neuroradiology 2000;42(7):509–14.

146. Chang SM, Lillis-Hearne PK, Larson DA, et al. Pineoblastoma in adults. Neurosurgery 1995;37(3): 383–90 [discussion: 390–1].

147. Chawla A, Emmanuel JV, Seow WT, et al. presurgical MRI features. Clin Radiol 2007;62(1): 43–52.

148. Rorke LB. The cerebellar medulloblastoma and its relationship to primitive neuroectodermal tumors. J Neuropathol Exp Neurol 1983;42(1):1–15.

149. Rorke LB, Trojanowski JQ, Lee VM, et al. Primitive neuroectodermal tumors of the central nervous system. Brain Pathol 1997;7(2):765–84.

150. Meyers SP, Kemp SS, Tarr RW. MR imaging features of medulloblastomas. AJR Am J Roentgenol 1992;158(4):859–65.

151. Koci TM, Chiang F, Mehringer CM, et al. Adult cerebellar medulloblastoma: imaging features with emphasis on MR findings. AJNR Am J Neuroradiol 1993;14(4):929–39.

152. Curati WL, Graif M, Kingsley DP, et al. Acoustic neuromas: Gd-DTPA enhancement in MR imaging. Radiology 1986;158(2):447–51.

153. Stack JP, Ramsden RT, Antoun NM, et al. Magnetic resonance imaging of acoustic neuromas: the role of gadolinium-DTPA. Br J Radiol 1988;61(729):800–5.

154. Elster AD, Challa VR, Gilbert TH, et al. Meningiomas: MR and histopathologic features. Radiology 1989;170(3 Pt 1):857–62.

155. Huson SM, Harper PS, Hourihan MD, et al. Cerebellar haemangioblastoma and von Hippel-Lindau disease. Brain 1986;109(Pt 6):1297–310.

156. Lee SR, Sanches J, Mark AS, et al. Posterior fossa hemangioblastomas: MR imaging. Radiology 1989; 171(2):463–8.

157. Ho VB, Smirniotopoulos JG, Murphy FM, et al. Radiologic-pathologic correlation: hemangioblastoma. AJNR Am J Neuroradiol 1992;13(5):1343–52.

158. Koeller KK, Smirniotopoulos JG, Jones RV. Primary central nervous system lymphoma: radiologic-pathologic correlation. Radiographics 1997;17(6): 1497–526.

159. Lee YY, Bruner JM, Van Tassel P, et al. Primary central nervous system lymphoma: CT and pathologic correlation. AJR Am J Roentgenol 1986; 147(4):747–52.

160. Louis DN, Ohgaki H, Wiestler OD, et al. The 2007 WHO classification of tumours of the central nervous system. Acta Neuropathol 2007;114(2):97–109.

161. Sumida M, Uozumi T, Kiya K, et al. MRI of intracranial germ cell tumours. Neuroradiology 1995;37(1): 32–7.

162. Jennings MT, Gelman R, Hochberg F. Intracranial germ-cell tumors: natural history and pathogenesis. J Neurosurg 1985;63(2):155–67.

163. Fujimaki T, Matsutani M, Funada N, et al. CT and MRI features of intracranial germ cell tumors. J Neurooncol 1994;19(3):217–26.

164. Liang L, Korogi Y, Sugahara T, et al. MRI of intracranial germ-cell tumours. Neuroradiology 2002; 44(5):382–8.

165. Sakamoto Y, Takahashi M, Korogi Y, et al. Normal and abnormal pituitary glands: gadopentetate dimeglumine-enhanced MR imaging. Radiology 1991;178(2):441–5.

166. Miki Y, Matsuo M, Nishizawa S, et al. Pituitary adenomas and normal pituitary tissue: enhancement patterns on gadopentetate-enhanced MR imaging. Radiology 1990;177(1):35–8.

167. Nakasu Y, Nakasu S, Ito R, et al. Tentorial enhancement on MR images is a sign of cavernous sinus involvement in patients with sellar tumors. AJNR Am J Neuroradiol 2001;22(8):1528–33.

168. Sorva R, Jaaskinen J, Heiskanen O. Craniopharyngioma in children and adults. Correlations between radiological and clinical manifestations. Acta Neurochir (Wien) 1987;89(1–2):3–9.

169. Yasargil MG, Curcic M, Kis M, et al. Total removal of craniopharyngiomas. Approaches and long-term results in 144 patients. J Neurosurg 1990;73(1):3–11.

170. Sartoretti-Schefer S, Wichmann W, Aguzzi A, et al. MR differentiation of adamantinous and squamous-papillary craniopharyngiomas. AJNR Am J Neuroradiol 1997;18(1):77–87.

171. Barajas RF Jr, Cha S. Imaging diagnosis of brain metastasis. Prog Neurol Surg 2012;25:55–73.

172. Nussbaum ES, Djalilian HR, Cho KH, et al. Brain metastases. Histology, multiplicity, surgery, and survival. Cancer 1996;78(8):1781–8.

173. Das A, Hochberg FH. Clinical presentation of intracranial metastases. Neurosurg Clin N Am 1996; 7(3):377–91.

174. Walker MT, Kapoor V. Neuroimaging of parenchymal brain metastases. Cancer Treat Res 2007; 136:31–51.

175. Cha S. Neuroimaging in neuro-oncology. Neurotherapeutics 2009;6(3):465–77.

176. Maroldi R, Ambrosi C, Farina D. Metastatic disease of the brain: extra-axial metastases (skull, dura, leptomeningeal) and tumour spread. Eur Radiol 2005;15(3):617–26.

177. Tyrrell RL 2nd, Bundschuh CV, Modic MT. Dural carcinomatosis: MR demonstration. J Comput Assist Tomogr 1987;11(2):329–32.

178. Chang YC, Huang CC, Wang ST, et al. Risk factor of complications requiring neurosurgical intervention in infants with bacterial meningitis. Pediatr Neurol 1997;17(2):144–9.

179. Kioumehr F, Dadsetan MR, Feldman N, et al. Post-contrast MRI of cranial meninges: leptomeningitis versus pachymeningitis. J Comput Assist Tomogr 1995;19(5):713–20.

180. Pui MH, Memon WA. Magnetic resonance imaging findings in tuberculous meningoencephalitis. Can Assoc Radiol J 2001;52(1):43–9.

181. Gupta RK, Gupta S, Singh D, et al. MR imaging and angiography in tuberculous meningitis. Neuroradiology 1994;36(2):87–92.

182. Falcone S, Post MJ. Encephalitis, cerebritis, and brain abscess: pathophysiology and imaging findings. Neuroimaging Clin N Am 2000;10(2):333–53.

183. Haimes AB, Zimmerman RD, Morgello S, et al. MR imaging of brain abscesses. AJR Am J Roentgenol 1989;152(5):1073–85.

184. Rauch RA, Jinkins JR. Infections of the central nervous system. Curr Opin Radiol 1991;3(1):16–24.

185. Tien RD, Felsberg GJ, Osumi AK. Herpesvirus infections of the CNS: MR findings. AJR Am J Roentgenol 1993;161(1):167–76.

186. Takasu A, Taneda M, Otuki H, et al. Gd-DTPA-enhanced MR imaging of cryptococcal meningoencephalitis. Neuroradiology 1991;33(5):443–6.

187. Mathews VP, Alo PL, Glass JD, et al. AIDS-related CNS cryptococcosis: radiologic-pathologic correlation. AJNR Am J Neuroradiol 1992;13(5):1477–86.

188. Yuh WT, Nguyen HD, Gao F, et al. Brain parenchymal infection in bone marrow transplantation patients: CT and MR findings. AJR Am J Roentgenol 1994;162(2):425–30.

189. Arndt S, Aschendorff A, Echternach M, et al. Rhino-orbital-cerebral mucormycosis and aspergillosis: differential diagnosis and treatment. Eur Arch Otorhinolaryngol 2009;266(1):71–6.

190. Srinivasan A, Goyal M, Al Azri F, et al. State-of-the-art imaging of acute stroke. Radiographics 2006; 26(Suppl 1):S75–95.

191. Provenzale JM, Jahan R, Naidich TP, et al. Assessment of the patient with hyperacute stroke: imaging and therapy. Radiology 2003;229(2):347–59.

192. Elster AD, Moody DM. Early cerebral infarction: gadopentetate dimeglumine enhancement. Radiology 1990;177(3):627–32.

193. Karonen JO, Partanen PL, Vanninen RL, et al. Evolution of MR contrast enhancement patterns during the first week after acute ischemic stroke. AJNR Am J Neuroradiol 2001;22(1):103–11.

194. Kimura K, Minematsu K, Wada K, et al. Lesions visualized by contrast-enhanced magnetic resonance imaging in transient ischemic attacks. J Neurol Sci 2000;173(2):103–8.

195. Hjort N, Wu O, Ashkanian M, et al. MRI detection of early blood-brain barrier disruption: parenchymal enhancement predicts focal hemorrhagic transformation after thrombolysis. Stroke 2008;39(3): 1025–8.

196. Kastrup A, Groschel K, Ringer TM, et al. Early disruption of the blood-brain barrier after thrombolytic therapy predicts hemorrhage in patients with acute stroke. Stroke 2008;39(8):2385–7.

197. Kim EY, Na DG, Kim SS, et al. Prediction of hemorrhagic transformation in acute ischemic stroke: role of diffusion-weighted imaging and early parenchymal enhancement. AJNR Am J Neuroradiol 2005;26(5):1050–5.

198. Latour LL, Kang DW, Ezzeddine MA, et al. Early blood-brain barrier disruption in human focal brain ischemia. Ann Neurol 2004;56(4):468–77.

199. Jensen-Kondering U, Knoss N, Dorner L, et al. Does routine MR contrast enhancement correlate with internal thrombosis in cerebral cavernous malformations? A radiological-histopathological correlation in a case series. Neurol Res 2011;33(5):558–9.

200. Lee RR, Becher MW, Benson ML, et al. Brain capillary telangiectasia: MR imaging appearance and clinicohistopathologic findings. Radiology 1997;205(3):797–805.

201. Wilms G, Marchal G, Van Hecke P, et al. Cerebral venous angiomas. MR imaging at 1.5 tesla. Neuroradiology 1990;32(2):81–5.

202. Sahraian MA, Eshaghi A. Role of MRI in diagnosis and treatment of multiple sclerosis. Clin Neurol Neurosurg 2010;112(7):609–15.

203. He J, Grossman RI, Ge Y, et al. Enhancing patterns in multiple sclerosis: evolution and persistence. AJNR Am J Neuroradiol 2001;22(4):664–9.

204. Kappos L, Moeri D, Radue EW, et al. Predictive value of gadolinium-enhanced magnetic resonance imaging for relapse rate and changes in disability or impairment in multiple sclerosis: a meta-analysis. Gadolinium MRI Meta-analysis Group. Lancet 1999;353(9157):964–9.

205. Sicotte NL, Voskuhl RR, Bouvier S, et al. Comparison of multiple sclerosis lesions at 1.5 and 3.0 Tesla. Invest Radiol 2003;38(7):423–7.

206. Srinivasan R, Sailasuta N, Hurd R, et al. Evidence of elevated glutamate in multiple sclerosis using magnetic resonance spectroscopy at 3 T. Brain 2005;128(Pt 5):1016–25.

207. Silver NC, Good CD, Barker GJ, et al. Sensitivity of contrast enhanced MRI in multiple sclerosis. Effects of gadolinium dose, magnetization transfer contrast and delayed imaging. Brain 1997;120(Pt 7):1149–61.

208. Pagani E, Filippi M, Rocca MA, et al. A method for obtaining tract-specific diffusion tensor MRI measurements in the presence of disease: application to patients with clinically isolated syndromes suggestive of multiple sclerosis. Neuroimage 2005;26(1):258–65.

209. Ge Y, Law M, Johnson G, et al. Dynamic susceptibility contrast perfusion MR imaging of multiple sclerosis lesions: characterizing hemodynamic impairment and inflammatory activity. AJNR Am J Neuroradiol 2005;26(6):1539–47.

210. Bellin MF. MR contrast agents, the old and the new. Eur J Radiol 2006;60:314–23.

211. Hesselink JR, Healy ME, Press GA, et al. Benefits of Gd-DTPA for MR imaging of intracranial abnormalities. J Comput Assist Tomogr 1988;12:266–74.

212. Dhermain FG, Hau P, Lanfermann H, et al. Advanced MRI and PET imaging for assessment of treatment response in patients with gliomas. Lancet Neurol 2010;9:906–20.

Contrast-Enhanced Magnetic Resonance Angiography

Tushar Chandra, MD[a], Bryan Pukenas, MD[b],*, Suyash Mohan, MD[b], Elias Melhem, MD, PhD[b]

KEYWORDS

- Magnetic resonance angiography • Contrast-enhanced MR angiography
- Time-of-flight MR angiography • Time-resolved MR angiography

KEY POINTS

- Magnetic resonance (MR) angiography is a powerful tool for evaluation of cervical and intracranial vasculature.
- Both noncontrast and contrast-enhanced MR angiography can provide exquisite vascular contrast and detail without the use of ionizing radiation.
- At present, the performance of contrast-enhanced 4-dimensional MR angiography is comparable with that of computed tomographic angiography.

INTRODUCTION

Contrast-enhanced (CE) magnetic resonance (MR) angiography has emerged as a noninvasive, robust, high-resolution imaging technique for the evaluation of vascular disease. CE MR angiography has been successfully applied to every vascular territory of the body using varying imaging strategies at multiple centers across the globe. The rapid evolution and success of this technique is reflected by its widespread acceptance in current clinical radiologic practice. The technique continues to progress, having evolved from noncontrast flow imaging techniques to the present-day dynamic CE 3-dimensional (3D) MR angiography at 3 T with high spatial and temporal resolution.

Recent improvements in hardware such as newer radiofrequency coils, higher field strength at 3 T, and newer imaging techniques such as time-resolved MR angiography, parallel imaging methods, and keyhole imaging have made MR angiography a nearly equipotent rival to computed tomographic (CT) angiography, without the radiation hazards of the latter. Although catheter digital subtraction (DS) angiography still remains the gold standard for

vascular imaging, it is expensive and the risk of arterial catheterization, iodinated contrast agents, and radiation hazard warrant safer imaging techniques.

As with all other MR imaging techniques, a thorough understanding of the underlying principles and diagnostic pitfalls of MR angiography is critical for optimal use of this tool. This article aims to acquaint the reader with basic principles of CE MR angiography and pertinent technical considerations, safety issues, and clinical applications in neuroradiology. The strengths and weaknesses of CE MR angiography in comparison with other noncontrast MR angiography techniques, and the recent technical innovations that continue to further enable the clinical utility of this robust imaging technique, are also discussed.

PRINCIPLES AND TECHNIQUES

CE MR angiography is based on the T1 shortening effect of intravenous paramagnetic contrast medium. By shortening the T1 relaxation time of blood, these contrast media help to produce images in which contrast is based on differences in T1 relaxation between arterial blood, venous

[a] Department of Radiology, Children's Hospital of Wisconsin, 9000 West Wisconsin Avenue, Milwaukee, WI, USA; [b] Department of Radiology, Perelman School of Medicine, University of Pennsylvania, 219 Dulles Building, 3400 Spruce Street, Philadelphia, PA, USA
* Corresponding author.
E-mail address: bryan.pukenas@uphs.upenn.edu

Magn Reson Imaging Clin N Am 20 (2012) 687–698
http://dx.doi.org/10.1016/j.mric.2012.08.007

blood, and surrounding tissue. The amount of contrast injected is sufficient to reduce the T1 relaxation time of arterial blood below the T1 relaxation time of stationary tissue. As a result, arterial blood appears brighter than other tissues and venous blood. The shortening of T1 relaxation time of arterial blood during the first pass is transient. Acquisition of 3D images is timed properly to use this effect maximally. Suppression of the background signal is achieved by application of a 3D radiofrequency spoiled gradient sequence. This action also helps to decrease the T2 contrast of the background tissue, resulting in higher T1-weighted images.

CE MR angiography is much less dependent on blood inflow or phase-shift effects, in contrast to earlier MR angiography techniques such as time-of-flight (TOF) MR angiography and phase-contrast (PC) MR angiography. Therefore, this technique is less affected by motion and flow-related artifacts. The T1 shortening of blood by the paramagnetic contrast (gadolinium chelates) combined with less dependency on inflow of blood allows for imaging in the plane of vessels, thereby decreasing the number of image sections required to cover a long vessel. This process allows for faster scan times.

The proper performance of CE MR angiography involves thorough understanding of the complex interplay between the contrast dose, acquisition timing, and postprocessing methods. As illustrated by Maki and colleagues,[1] for optimal CE MR angiography, patient-specific parameters, contrast dynamics, and pulse-sequence configuration should be considered. Patient-specific parameters such as breath-hold timing and contrast delay should be precisely ascertained. Contrast dynamics such as dose, contrast injection rate, and proper timing with respect to k-space acquisition should be determined. Finally, pulse sequence should be properly configured with proper selection of repetition time (TR), echo time (TE), flip angle, readout bandwidth, number of acquisitions, and so forth. These considerations are briefly discussed here.

PATIENT-SPECIFIC CONSIDERATIONS

Certain patient-specific parameters need to be addressed for optimal imaging, and include ascertaining which vascular structures need to be visualized, preventing patient movement during acquisition, and accurately determining the contrast travel time from the site of venous injection to the vascular structure of interest. Predicting the duration of breath hold is also important, more so for abdominal and chest studies.

Timing of Injection and Acquisition: k-Space Considerations

Proper timing of the bolus injection and the image acquisition is vital, as the T1 shortening of the contrast is transient. It is also important to understand the concept of k space and its relevance in image-acquisition strategies. The appropriate scan delay between beginning of the injection and beginning of the scan should be ascertained, given by the following equation:

$$\text{Scan delay} = \text{Contrast travel time} + \text{Injection time}/2 - \text{Scan time}/2.$$

Contrast travel time can be ascertained by different strategies. "Best-guess" technique involves making an educated best guess based on injection site, vascular territory involved, and patient characteristics such as age and cardiac output. "Test bolus" involves injecting 1 to 2 mL of gadolinium before the actual scan at the same rate as that planned for the actual injection. The contrast travel time is then determined visually or by using region-of-interest analysis. This time can then be used to calculate scan delay for the actual study, as per the equation above. "Automated bolus detection" involves visually monitoring a vascular structure for arrival of contrast material followed by "triggering" of centric acquisition once contrast arrival is detected.

The k space

MR images are collected as spatial frequencies placed in a 2-dimensional (2D) array known as the k space. The Fourier transformation is then applied to these spatial frequencies to produce an image. Hence, k space represents an array of data representing the Fourier transformation of an object. It is a mathematical construct that facilitates the visualization of different MR imaging techniques.[2] The center of k space represents low spatial frequency data that determine image contrast, while the periphery of k space represents high spatial frequency data that determine image detail. By proper timing of the contrast injection, it is possible to have the maximum arterial gadolinium concentration at the time of central k-space filling, thereby maximizing contrast-to-noise ratio and signal-to-noise ratio. For a given gadolinium dose, the injection strategy is a trade-off between a fast injection (shorter T1, more intravascular signal) and long injection (more uniform T1, fewer artifacts).[1]

Phase encoding is used to spatially encode the data acquired. For 3D imaging, there are 2 phase-encoding directions and a single frequency direction, and all the data are collected before reconstructing individual images. There are different ways in which this is done. Linear or sequential phase encoding refers to acquiring k-space data sequentially, beginning at the periphery of the k space so that central k-space data are acquired at the midpoint of the scan (**Fig. 1**). Centric phase encoding refers to acquiring central k-space data at the beginning of the scan.[3,4] The image contrast in centric 3D data acquisition is determined by signals at the beginning of acquisition. Centric phase encoding is more suited for CE MR angiography, as it is less prone to incomplete breath-hold artifacts.[5] Elliptical centric phase encoding involves concentrating the center of k space into a shorter period of time than with centric k-phase encoding. This process further improves suppression of venous signals, and reduces respiratory and motion artifacts. Another modification of this technique is recessed centric encoding, whereby absolute center of the k space is recessed a few seconds after initiating the scan, helping to avoid the ringing artifacts caused by data acquisition at the center of the k space as the contrast bolus arrives, as seen with elliptical centric phase–encoding methods.[6]

Contrast Dose

The T1 shortening effect of gadolinium is proportional to its blood concentration according to the following equation:

$$1/T1 = 1/1200 \text{ ms} + R1 \text{ [Gd]}$$

where *R1* is *T1* relaxivity of gadolinium chelate and [Gd] is gadolinium concentration in the blood.

Of all background tissues, fat has the shortest T1 relaxation time (270 ms at 1.5 T). Therefore, the amount of contrast chosen should be sufficient to decrease the T1 of blood to less than 270 ms. This goal is usually achieved by 0.05 to 0.3 mmol/kg of intravenous gadolinium injected at 0.5 to 4 mL/s. With newer MR angiography techniques at 3 T, the contrast dose required to produce the same image

contrast is much less than that needed with conventional CE MR angiography at 1.5 T. This method is discussed in further detail later.

Contrast Injection Rate

Contrast injection rate determines the arrival time of the contrast at the targeted vascular bed. The trade-off is between fast contrast injection to achieve maximal arterial signal and slower injection to minimize artifacts from rapid intravascular signal changes. A double-dose contrast (0.2 mmol/kg of Gd) with an injection rate of about 2 mL/s is considered a good compromise for routine CE MR angiography.

Selection of TR, TE, Readout Bandwidth, and Flip Angle

TR
The TR should be kept as short as possible (<4 ms) without increasing the bandwidth. Decreasing the TR results in shorter acquisition time, which allows for multiphase imaging or increased spatial resolution. However, the signal-to-noise ratio decreases as TR is shortened. This effect can be compensated by faster injection rate that concentrates the contrast bolus.

TE
TE should also be as short as possible. Decreasing the TE results in less dephasing of protons, which in turn decreases the artifactual loss of signal. However, decreasing TE also tends to decrease the signal-to-noise ratio by widening the readout bandwidth. The TE routinely used in clinical CE MR angiography is usually less than 2 ms.

Readout bandwidth
Adjusting the readout bandwidth can alter TR, TE, and signal-to-noise ratio. High readout bandwidths allow for shorter TR and TE at the expense of signal-to-noise ratio (see **Fig. 1**). The bandwidth used for clinical CE MR angiography is usually 32 or 64 kHz.

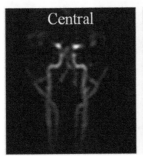 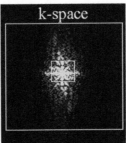 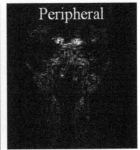

Fig. 1. Example of k-space acquisition, with image detail determined by central low spatial frequency high-contrast data and peripheral high spatial frequency data.

Flip angle

Flip angle in the range of 20° to 60° is acceptable. Low flip angles are more suited for lower contrast doses, slow injection rates, and imaging with very low TR. For higher contrast doses and imaging with higher TR, higher flip angles are better. Usually flip angles in the range of 30° to 45° are used in clinical CE MR angiography (**Figs. 2** and **3**).

NONCONTRAST MR ANGIOGRAPHY TECHNIQUES

Noncontrast MR angiography techniques have been routinely used for intracranial imaging since the advent of MR imaging. These techniques are still relied on widely at various centers around the world, especially for initial evaluation of intracranial and neck vessels. Their use is limited by long acquisition times and multiple flow-related artifacts. However, there has been a renewed interest in these techniques because of concerns over safety of gadolinium-based contrast media in patients at high risk for nephrogenic systemic fibrosis (NSF). These techniques are also used in cases where intravenous access is difficult, in pregnant patients, or when gadolinium is contraindicated. The major noncontrast MR angiography techniques are discussed here.

Time-of-Flight MR Angiography

3D TOF MR angiography is the most commonly used MR angiography technique, especially for imaging intracranial and neck vessels. TOF MR angiography relies on suppression of background signal by slice-selective radiofrequency excitation pulses so that in tissue planes with high flow velocity, the incoming blood that is free of the excitation pulse results in increased signal intensity.[7,8] Selective arteriograms or venograms are possible by applying a presaturation pulse to eliminate signal from a specific direction. TOF MR angiography can be used in 2D or 3D format; the former is more suitable for imaging of veins and the latter for intracranial and neck arteries. 3D format allows for isotropic voxels, but the time of acquisition is long. Because of the long acquisition time, the use of 3D TOF MR angiography is largely limited to intracranial and head and neck vessels, where respiratory artifacts are minimal (**Fig. 4**).

MOTSA (Multiple Overlapping Thin Slice Angiography) is a hybrid of sequential 2D MR angiography and single-slab 3D TOF MR angiography, which results in isotropic high-resolution images and allows for larger anatomic coverage. Each overlapping subvolume is acquired sequentially and is then fused with other subvolumes to form the complete 3D volume.[9] This technique is especially useful for evaluation of large anatomic regions in high resolution. One of the major drawbacks of TOF methods, apart from the long acquisition times, is the artifactual loss of flow signals or pseudo-occlusion in regions of complex flow or flow reversal, such as in subclavian steal.

Phase-Contrast MR Angiography

PC MR angiography is a technique whereby contrast is generated by exploiting the inherent

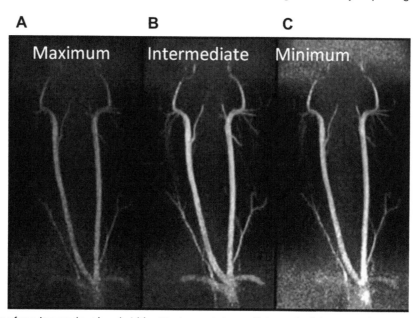

Fig. 2. Effects of varying readout bandwidths. Maximum, intermediate, and minimum readout bandwidths affect signal-to-noise ratios and image quality.

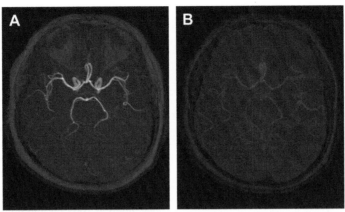

Fig. 3. Effects of varying flip angles. Changing the flip angle from 25° (*A*) to 10° (*B*) alters background suppression and signal-to-noise ratios.

differences in transverse magnetization that occur between stationary and moving tissues,[10,11] resulting in a phase shift. The phase shift is proportional to the flow velocity in the vessel. The velocity-induced phase shift can also be quantified. PC MR angiography uses a flow-encoding gradient along multiple planes to visualize flow. Owing to the need for multiple flow-encoding gradients, the acquisition time is higher than similar 3D TOF acquisitions. PC MR angiography also requires preselection of velocity-encoding factor (Venc), based on whether faster moving arterial blood or slower moving venous blood has to be imaged. If the Venc chosen is too low, velocity aliasing occurs, whereas if the Venc chosen is too high, the vascular contrast-to-noise ratio is low. However, the strength of PC MR angiography is in providing directional information and in quantitatively assessing flow. PC MR angiography is probably the most useful noncontrast MR angiography technique for imaging intracranial veins. For instance, the use of PC MR angiography is critical in cases when there is a subacute thrombus in the venous sinuses, as this can be incorrectly interpreted as blood using TOF MR angiography.

Steady-State Free-Procession MR Angiography

Steady-state free-procession MR angiography is a technique that has applications in evaluation of thoracic, abdominal, and cardiac vessels. The technique generates contrast that does not depend on flow; rather, the T2/T1 ratio of blood is exploited. Very short TR times (<3 ms) are used, so images can be generated in less than 1 second and breath holding is not required. However, the images are prone to spin dephasing and off-resonance artifacts. The technique has been used for the evaluation of coronary vessels, in breath-holding as well as free-breathing formats.[12,13] It has also been used for the evaluation of carotid vessels.[14]

ADVANCED TECHNIQUES OF CE MR ANGIOGRAPHY
Time-Resolved MR Angiography

The lack of dynamic flow information was a serious limitation of CE MR angiography before the evolution of time-resolved techniques. Time-resolved

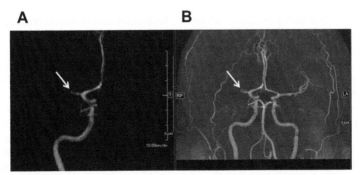

Fig. 4. Coronal CE MR angiography maximum-intensity projection (MIP) image (*A*) and coronal MIP 3-dimensional (3D) time-of-flight image (*B*) demonstrating occlusion of the right middle cerebral artery (*arrow*).

MR angiography provides high temporal resolution while maintaining sufficient signal-to-noise ratio and spatial resolution. With time-resolved MR angiography it is possible to distinguish arterial from venous structures and determine the direction of circulation. This hemodynamic flow information is possible as a result of temporal and spatial k-space data interpolation. Another advantage of this technique is that precise bolus timing calculation is not necessary, as multiple vascular phases can be obtained.

Time-resolved MR angiography has emerged as an effective means of imaging circulation, with high spatial and temporal resolution. Although DS angiography still remains the gold standard for assessing the intracranial circulation, time-resolved MR angiography provides a useful, less invasive alternative. Time-resolved MR angiography allows for detection of complex flow patterns, which is not possible with other techniques. In addition, 3D volume acquisition is possible, which provides greater anatomic coverage as well as higher signal-to-noise ratio. Time-resolved MR angiography also provides for development of innovative techniques for vessel segmentation based on temporal characteristics.[15,16] Various time-resolved MR angiography techniques have been developed, including time-resolved imaging of contrast kinetics (TRICKS),[17] time-resolved echo-shared angiographic technique (TREAT),[18] time-resolved imaging with stochastic trajectories (TWIST), and 4-dimensional (4D) time-resolved angiography using keyhole (4D-TRAK).[19]

2D-projection MR angiography

2D imaging has an advantage of being faster than 3D imaging because there is no need for phase encoding in the direction of slice selection. The high subsecond temporal resolution provides for imaging the vascular anatomy with a single, thick 2D slice. 2D MR DS angiography is performed by having a slice of sufficient thickness to image the entire vascular territory. The same image is acquired repeatedly following the injection of contrast. DS angiography, like serial images, can be produced by using a precontrast mask image and subtraction techniques. MR fluoroscopy can be performed by reconstructing and displaying images immediately after data acquisition. There is some time lag, which can be decreased to less than 1 second by oversampling the center of k space and using thicker slabs.[6]

3D TRICKS

As mentioned earlier, most of the information to create an image is present in the central region of the k space. TRICKS is a technique whereby

central k-space data are acquired more often than those from peripheral regions. The central-phase values are retrospectively combined with high spatial frequency data acquired later in time. Therefore, with TRICKS higher frame rates are possible without sacrificing the spatial resolution. TRICKS has been used successfully to increase the frame rate of 3D multiphase examinations by factors of 3 or 4. These rapid frame rates are useful to capture an arterial time frame, even in areas such as the carotid bifurcation where rapid venous opacification has been problematic.[20]

Keyhole imaging

Described in 1993 by Van Vaals and colleagues,[21] keyhole imaging is a modification of TRICKS whereby the highest spatial frequencies that contribute to edge depiction are acquired at the end of the examination. Keyhole imaging is essentially a modification of TRICKS whereby the highest spatial frequencies that contribute to edge depiction are acquired only at the end of examination. As a consequence, the arterial sampling rate is rapid, and the recirculation of gadolinium leads to increased intravascular T1 shortening and improved signal-to-noise ratio. There is a tendency of ringing artifacts if the time between acquisition of central and peripheral k-space data is too high.

CENTRA

A technique of randomly segmented k-space ordering is used in contrast-enhanced time-robust angiography (CENTRA). In this technique, the central sphere of k space is randomly sampled during the full arterial window. The acquisition of data can extend beyond the time of passage of the bolus of contrast material through the arteries, so that high spatial resolution over a large field of view is achieved.[22]

Non-Cartesian imaging strategies

Traditional Fourier encoding techniques sample k space in a rectilinear or Cartesian fashion. Newer methods sample Fourier data in a nonrectilinear fashion and are hence termed non-Cartesian. A technique called undersampled projection reconstruction (PR) samples k space in a radial fashion. Both the central and peripheral k space is sampled in a radial fashion for every echo. Undersampling is achieved by decreasing the number of angular samples. As a result, the acquisition time decreases. This technique has been combined with TRICKS to produce PR-TRICKS. A newer modification, VIPR (vastly undersampled isotropic projection reconstruction), samples k-space data using 3D radial trajectories, resulting in isotropic spatial resolution and large coverage.[23] With this technique, reprojection of images in any plane is possible, owing to isotropic resolution. Acquisition of high-resolution data sets can be obtained within a single breath hold.

Parallel imaging techniques

The time required for sampling of k-space data in the phase-encoding direction is far greater than that required for frequency encoding. Therefore, reduction in phase-encoding k-space sampling time can lead to faster image acquisition; this is the basic principle behind parallel imaging. Parallel imaging techniques involve collecting multiple k-space coefficients simultaneously using coil arrays. The inherent spatial sensitivity of phased-array coils is used to provide some of the spatial information in the image that would otherwise be obtained in the traditional manner of Fourier transform MR imaging.

Simultaneous acquisition of spatial harmonics (SMASH) was described by Sodickson and Manning,[24] whereby the missing k-space lines are restored before the Fourier transform by linear combination of multiple-coil sample values obtained in a reduced number of phase-encoding steps. GRAPPA (generalized autocalibrating partially parallel acquisition) is a variant of SMASH whereby a small number of additional lines of k space are acquired during the acquisition, which results in better signal-to-noise ratio and decreased artifacts. Pruessmann and colleagues[25] described a technique called sensitivity encoding (SENSE). As mentioned earlier, the time required for acquisition of phase-encoding data is much higher than the time needed for frequency encoding. SENSE is a technique whereby the image acquisition time is shortened by undersampling k space in the phase-encoding direction. However, as a result of undersampling, the field of view is reduced in the phase-encoding direction, which results in aliasing. This effect is usually offset by using multiple passed array coils. The increase in speed is proportional to the number of coils in the coil array.

Parallel imaging results in increased resolution, decreased scan time, or a combination of the two (Fig. 5). Motion and timing artifacts are also minimized. The use of parallel imaging techniques has improved time-resolved MR angiography either by increasing temporal resolution at a constant spatial resolution or by allowing high-resolution imaging at an unchanged acquisition time.[26] However, limitations include reduced signal-to-noise ratio and reconstruction artifacts.[27]

4D TRAK

4D time-resolved angiography using keyhole acquisition (4D-TRAK) has been introduced by combining CENTRA with SENSE, partial Fourier, and keyhole techniques. 4D-TRAK allows for more than 60-times accelerated MR angiography with high spatial resolution. Using this technique the temporal performance of dynamic high-resolution 3D MR angiography is closer to that of catheter DS angiography and is faster than that achieved with conventional MR angiography techniques. Using 4D TRAK, high temporal resolution ranging from 1.6 to 3 seconds in the brain and 1.9 to 4.8 seconds in the carotids has been achieved.[28]

Higher Field Strength: CE MR Angiography at 3 T

The greatest advantage of 3-T CE MR angiography is a theoretical 2-fold increase in signal-to-noise ratio. This increased ratio can in turn be used to increase the spatial resolution and decrease acquisition time, or a combination of the two. In addition, The T1-shortening effect of gadolinium is more pronounced at 3 T, resulting in higher contrast. Therefore, a lesser dose of gadolinium is required to produce images of similar quality in comparison with imaging at 1.5 T.[29] At 3 T, the contrast dose used in CE MR angiography in current practice is likely higher than needed, and can be lowered without negatively affecting overall image quality.[30] There are some limitations of CE MR angiography at 3 T, including a 4-fold increase in specific absorption rate (SAR) and higher field inhomogeneity compared with imaging at 1.5 T. The SAR increases as the square of the increased field strength. Increased SAR reflects higher heat production within the patient's body and may have detrimental side effects. Furthermore, increased SAR at higher field limits the maximum flip angle, which limits the gain in signal-to-noise ratio. However, there is still a net gain in signal with 3-T imaging compared with 1.5-T imaging (Fig. 6).

CLINICAL APPLICATIONS
Stroke

Stroke is a major cause of morbidity and mortality in the Western population. Arterial steno-occlusive disease accounts for the vast majority of ischemic strokes seen in clinical practice. MR angiography serves as the primary noninvasive imaging modality for evaluation of carotid and intracranial arteries in these patients. As discussed earlier, TOF MR angiography is limited in its evaluation of these vessels because of artifacts arising from intravoxel dephasing owing to turbulent flow and proximity of the vessels to skull base, causing susceptibility artifacts. CE MR angiography provides more precise information about the

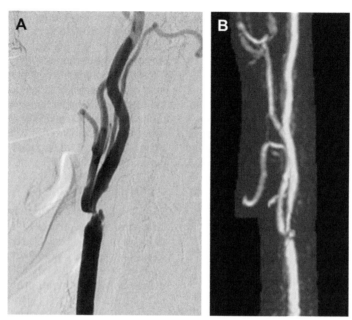

Fig. 5. Lateral digital subtraction angiography (*A*) and corresponding 3D MR angiography MIP image (*B*) using parallel imaging, demonstrating comparable image quality and resolution.

extent and severity of stenosis (see **Fig. 4**). CE MR angiography with TRICKS has been successfully used for the evaluation of carotid vessels. Despite rapid opacification of the jugular vein, angiograms obtained with the TRICKS sequence have minimal venous contamination.[31] In the intracranial circulation, time-resolved MR angiography provides information about the presence and direction of flow in the pial collateral vessels, which is important in acute ischemic stroke for risk stratification and therapeutic decision making. Identification of retrograde flow within a vessel is also possible, which may be of critical importance in cases such as vertebrobasilar insufficiency caused by subclavian steal.

In a recent study comparing CE MR angiography with TOF MR angiography and DS angiography for assessment of carotid stenosis, Anzalone and colleagues[32] reported that the overall accuracy for the detection of hemodynamically relevant stenoses was 95.2% for contrast-enhanced MR angiography, 91.6% for 3D TOF MR angiography, and 94.0% for conventional DS angiography. Moreover, the positive predictive value of CE MR angiography for the detection of severe stenosis was greater than that of 3D TOF MR angiography (96.6% vs 90.3%). Elgersma and colleagues[33] pointed out that because carotid narrowing occurs asymmetrically, DS angiography with only 2 projectional views tends to

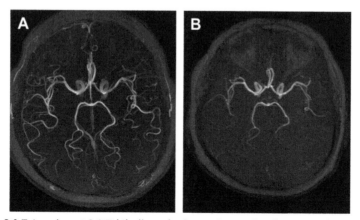

Fig. 6. 1.5 T versus 3.0 T. Imaging at 3.0 T (*A*) allows for better image detail compared with 1.5 T (*B*).

underestimate the severity of stenosis. Therefore, it has been suggested by some investigators that CE MR angiography rather than conventional DS angiography should be considered the technique of choice for evaluation of carotid vessels.[32]

Intracranial Aneurysms

With the evolution of time-resolved MR angiography techniques and 3-T imaging, CE MR angiography has emerged as a reliable modality for initial assessment and follow-up of intracranial aneurysms (**Fig. 7**). DS angiography is still considered the gold standard in the investigation of intracranial aneurysms. However, it is invasive, involves radiation exposure, and has a small risk of associated neurologic complications.[34,35] Therefore, catheter DS angiography is no longer routinely performed in patients with suspected intracranial aneurysms for screening or repeated follow-up. For evaluation of intracranial aneurysms, precise information about aneurysm location, orientation, size, morphologic features, and relation to the parent vessels are crucial for therapeutic decision making. CT angiography uses ionizing radiation and potentially nephrotoxic contrast agent, limiting its utility. Nael and colleagues[36] compared CE MR angiography at 3 T with CT angiography, and concluded that CE MR angiography can be used

to reliably evaluate intracranial aneurysms, with high correlation with the findings on CT angiography. Kaufmann and colleagues[37] compared CE MR angiography and TOF MR angiography at 3 T and 1.5 T for follow-up of coiled aneurysms, and found that CE MR angiography is more likely than TOF MR angiography to appropriately classify larger aneurysm remnants. The investigators recommended performing both CE MR angiography and TOF MR angiography in the follow-up of coiled intracranial aneurysms, and at 3 T if available. The accuracy of CE MR angiography in the evaluation of intracranial aneurysms is limited by venous enhancement, particularly within the cavernous sinus and enhancement of the aneurysm wall. Another pitfall is that a subacute thrombus within an aneurysmal remnant may mimic flow, both on TOF and CE MR angiography.

Arteriovenous Malformations and Arteriovenous Fistulas

For evaluation of arteriovenous malformations, catheter DS angiography has been the study of choice. Information about the direction, speed, and order of filling of intracranial vessels is of critical importance in these cases. Noncontrast MR angiography techniques are limited by of lack of dynamic information and temporal resolution. These techniques do not provide precise information about the nidus and the draining veins. Use of CE MR angiography with time-resolved techniques provides optimal evaluation of the complex flow patterns of these vascular malformations. Using 4D MR angiography facilitates visualization of the arterial feeders, the nidus, and the draining vein.[38] Recently, Riederer and colleagues[39] described a novel method of obtaining time-of-arrival maps that may facilitate the differentiation between arterial and venous structures in a 3D volume. This method may further improve the temporal resolution of CE MR angiography and provide quantitative information. Evaluation of arteriovenous fistulas is possible even in cases where direct visualization of a fistula is not possible, because early opacification of draining veins or the venous sinus can be detected, owing to the high temporal resolution of this technique.[28]

Vasculitis

Vasculitis typically tends to affect the medium-sized vessels, therefore TOF MR angiography is poor in evaluation of these cases. Traditionally, catheter DS angiography is done in such cases when clinical suspicion warrants its use after a negative TOF MR angiography. CE MR angiography at 3 T increases the conspicuity of the

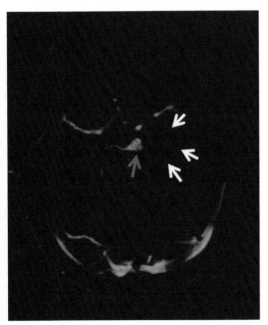

Fig. 7. Axial CE MR angiography image demonstrating partial recanalization (*red arrow*) of a previously embolized left superior cerebellar artery aneurysm (*white arrows*).

medium and small cerebral arteries, and can be used as a safer technique in selected cases. CE MR angiography has been used in moyamoya syndrome to provide assessment of the severity of stenosis and the degree of collateralization. Furthermore, in conditions like Takayasu arteritis, the increased anatomic coverage allows for evaluation of all the vessels from the arch of aorta to the circle of Willis (see **Fig. 4**). Garg and colleagues[40] found a very strong and statistically significant correlation between DS angiography and 3D CE MR angiography in detection and grading of characteristic steno-occlusive lesions of Takayasu arteritis (**Fig. 8**). Yamada and colleagues[41] also found CE MR angiography as a reliable modality for the evaluation of Takayasu arteritis.

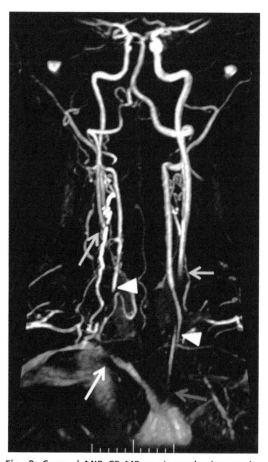

Fig. 8. Coronal MIP CE MR angiography image demonstrating innominate and right subclavian artery stenosis (*white arrow*), left common carotid artery stenosis (*red arrow*), bilateral vertebral artery occlusion with distal reconstitution (*white arrowheads*), and bilateral distal common carotid artery occlusions with distal reconstitution (gray arrows). Findings are consistent with Takayasu arteritis.

OTHER APPLICATIONS

There are many other applications of CE MR angiography in neuroradiology. Time-resolved MR angiography has been used for evaluation of cerebral veins in cases of cerebral venous thrombosis, a scenario in which TOF or PC MR angiography is traditionally used. Time-resolved CE MR angiography provides additional information about the venous flow pattern and collateral circulation. Kirchhof and colleagues[42] found that CE MR venography depicts some venous structures better than TOF and PC MR angiographic examinations. 3D CE MR angiography with parallel imaging techniques has also been successfully used for postoperative evaluation of ECA-ICA bypass surgery in patients with ischemic cerebrovascular disease.[43] CE MR angiography is also useful in studying the vascularization pattern of various intracranial neoplasms. Another application is preoperative assessment of the artery of Adamkiewicz before thoracoabdominal surgery for patients with aortic aneurysm. Yoshioka and colleagues[44] found that CE MR angiography is superior to CT angiography for depiction of the artery of Adamkiewicz, especially when it arises from the false lumen of a dissecting aneurysm. Such precision can help in minimizing spinal cord ischemia following surgery.

SAFETY ISSUES

Recently, gadolinium has been shown to cause a potentially fatal disease, NSF, in patients with renal disease, the vast majority of whom are on dialysis.[45] Patients with acute kidney injury (AKI) or chronic kidney disease (stages 4 or 5, glomerular filtration rate <30 mL/min/1.73 m^2) are also at increased risk after gadolinium exposure. NSF is also directly related to the cumulative dose of gadolinium administered during multiple studies.[45] The exact cause of this disease is unknown, but it is thought to be caused by dissociation of gadolinium from its chelate, resulting in free gadolinium. As per American College of Radiology Blue Ribbon Panel on safe MR practices in 2007, for all patients with stage 3, 4, or 5 kidney disease or those with AKI, it is recommended that one consider refraining from administering any gadolinium-based contrast agents unless a risk-benefit assessment for that particular patient indicates that the benefit of doing so clearly outweighs the potential risk(s).[46]

In pregnant patients, studies have demonstrated that gadolinium-based MR contrast agents pass through the placental barrier and enter the fetal circulation. Therefore, MR contrast agents should not be routinely administered to pregnant patients.[46] These agents should be avoided in patients with previous anaphylactoid reaction to gadolinium, and cautiously used in those with a history of asthma. Otherwise, gadolinium-based contrast media are generally safe and free from major side effects.

SUMMARY

CE MR angiography has rapidly evolved over the last decade. It is a safe, reliable, and versatile technique for the evaluation of all vascular territories, including intracranial as well as head and neck vessels. With the advent of time-resolved MR angiography and parallel imaging techniques, the spatial and temporal resolution of CE MR angiography is better than ever. At present, the performance of CE 4D MR angiography is comparable with that of CT angiography. The technique continues to evolve, and with further improvements may replace catheter DS angiography for diagnostic studies in the near future.

REFERENCES

1. Maki JH, Prince MR, Chenevert TC. Optimizing three-dimensional gadolinium-enhanced magnetic resonance angiography. Original investigation. Invest Radiol 1998;33(9):528–37.

2. Bradley WG, Chen DY, Atkinson DJ, et al. Fast spin-echo and echo-planar imaging. In: Stark DD, Bradley WG, editors. Magnetic resonance imaging. 3rd edition. St Louis (MO): Mosby; 1999. p. 125–58.

3. Bampton AE, Riederer SJ, Korin HW. Centric phase-encoding order in three-dimensional MP-RAGE sequences: application to abdominal imaging. J Magn Reson Imaging 1992;2:327–34.

4. Wilman AH, Riederer SJ. Improved centric phase encoding orders for three-dimensional magnetization-prepared MR angiography. Magn Reson Med 1996;36:384–92.

5. Maki JH, Prince MR, Chenevert TL. The effects of incomplete breath-holding on 3D MR image quality. J Magn Reson Imaging 1997;7:1132–9.

6. Prince MR, Grist TM, Debatin JF. 3D contrast MR angiography. 3rd edition. Berlin: Springer-Verlag; 2003.

7. Miyazaki M, Lee VS. Nonenhanced MR angiography. Radiology 2008;248:20–43.

8. Laub GA. Time-of-flight method of MR angiography. Magn Reson Imaging Clin N Am 1995;3:391–8.

9. Melhem ER, Poon EK, Weinreich EM, et al. Comparison of 2D- and 3DFT multiple overlapping thin-slab acquisition TOF MR angiography in carotid disease. J Neuroimaging 1998;8:3–7.

10. Dumoulin CL, Hart HJ. Magnetic resonance angiography. Radiology 1986;161:717–20.

11. Nyler GL, Firmin DN, Longmore DB. Blood flow imaging by cine magnetic resonance. J Comput Assist Tomogr 1986;10:715–22.

12. Deshpande VS, Shea SM, Laub G, et al. 3D magnetization-prepared true-FISP: a new technique for imaging coronary arteries. Magn Reson Med 2001;46:494–502.

13. Bi X, Deshpande V, Carr JC, et al. Coronary artery magnetic resonance angiography (MRA): a comparison between the whole-heart and volume-targeted methods using a T2-prepared SSFP sequence. J Cardiovasc Magn Reson 2006;8:703–7.

14. Zavodni AE, Emery DJ, Wilman AH. Performance of steady-state free precession for imaging carotid artery disease. J Magn Reson Imaging 2005;21:86–9.

15. Klisch J, Strecker R, Hennig J, et al. Time-resolved projection MRA: clinical application in intracranial vascular malformations. Neuroradiology 2000;42: 104–7.

16. Bock M, Schoenberg SO, Flomer F, et al. Separation of arteries and veins in 3D MR angiography using correlation analysis. Magn Reson Med 2000;43:481–7.

17. Korosec FR, Frayne R, Grist TM, et al. Time-resolved contrast-enhanced 3D MR angiography. Magn Reson Med 1996;36(3):345–51.

18. Pinto C, Hickey R, Carroll TJ, et al. Time-resolved MR angiography with generalized auto-calibrating partially parallel acquisition and time-resolved echo-sharing angiographic technique for hemodialysis arteriovenous fistulas and grafts. J Vasc Interv Radiol 2006;17:1003–9.

19. Willinek WA, Hadizadeh DR, von Falkenhausen M, et al. 4D time-resolved MR angiography with keyhole (4D-TRAK): more than 60 times accelerated MRA using a combination of CENTRA, keyhole, and SENSE at 3.0T. J Magn Reson Imaging 2008;27(6):1455–60.

20. Carroll TJ, Korosec FR, Petermann GM, et al. Carotid bifurcation: evaluation of time-resolved three-dimensional MR angiography. Radiology 2001;220:525–32.

21. Van Vaals JJ, Brummer ME, Dixon WT, et al. "Keyhole" method for accelerating imaging of contrast agent uptake. J Magn Reson Imaging 1993;3:671–5.

22. Willinek WA, Gieseke J, Conrad R, et al. Randomly segmented central k-space ordering in high spatial resolution contrast-enhanced MR angiography of the supra-aortic arteries: initial experience. Radiology 2002;225:583–8.

23. Du J, Carroll TJ, Brodsky E, et al. Contrast-enhanced peripheral magnetic resonance angiography using time-resolved vastly undersampled isotropic projection reconstruction. J Magn Reson Imaging 2004;20:894–900.

24. Sodickson DK, Manning WJ. Simultaneous acquisition of spatial harmonics: fast imaging with radiofrequency coil arrays. Magn Reson Med 1997; 38:591–603.

25. Pruessmann KP, Weiger M, Boesiger P. Sensitivity encoded cardiac MRI. J Cardiovasc Magn Reson 2001;3:1–9.

26. Taschner CA, Gieseke J, Le Thuc V, et al. Intracranial arteriovenous malformation: time-resolved contrast-enhanced MR angiography with combination of parallel imaging, keyhole acquisition, and k-space sampling techniques at 1.5 T. Radiology 2008; 246(3):871–9.

27. Glockner JF, Hu HH, Stanley DW, et al. Parallel MR imaging: a user's guide. Radiographics 2005;25(5): 1279–97.

28. Parmar H, Ivancevic MK, Dudek N, et al. Dynamic MRA with four-dimensional time-resolved angiography using keyhole at 3 tesla in head and neck vascular lesions. Magn Reson Imaging Clin N Am 2009;17(1):63–75.

29. Huang BY, Castillo M. Neurovascular imaging at 1.5 tesla versus 3.0 tesla. Magn Reson Imaging Clin N Am 2009;17:29–44.

30. Hartung MP, Grist TM, François CJ. Magnetic resonance angiography: current status and future directions. J Cardiovasc Magn Reson 2011;13:19.

31. Korosec FR, Turski PA, Carroll TJ, et al. Contrast-enhanced MR angiography of the carotid bifurcation. J Magn Reson Imaging 1999;10(3):317–25.

32. Anzalone N, Scomazzoni F, Castellano R, et al. Carotid artery stenosis: intraindividual correlations of 3D time-of-flight MR angiography, contrast-enhanced MR angiography, conventional DSA, and rotational angiography for detection and grading. Radiology 2005;236(1):204–13.

33. Elgersma OE, Buijs PC, Wust AF, et al. Maximum internal carotid arterial stenosis: assessment with rotational angiography versus conventional intra-arterial digital subtraction angiography. Radiology 1999;213:777–83.

34. Hankey GJ, Warlow CP, Sellar RJ. Cerebral angiographic risk in mild cerebrovascular disease. Stroke 1990;21(2):209–22.

35. Heiserman JE, Dean BL, Hodak JA, et al. Neurological complications of cerebral angiography. AJNR Am J Neuroradiol 1994;15(8):1401–7 [discussion: 1408–11].

36. Nael K, Villablanca JP, Mossaz L, et al. 3-T contrast-enhanced MR angiography in evaluation of suspected intracranial aneurysm: comparison with MDCT angiography. AJR Am J Roentgenol 2008; 190(2):389–95.

37. Kaufmann TJ, Huston J 3rd, Cloft HJ, et al. A prospective trial of 3T and 1.5T time-of-flight and contrast-enhanced MR angiography in the follow-up of coiled intracranial aneurysms. AJNR Am J Neuroradiol 2010;31(5):912–8.

38. Oleaga L, Dalal SS, Weigele JB, et al. The role of time-resolved 3D contrast-enhanced MR angiography in the assessment and grading of cerebral arteriovenous malformations. Eur J Radiol 2010; 74(3):e117–21.

39. Riederer SJ, Haider CR, Borisch EA. Time-of-arrival mapping at three-dimensional time-resolved contrast-enhanced MR angiography. Radiology 2009;253(2):532–42.

40. Garg SK, Mohan S, Kumar S. Diagnostic value of 3D contrast-enhanced magnetic resonance angiography in Takayasu's arteritis—a comparative study with digital subtraction angiography. Eur Radiol 2011;21(8):1658–66.

41. Yamada I, Nakagawa T, Himeno Y, et al. Takayasu arteritis: diagnosis with breath-hold contrast-enhanced three-dimensional MR angiography. J Magn Reson Imaging 2000;11(5):481–7.

42. Kirchhof K, Welzel T, Jansen O, et al. More reliable noninvasive visualization of the cerebral veins and dural sinuses: comparison of three MR angiographic techniques. Radiology 2002;224(3):804–10.

43. Tsuchiya K, Honya K, Fujikawa A, et al. Postoperative assessment of extracranial-intracranial bypass by time-resolved 3D contrast-enhanced MR angiography using parallel imaging. AJNR Am J Neuroradiol 2005;26(9):2243–7.

44. Yoshioka K, Niinuma H, Ehara S, et al. MR angiography and CT angiography of the artery of Adamkiewicz: state of the art. Radiographics 2006;26(Suppl 1): S63–73.

45. Weinreb JC, Abu-Alfa AK. Gadolinium-based contrast agents and nephrogenic systemic fibrosis: why did it happen and what have we learned? J Magn Reson Imaging 2009;30(6):1236–9.

46. Kanal E, Barkovich AJ, Bell C, et al, ACR Blue Ribbon Panel on MR Safety. ACR guidance document for safe MR practices: 2007. AJR Am J Roentgenol 2007;188:1447–74.

Advanced Techniques Using Contrast Media in Neuroimaging

Jean-Christophe Ferré, MD, PhD[a,b,*], Mark S. Shiroishi, MD[a], Meng Law, MD[a]

KEYWORDS

• Perfusion • Permeability • Contrast agent • Brain tumor • Stroke

KEY POINTS

• Studying brain perfusion and permeability is possible without an additional dose of gadolinium-based contrast agent.
• Dynamic susceptibility contrast magnetic resonance (MR) imaging) using T2- or T2*-weighted imaging is the most commonly used MR perfusion technique of the brain.
• Dynamic relaxivity contrast-enhanced MR imaging using T1-weighted relaxivity imaging is the most commonly used MR permeability technique.
• Dynamic susceptibility contrast and dynamic relaxivity contrast-enhanced MR imaging can provide clinically useful physiologic information to complement conventional contrast-enhanced MR imaging, particularly of brain tumors and stroke.

INTRODUCTION

Contrast agent injection is essential to characterize abnormalities in neuroimaging (see the articles by Guttierrez and colleagues, Kim and colleagues elsewhere in this issue for further exploration of this topic). However, contrast enhancement is nonspecific reflection of blood-brain barrier (BBB) disruption. The injection of gadolinium-based contrast agents (GBCAs) allows characterization of the brain's hemodynamic processes (ie, brain perfusion) and the BBB leakage-permeability. It is now recognized that advance MR imaging techniques, such as those used to study perfusion and permeability, provide physiologic instead of simply the morphologic data obtained with conventional magnetic resonance (MR) imaging.[1]

Dynamic contrast imaging can be separated into 2 main categories according to the contrast agent properties: the dynamic susceptibility contrast (DSC) MR imaging using T2- or T2*-weighted imaging and the dynamic relaxivity contrast-enhanced (DCE) MR imaging) using T1-weighted relaxivity imaging. Both perfusion and permeability measurements could be extracted from these 2 technique categories, but DSC-MR imaging is commonly referred to as "perfusion" imaging and DCE-MR imaging is commonly referred to as "permeability" imaging.

Funding sources: Dr Ferré: French Society of Radiology (SFR) research grant, French Society of Neuroradiology (SFNR) research grant. Dr Shiroishi: GE Healthcare/RSNA Research Scholar Grant. Dr Law: NIH CTSA Grant 1UL1RR031986-01, NIH 1R21EB013456 and Bayer Healthcare.
Conflicts of interest: Dr Ferré: none. Dr Shiroishi: Consultant, Bayer Healthcare. Dr Law serves on the scientific advisory boards for Bayer HealthCare, Toshiba Medical, has received speaker honoraria from Siemens Medical Solutions, iCAD Inc, Bayer HealthCare, Bracco, Prism Clinical Imaging.
[a] Division of Neuroradiology, Department of Radiology, Keck Medical Center of University of Southern California, 1520 San Pablo Street, Los Angeles, CA 90033, USA; [b] CHU Rennes, Department of Radiology, University Hospital, 2 rue Henri Le Guilloux, Rennes 35000, France
* Corresponding author.
E-mail address: Jean-christophe.ferre@chu-rennes.fr

Magn Reson Imaging Clin N Am 20 (2012) 699–713
http://dx.doi.org/10.1016/j.mric.2012.07.007
1064-9689/12/$ – see front matter © 2012 Elsevier Inc. All rights reserved.

DSC-MR imaging is the most used technique in clinical imaging of brain tumor and stroke. This technique can provide hemodynamic metrics such as cerebral blood flow (CBF), cerebral blood volume (CBV), and mean transit time (MTT). Compared with DSC-MR imaging, DCE-MR imaging has less widespread use, likely owing to more stringent acquisition and complex requirements to explore BBB permeability.

The aim of this review is to give an overview of the basic principles and common neuroimaging applications of these 2 advanced techniques using contrast media.

IMAGING TECHNIQUE
Perfusion: DSC-MR Imaging

Principle
DSC-MR imaging, also known as perfusion-weighted MR imaging, MR perfusion, or bolus-tracking MR imaging, is a technique to track the first-pass of an exogenous, paramagnetic,

nondiffusible contrast agent, typically a GBCA through the tissue. Since it was first described by Villringer and colleagues[2] in 1988, DSC-MR imaging has emerged as a dominant method to study the brain microvascular component. To record the signal loss caused by susceptibility effects during the first passage of a GBCA through the tissue of interest, T2- or T2*-weighted images should be dynamically acquired at a rate faster than the time it takes the bolus to pass through the tissue. With the application of tracer kinetic models for intravascular tracers and the use of the central volume theorem, the major perfusion parameters CBV, CBF, and MTT can be estimated (**Fig. 1**).[3,4]

Images acquisition
A single-shot echo planar imaging (EPI) is generally used because it provides a means for very rapid image acquisition. EPI is generally performed in conjunction with multislice gradient-echo (GRE) or spin-echo (SE)-EPI techniques.

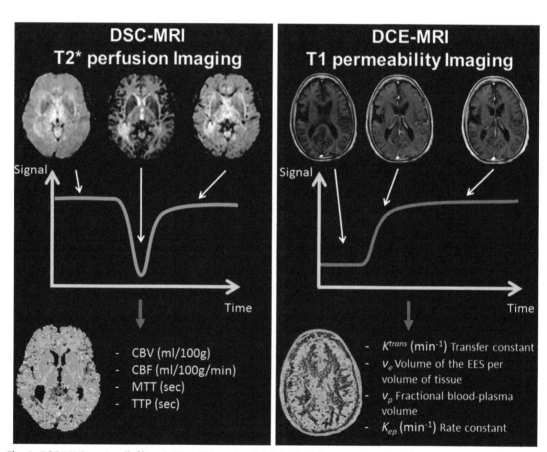

Fig. 1. DSC-MR imaging (*left*) and DCE-MR imaging (*right*) principles overview. Sample time-series images during the passage of the contrast agent (*first row*) and the resulting time signal course (*second row*). The image processing based on the time curve allows extraction of qualitative or quantitative metrics of perfusion (DSC-MR imaging) and/or permeability (DCE-MR imaging) and parametric maps to be obtained.

GRE-EPI methods (T2*-weighted images) are able to provide better spatial coverage of the brain, are sensitive to both large and small vessels with better signal-to-noise ratio, and require half the dose of a GBCA compared with multislice SE (T2-weighted images). Compared with GRE, SE techniques seem to be more sensitive to smaller vessels (capillaries) and have less image distortion and artifacts at the brain–bone interface.[5,6] Despite these advantages, studies have shown that GRE sequences are superior in their ability to predict glioma grade compared with SE sequences.[7,8] Even if combinations of the 2 techniques have been reported,[6] the GRE-EPI method is the most widely used technique. Both 2-dimensional (2D) EPI and 3-dimensional sequences are used; however, 2D sequences are usually preferably compared because of their ability to achieve better spatial resolution and shorter repetition times (TR) and provide a more accurate characterization of bolus passage.[9] The typical acquisition time for the first-pass T2* DSC-MR imaging acquisition is on the order of 90 seconds. A temporal resolution on the order of 1 to 2 seconds is desired to obtain the correct shape of the concentration–time curve. The recommended matrix resolution is 128 × 128. Slice thickness could range between 2 and 5 mm depending on the need for whole brain volume coverage. A combination of a phase-array coil and parallel imaging, in particular at 3 T, offers a good compromise in the quality of images.[10]

Injection protocol

A GBCA bolus injection should commence within 20 seconds after the start of the T2* DSC sequence to establish a precontrast baseline. A power injector is used to inject at a minimum rate of 4 mL/s, followed by a saline flush at the same rate, through an 18- to 22-gauge peripheral intravenous line. A 0.1 mmol/kg dose of GBCA is generally recommended. When the possibility of contrast agent extravasation exists (ie, evaluation of brain tumors), a preload-correction approach is recommended.[11] Although the optimal amount of preload dosing of GBCA is not entirely clear, work by Hu and colleagues[12] found that at 3 T, a preload dose of 0.1 mmol/kg administered 6 minutes before the DSC acquisition injection seemed to provide correction for leakage effects and to obtain the highest accuracy of CBV. If combined permeability and perfusion MR imaging is being performed, then it is recommended that the dose be split into 2 equivalent 0.05 mmol/kg doses.[13]

There is no clear consensus in the choice of GBCA. High relaxivity contrast agents such as gadobenate dimeglumine allows high-quality (relative

CBV [rCBV]) maps.[14] Gadobenate dimeglumine and high-concentration GBCA gadobutrol give similar high-quality perfusion maps at a dose of 0.1 mmol/kg at 1.5 T,[15] although at 3 T gadobutrol seems to offer advantages over gadobenate dimeglumine.[16] A recent study concluded that DSC-MR imaging with a blood pool agent such as ferumoxytol may provide a better monitor of tumor rCBV than DSC-MR imaging with gadoteridol.[17]

Image processing

First, the GBCA concentration–time curve is calculated based on the susceptibility signal intensity–time curve. GBCA concentration is assumed to be proportional to the change in relaxation rate ΔR2* (or ΔR2 if SE sequence is used), which can be calculated from the signal intensity[18] via use of Equation 1:

$$\Delta R2^* = [-\ln(S(t)/S0)]/TE \qquad [1]$$

where S(t) is the signal intensity in the voxel at time t and S0 is the baseline signal intensity before the bolus arrives.

A gamma-variate function is then generally fitted to the curve to eliminate contribution of tracer recirculation.[19]

The most common processing methods used in clinical work give qualitative parametric maps assuming a constant arterial input function in all the pixels. rCBV is calculated from the area under the curve, realtive MTT (rMTT) is calculated from the first moment of the measured efflux concentration–time curve (ie, the weighted arithmetic mean of the time values represented in the concentration–time curve), and rCBF is equal to rCBV/rMTT according to the central volume principle.[20] These maps do not afford quantitative assessment of brain hemodynamics but provide indicators of hemodynamic disturbances that are very useful in a clinical setting. They can be interpreted visually or semiquantitatively by calculating the ratio or difference between the values in a region of interest (ROI) placed in the abnormal area and a contralateral ROI placed in the area considered as a normal reference.

To quantitatively determine CBF (mL/100 g/min) and MTT (seconds), the arterial input function (AIF) must be known to correct for bolus delay and dispersion. Following deconvolution of the concentration–time curve with the AIF, MTT and CBF can be determined from the tissue residue function: CBF is the peak of the residue function and MTT is the weighted arithmetic mean of the time of transit values.[20–22] CBV (in mL/100 g) is then equal to CBF × MTT according to the central volume principle.

As opposed to the relationship between attenuation and contrast agent concentration in CT perfusion, there may not always exist a linear relationship between MR signal intensity and tissue contrast agent concentration in DSC-MR imaging.[23] In clinical context, this nonlinear relationship is often ignored; this can lead to substantial errors in absolute quantification of DSC-MR imaging.[24]

Permeability: DCE-MR Imaging

Principle

DCE-MR imaging is used to characterize the functional integrity of the BBB via estimation of microvascular permeability parameters. During T1-weighted DCE-MR imaging, the contrast agent accumulation results in T1-shortening and positive enhancement. Through pharmacokinetic modeling of contrast agent accumulation into the extravascular-extracellular space (EES), several parameters can be determined (see **Fig. 1**)[25]:

- Transfer constant (K^{trans}), frequently called vascular permeability, is a combination of capillary wall permeability surface area product per unit volume of tissue (PS) and capillary blood flow (F)
- Volume of the EES per volume of tissue (v_e)
- Fractional blood-plasma volume (v_p)
- Rate constant between EES and blood plasma (k_{ep}, where $k_{ep} = K^{trans}/v_e$)

Image acquisition

Baseline T1 mapping is performed before the acquisition of the DCE images. This is necessary to apply pharmacokinetic modeling because the relationship between the measured signal intensity and contrast agent concentration is nonlinear.[26] The most commonly used method is a multiple flip angle gradient echo acquisition but inversion or saturation recovery techniques could also be used.[27,28]

Then rapid repeated T1-weighted images are acquired before, duringm and after bolus GBCA administration for several minutes. This is commonly performed using gradient-echo sequence (spoiled gradient echo [SPGR], volume interpolated gradient echo [VIBE], magnetization-prepared rapid acquisition with gradient echo [MPRAGE]) that provides adequate compromise between temporal resolution, volume coverage and sensitivity to T1 effects.[29] Although 2D sequences could be used, 3-dimensional sequences are the preferred technique because of its better signal-to-noise-ratio and less severe distortions.

The acquisition time for the dynamic acquisition should be at least 3 to 5 minutes, and a temporal resolution of between 3.5 and 6 seconds would be optimal. The recommended matrix resolution is 128 × 128. Slice thickness could range between 2 to 7 mm depending on the need for volume coverage. To improve temporal and/or spatial resolution, parallel imaging methods or other undersampling methods such as highly constrained back-projection or compressed sensing methods can be used.[30,31]

Injection protocol

GBCA bolus injection should commence within 20 seconds after the start of the T1 DCE sequence to establish a precontrast baseline. A power injector is used to inject through an 18- to 22-gauge peripheral intravenous line, at a rate of 2 to 5 mL/s, followed by a saline flush at the same rate. A 0.1 mmol/kg dose of contrast agent is generally recommended. If combined permeability and DSC-MR imaging is being performed, then it is recommended that the dose be split into 2 equivalent 0.05 mmol/kg doses followed by a 10-mL saline flush.

Image processing

Many methods have been described to analyze DCE-MR imaging, from simple measurement of MR signal changes to physiologic methods using pharmacokinetic models.

Descriptive methods examine simple descriptions of the signal intensity–time curve, such as percentage of enhancement, curve shape, wash-in and wash-out slopes, or time to 90% enhancement.[32] To improve reproducibility and repeatability, determination of the contrast-concentration curve could be derived from signal intensity–time curve. A simple descriptor as the initial area under the contrast agent concentration–time curve can be calculated without pharmacokinetic modeling. It is widely used in drug trials and seems to have fair reproducibility. However, what it represents physiologically is unclear because it is a combination of blood volume, flow, permeability, and EES volume.[25]

Permeability metrics can also be extracted from the concentration–time curve using pharmacokinetic models, which in theory should limit individual patient variation, scanner type, or imaging technique. Most of pharmacokinetic models applied to DCE-MR imaging are compartmental models. A simplification of the pharmacokinetic model was proposed by Patlak and colleagues,[33] to estimate K^{trans} with a graphic approach in case of limited permeability. Models proposed by Toft and Kernode and Larson and colleagues[34] define K^{trans} (min^{-1}) and v_e neglecting the contribution of the intravascular compartment.[35] However, when here is a large increase in blood volume (ie, in high-grade tumor), ignoring the contribution of the intravascular tracer may be problematic.[36] Extensions of this model that take into consideration the contribution the intravascular contrast have been developed that allow modeling of v_p in addition to K^{trans} and v_e. These models provide a more accurate calculation of K^{trans} and v_e.[37] Because K^{trans} is a composite parameter depending on the relationship between flow and PS, more complex models, such as the adiabatic tissue homogeneity model, separate flow and PS.[38] However, these models demand a very high temporal resolution and a high quality of data.

An AIF is needed for the models just described. Ideally, the AIF should be determined in an artery local to the tissue of interest for each examination. But an accurate measurement is challenging.[39] Several techniques have been proposed, but many groups use an idealized mathematical function, based on population-averaged AIF.[35,40]

LIMITATIONS OF DSC-MR AND DCE-MR IMAGING

Quantification of perfusion and permeability metrics is based on several approximations and assumptions. Moreover, many acquisition, processing, and interpretation methods are used for DSC-MR and DCE-MR imaging, without standardization across centers. These imply difficulties in comparing and in using the reported values in the literature.

Because the main DSC-MR imaging acquisition techniques are T2*-weighted methods, susceptibility artifacts can confound perfusion measurements, particularly in the posterior fossa, temporal and frontal lobes, and hemorrhagic lesions and in the surgical setting, where there can be blood products.[13,41] Several solutions include decreasing slice thickness and shortening echo time (TE) with the use of parallel imaging.[10]

T2*-weighted methods have also significant T1 sensitivity. When the BBB is disrupted, as is often the case with brain tumors, the leakage of GBCA results in enhanced T1 relaxation effects. These effects produce an elevation in the signal curve mask signal that can result in underestimation of rCBV.[42,43] Acquisition method with low flip angle and short TE can minimize the T1 effects.[42] Moreover, the leakage effect can be reduced using GBCA preloading to saturate the extravascular space and mathematical correction.[11,12]

DCE-MR imaging metrics could be easily extracted in brain area with high leakage of gadolinium in the post gadolinium-enhanced part of the brain, with a relatively short acquisition time.

Measuring permeability in nonenhanced brain is more challenging: a longer acquisition and an adaptation of quantification model are needed.

IMAGING FINDINGS/PATHOLOGIC CONDITIONS

This section highlights the current and future potential clinical applications of DSC-MR and DCE-MR imaging in neuroimaging. Several recent review articles have previously detailed the use of these techniques.[13,44–46]

Brain Tumor

The usefulness of DSC-MR and DCE-MR imaging in brain tumor imaging is based on the detection of intratumoral microvascular abnormalities: The disorganized angiogenesis is associated with vascular permeability induced by the vascular endothelial growth factor A in high-grade tumor.[47] CBV and K^{trans} are respectively correlated with these histopathologic findings in high-grade tumor.[48,49]

The most widely used parameter is the rCBV ratio (tumoral rCBV/contralateral normal brain rCBV). Several different methods exist to determine the ROIs used to extract rCBV values. A more accurate measurement of tumoral rCBV is the maximal rCBV chosen among several ROIs placed in several hot spots.[50]

Differential diagnosis of intracranial lesions
Differentiation of brain abscess versus cystic brain tumor Distinguishing a pyogenic brain abscess from a cystic brain tumor is sometimes difficult using conventional MR imaging, for which both conditions can present as rim-enhancing masses. Diffusion imaging is very helpful to making a distinction when an abscess is classically associated with internal diffusion restriction. However, small abscesses and nonpyogenic abscesses, such as toxoplasmosis, can display increased diffusion.[51] A few studies have demonstrated a significantly lower rCBV ratio (<0.95) in the abscess wall than in tumor wall (**Fig. 2**).[52,53] One study demonstrated that K^{trans} and v_e could also be helpful for this distinction.[54]

Tumefactive demyelinating lesion versus glioma A tumefactive demyelinating lesion can seem similar to a brain tumor not only on conventional imaging but also on histopathologic examination, when hypercellularity and atypical reactive astrocytes can mimic high-grade glioma (HGG). Cha and colleagues[55] have demonstrated that rCBV ratio was useful in differentiating tumefactive demyelinating lesion from intracranial neoplasms, with

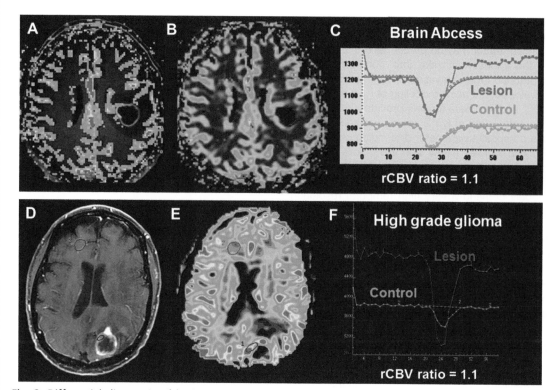

Fig. 2. Differential diagnostic of brain tumor using DSC-MR imaging. Both patients presented with a mass demonstrating central necrosis and peripheral enhancement (*A, D*). In a brain abscess (*upper row*), DSC-MR imaging demonstrates a low rCBV ratio (*C*) without visible increased perfusion on the rCBV color map (*B*), whereas in a brain tumor, in this case a metastasis (*lower row*), DSC-MR imaging demonstrates an increase perfusion within enhanced parts of the lesion (*E*) with a high rCBV ratio (*F*).

values of 0.88 and 6.47, respectively (**Fig. 3**). However, some contrast-enhanced lesions in multiple sclerosis can have an increased CBV (see later).[56]

Differentiation of cerebral lymphoma versus glioma A lower rCBV ratio was found in primary lymphoma than in HGG (**Fig. 4**) because an important pathologic finding in primary lymphoma is the tumor infiltration along the capillaries and not an important tumor neoangiogenesis like in HGG. A threshold value of 1.2 for rCBV ratio gave a positive predictive value of 94% and a negative predictive value of 89% to differentiate these tumors.[57] In this study, metrics extracted from DCE were not significantly different between lymphomas, HGGs, and metastases.[57]

Using a BBB leakage correction algorithm, but not a GBCA preloading, Mangla and colleagues[58] reported that percentage signal recovery derived from the DSC-MR imaging signal–time curve was superior to the rCBV ratio to differentiate lymphoma, HGG, and metastasis. Mean percentage signal recovery was high in lymphoma (113.1 ± 41.6),

intermediate in glioblastoma (78.2 ± 14.3), and low in metastases (53.5 ± 12.9).

Glioma
Predicting glioma grade Compared with biopsy or surgery, MR imaging has the advantage of being able to evaluate the entire glioma and the surrounding brain parenchyma, which is typically neither resected nor biopsied. However, despite numerous shortcomings such as reproducibility and sampling error, the World Health Organization (WHO) classification remains the standard reference for predicting prognosis and guiding therapy in patients with brain tumors. Therapy for HGG (WHO grades III and IV) typically consists of surgery and adjuvant chemoradiation, whereas management for low-grade glioma (LGG; WHO grades I and II) is less invasive.

Compared with conventional contrast-enhanced MR imaging, perfusion MR using rCBV ratio increases the sensitivity and predictive value in predicting glioma grade.[59] However, reported threshold values vary because of the absence of

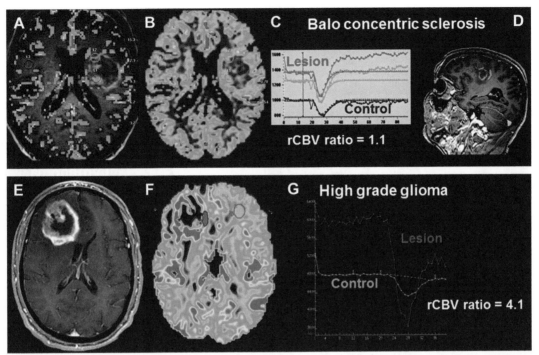

Fig. 3. Differential diagnosis of an intracranial mass using DSC-MR imaging. Both patients presented with a peripherally enhancing, centrally necrotic mass (*A, E*). In Balo concentric sclerosis (*upper row*), DSC-MR imaging demonstrates a low rCBV ratio (*C*) without visible increased perfusion on the rCBV color map (*B*). Concentric enhancement of the lesion is seen on sagittal postcontrast T1-weighted image (*D*). In an HGG (*lower row*), DSC-MR imaging demonstrates increased perfusion within the enhancing portions of the lesion (*F*) with a high rCBV ratio (*G*).

standardization for acquisition parameters and processing methods. Maximal rCBV values of LGG range between 1.11 to 2.14, whereas maximal rCBV values of HGG are higher, between 3.54 and 7.32.[59–62] Law and colleagues[59] demonstrated that a threshold value of 1.75 provides a sensitivity of 95%, a specificity of 57.5%, a predictive positive value of 87%, and a negative predictive value of 79.3% (**Fig. 4**).

K^{trans} values derived from DCE-MR imaging have also been found to correlate with glioma grade and the histologic proliferative marker MIB-1.[63] Using K^{trans} extracted from DSC-MR imaging, the correlation between K^{trans} and tumor grade was less important than the correlation between rCBV and tumor grade.[64] However, using DCE-MR imaging, K^{trans} has been found to discriminate LGG from HGG with a sensitivity and specificity greater than 90%.[65,66] Also, rCBV and K^{trans} were correlated for tumor grading, but regions of increased rCBV were different from regions of increased permeability, likely reflecting the heterogeneity of the glioma vasculature.[64,67]

Predicting prognosis and therapeutic response DSC-MR and DCE-MR imaging can help in predicting the prognosis of gliomas. Bisdas and colleagues[68] determined that an rCBV ratio greater than 4.2 was predictive of recurrence and an rCBV ratio of 3.8 or less was predictive of 1-year survival. In patients with HGG, Hirai and colleagues[69] demonstrated that an rCBV ratio greater than 2.3 was an independent prognostic biomarker for predicting survival. They found that 2-year survival was significantly higher for patients with low (≤2.3) than for those with high (≥2.3) maximum rCBV ratio. Cao and colleagues[70] demonstrated that permeability assessed by DCE-MR imaging in HGG, although not a predictor for survival, was a predictor for time to progression.

Using clinical outcome and not the WHO classification scheme as reference, Law and colleagues[71] compared the value of rCBV in 189 patients with glioma. They show that patients with glioma who have high baseline rCBV (>1.75) had a significantly more rapid time to progression than did patients with low rCBV (<1.75), regardless of whether the grade was

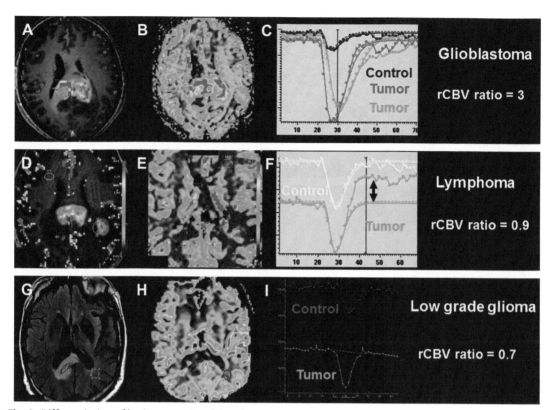

Fig. 4. Differentiation of brain tumors involving the corpus callosum using DSC-MR imaging: glioblastoma (*upper row*), primary central nervous system lymphoma (*middle row*), and LGG (*lower row*). Contrast enhancement within the tumor seen on axial T1-weighted image postgadolinium does not discriminate glioblastoma (*A*) from lymphoma (*D*). rCBV color maps demonstrates increased perfusion within glioblastoma (*B*) but not within lymphoma (*E*). The rCBV ratio (tumoral rCBV/normal brain rCBV) is elevated (>1.75) for glioblastoma and low for lymphoma. The nonenhancing LGG, seen with increased signal on fluid-attenuated inversion recovery (FLAIR) images (*G*), has decreased perfusion on rCBV map (*H*) with a low rCBV ratio. Visual inspection of the curve demonstrates a high percentage signal recovery within lymphoma (*F, double arrow*), not visible for LGG (*I*).

high or low.[71] These results suggest that rCBV from DSC-MR imaging may overcome some of the limitations of the current histologic methods to provide an additional prognostic factor for tumor biology.

Guiding biopsy and radiosurgery Tumor biopsy and radiosurgery are usually guided with enhancement on postcontrast T1-weighted images.[72] The most malignant region of a tumor could be outside the enhancing of a glioma; DSC-MR and DCE-MR imaging may be useful to guide the surgeon toward the most vascular and malignant portion of the mass.[13]

Follow-up of Brain Tumor

Predicting malignant transformation of LGG
Patients with LGG often undergo regular follow-up MR imaging to detect malignant transformation at the earliest stage possible. DSC-MR imaging

perfusion imaging could be helpful. Indeed, studies have demonstrated that high rCBV (>1.75) in LGG is associated with poor prognosis.[71] Moreover, significant increases in rCBV can be detected up to 12 months before contrast enhancement is noted on conventional postcontrast T1-weighted images.[73]

Therapeutic monitoring
DSC-MR and DCE-MR imaging may help monitor treatment response and recurrence in the posttherapeutic brain because the appearance of contrast enhancement is nonspecific.[1] DSC-MR[74] and DCE-MR imaging could be helpful to differentiate residual or recurrent tumor from therapy-induced changes as late necrosis induced by radiotherapy, pseudoprogression (ie, early necrosis induced by combined chemoradiotherapy), or pseudoresponse (ie, "masked" disease progression after antiangiogenic treatment).

Delayed radiation necrosis and recurrent tumor Although recurrent tumor demonstrates increased vascular proliferation and angiogenesis, delayed radiation necrosis (DRN) is an occlusive vasculopathy. Both conditions can appear as regions contrast enhancement and sometimes the 2 conditions can be present simultaneously. rCBV is decreased and permeability is mildly elevated in DRN, whereas in residual/recurrent tumor, both rCBV and permeability are significantly elevated.[13]

Several studies have demonstrated good results of DSC-MR imaging in the differentiation between DRN and tumor recurrence.[41,75] Although threshold rCBV values vary according the studies, the rCBV in DRN are lower than the rCBV of normal white matter, whereas in tumor recurrence, rCBV is generally higher than the rCBV of normal white matter. K^{trans} is reduced in DRN because the enhancement is typically slow, without a rapid vascular phase. On the other hand, K^{trans} is elevated in recurrent tumor, in association with a very rapid initial increase in the vascular permeability curve, compatible with a rapid vascular phase.[13,76]

Pseudoprogression Pseudoprogression is an increase of size and enhancement in HGGs attributed to the use of combined chemoradiotherapy with temozolomide. This therapy-induced necrosis appears in the first 3 to 6 months of treatment and occurs more dramatically than that seen with radiotherapy alone.[74,77]

The use of conventional contrast-enhanced MR to distinguish true early progression from pseudoprogression seems to be limited.[78,79] Preliminary findings of pseudoprogression using DSC-MR and DCE-MR imaging suggest a decrease in rCBV and a moderate increase in vascular permeability **(Fig. 5)**.[80,81]

Pseudoresponse Antiangiogenic agents, such as bevacizumab or cediranib, are now administered in patients with recurrent HGGs.[82] The term

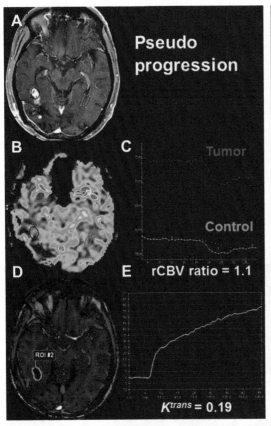
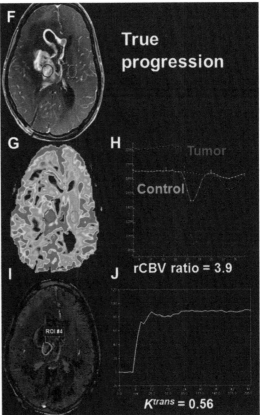

Fig. 5. Posttherapeutic evaluation of HGG using DSC-MR and DCE-MR imaging. Both patients demonstrate increased contrast enhancement 3 months after combined chemoradiotherapy with temozolomide (A, F). Pseudoprogression may demonstrate decreased perfusion with a low rCBV ratio using DSC-MR imaging (B, C) and moderate vascular permeability (D, E) with a progressive enhancement (E) using DCE-MR imaging. True early progression may demonstrate increased perfusion with a high rCBV ratio (G, H) with high permeability and rapid enhancement (I, J).

"pseudoresponse" is applied to the rapid decrease in enhancement following treatment with antiangiogenic agents.[83] The decreased enhancement may at least partially result from decreased vessel permeability and not necessarily from antitumor effects. Some patients clinically progress despite the absence of enhancing tumor progression on MR imaging.[82] In our preliminary experience, those patients with true response to bevacizumab seem to demonstrate a decrease in rCBV and permeability.[13] The decrease in K^{trans} can be seen even after a single dose of cediranib, and this effect is reversible when the drug is withdrawn.[83] Using a "vascular normalization index," including in K^{trans}, microvessel volume, and circulating collagen intravenously, was found to be associated with overall survival and progression-free survival in patients given a single dose of cediranib.[84]

OTHER PATHOLOGIC CONDITIONS
Stroke

Preliminary studies using DSC-MR imaging in acute ischemic stroke have demonstrated its usefulness in establishing diagnosis and predicting prognosis. The perfusion/diffusion mismatch (hypoperfusion volume greater than diffusion-weighted imaging (DWI) ischemic lesion volume) is considered to represent the tissue at risk for infarction without arterial recanalization.[85–87] Baseline volume DSC-MR imaging hypoperfusion demonstrates a better correlation with the National Institutes of Health Stroke Scale at baseline or clinical outcome than the volume of DWI lesions,[88,89] regardless of the perfusion parameter used: TTP,[88] CBF, or MTT (**Fig. 6**).[85,86]

The most widely used therapy for acute stroke reperfusion is recombinant tissue plasminogen activator. Initially, it was proved to improve patients' outcome if used within 3 hours of symptom onset (National Institute of Neurological Disorders and Stroke rt-PA stroke study).[90] More recently, the time window was extended to 4.5 hours in a select stroke population (European Cooperative Acute Stroke Study III - ECASS III).[91] However, this time window ignores the variation among individual patients with stroke. Several studies demonstrated a benefit of thrombolysis outside of the usual time window up to 6 or 9 hours after clinical onset using a different definition of DWI/DSC-MR imaging mismatch.[92–95] Several perfusion thresholds were used to differentiate "at-risk tissue" versus "not at-risk tissue."[96] For a wider clinical use of perfusion imaging in this context, a greater consistency of threshold definitions is needed. Using automatic software is suggested as a way to improve the determination of patients who could benefit from recanalization.[45]

An early reperfusion response based on MTT has been found to be predictive of clinical recovery with standard intravenous recombinant tissue plasminogen activator therapy. A decrease of 30% or greater in the volume of hypoperfusion on MTT maps 2 hours after treatment was a strong predictor of clinical outcome.[97]

PERMEABILITY

Some studies suggested that permeability imaging may be helpful to predict hemorrhagic transformation (HT) in patients with acute ischemic stroke. In a study of 10 patients with acute ischemic stroke, Kassner and colleagues[98] found

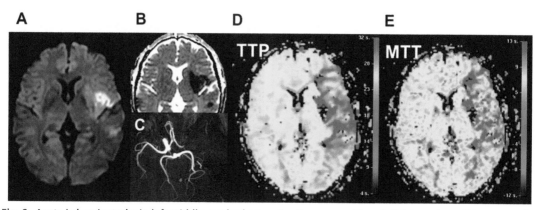

Fig. 6. Acute ischemic stroke in left middle cerebral artery territory, caused by a left internal carotid artery occlusion (*C*). Diffusion-weighted image (*A*) and apparent diffusion coefficient (ADC) map (*B*) demonstrates an ischemic core smaller than the hypoperfused territory seen on TTP (*D*) or MTT (*E*) maps (*red area*). The perfusion/diffusion mismatch (difference between these 2 volumes) is considered as the tissue at risk to infarction without arterial recanalization.

significantly increased permeability in 3 patients who went on to HT within 48 hours after clinical onset using DCE-MR imaging with the Patlak model. With this technique, a minimal DCE acquisition duration of 3 minutes 30 seconds seemed to be necessary to discriminate between patients with and without HT.[99] Permeability maps extracted from DSC-MR imaging may also identify patients at risk for HT.[100]

Dementia

DSC-MR imaging has been rarely used to study patient with dementia. Nuclear medicine techniques or arterial spin labeling techniques are preferred because injection of GBCA is not recommended to evaluate dementia patients with MR imaging.

However, recent reports showed that reduction in flow, hypoxia, and BBB dysfunction might initiate or contribute to neuronal degeneration, notably in Alzheimer disease.[101] Some studies using MR imaging have shown increased BBB permeability with normal aging and an increased permeability in patients with vascular dementia compared with age-matched controls.[102] Starr and colleagues[103] demonstrated no significant permeability difference for subjects with Alzheimer disease versus control subjects or for patients with mild cognitive impairment (MCI) versus controls.[104] However, these studies used only descriptive methods to estimate permeability without calculating K^{trans} or PS. Improvement of DCE-MR imaging techniques may permit accurate estimation of permeability in the hippocampus in the near future.[105]

Multiple Sclerosis

DSC-MR imaging has demonstrated an increased perfusion in acute multiple sclerosis (MS) lesions and decreased CBF and CBV in most nonenhancing MS lesions.[56] A decreased CBF was also found in normal-appearing white matter and in gray matter.[106–108] Cortical hypoperfusion seems to appear early in disease progression. Deep gray matter hypoperfusion is found in patients with relapsing-remitting and primary progressive MS and is correlated with fatigue score and neuropsychological dysfunction.[107] Decreased perfusion in patients with MS could be explained by the presence of lesions in gray matter, degeneration of axons, and neuronal loss secondary to demyelination, Hypoperfusion, or Wallerian degeneration. A recent study using DCE-MR imaging demonstrated the feasibility of DCE-MR imaging for the quantitative assessment of PS in normal-appearing white matter (NAWM) as well as in focal lesions.[109]

SUMMARY

DSC-MR and DCE-MR imaging can provide imaging biomarkers that reflect brain hemodynamic processes and permeability. These techniques provide physiologic information to complement conventional contrast-enhanced MR imaging, and their added value is now recognized, especially in of the evaluation of brain tumors and stroke. However, standardization of acquisition and processing is needed to increase their clinical benefit and allow widespread use.

REFERENCES

1. Essig M, Anzalone N, Combs SE, et al. MR imaging of neoplastic central nervous system lesions: review and recommendations for current practice. AJNR Am J Neuroradiol 2012;33:803–17.
2. Villringer A, Rosen BR, Belliveau JW, et al. Dynamic imaging with lanthanide chelates in normal brain: contrast due to magnetic susceptibility effects. Magn Reson Med 1988;6:164–74.
3. Calamante F, Thomas DL, Pell GS, et al. Measuring cerebral blood flow using magnetic resonance imaging techniques. J Cereb Blood Flow Metab 1999;19:701–35.
4. Zaharchuk G. Theoretical basis of hemodynamic MR imaging techniques to measure cerebral blood volume, cerebral blood flow, and permeability. AJNR Am J Neuroradiol 2007;28:1850–8.
5. Simonsen CZ, Ostergaard L, Smith DF, et al. Comparison of gradient- and spin-echo imaging: CBF, CBV, and MTT measurements by bolus tracking. J Magn Reson Imaging 2000;12:411–6.
6. Fisel CR, Ackerman JL, Buxton RB, et al. MR contrast due to microscopically heterogeneous magnetic susceptibility: numerical simulations and applications to cerebral physiology. Magn Reson Med 1991;17:336–47.
7. Donahue KM, Krouwer HG, Rand SD, et al. Utility of simultaneously acquired gradient-echo and spin-echo cerebral blood volume and morphology maps in brain tumor patients. Magn Reson Med 2000;43:845–53.
8. Sugahara T, Korogi Y, Kochi M, et al. Perfusion-sensitive MR imaging of gliomas: comparison between gradient-echo and spin-echo echo-planar imaging techniques. AJNR Am J Neuroradiol 2001; 22:1306–15.
9. van Gelderen P, Grandin C, Petrella JR, et al. Rapid three-dimensional MR imaging method for tracking a bolus of contrast agent through the brain. Radiology 2000;216:603–8.

10. Lupo JM, Lee MC, Han ET, et al. Feasibility of dynamic susceptibility contrast perfusion MR imaging at 3T using a standard quadrature head coil and eight-channel phased-array coil with and without SENSE reconstruction. J Magn Reson Imaging 2006;24:520–9.

11. Paulson ES, Schmainda KM. Comparison of dynamic susceptibility-weighted contrast-enhanced MR methods: recommendations for measuring relative cerebral blood volume in brain tumors. Radiology 2008;249:601–13.

12. Hu LS, Baxter LC, Pinnaduwage DS, et al. Optimized preload leakage-correction methods to improve the diagnostic accuracy of dynamic susceptibility-weighted contrast-enhanced perfusion MR imaging in posttreatment gliomas. AJNR Am J Neuroradiol 2010;31:40–8.

13. Lacerda S, Law M. Magnetic resonance perfusion and permeability imaging in brain tumors. Neuroimaging Clin N Am 2009;19:527–57.

14. Cotton F, Hermier M. The advantage of high relaxivity contrast agents in brain perfusion. Eur Radiol 2006;16(Suppl 7):M16–26.

15. Essig M, Lodemann KP, Le-Huu M, et al. Intraindividual comparison of gadobenate dimeglumine and gadobutrol for cerebral magnetic resonance perfusion imaging at 1.5 T. Invest Radiol 2006;41: 256–63.

16. Giesel FL, Mehndiratta A, Risse F, et al. Intraindividual comparison between gadopentetate dimeglumine and gadobutrol for magnetic resonance perfusion in normal brain and intracranial tumors at 3 Tesla. Acta Radiol 2009;50:521–30.

17. Gahramanov S, Raslan AM, Muldoon LL, et al. Potential for differentiation of pseudoprogression from true tumor progression with dynamic susceptibility-weighted contrast-enhanced magnetic resonance imaging using ferumoxytol vs. gadoteridol: a pilot study. Int J Radiat Oncol Biol Phys 2011;79:514–23.

18. Rosen BR, Belliveau JW, Vevea JM, et al. Perfusion imaging with NMR contrast agents. Magn Reson Med 1990;14:249–65.

19. Thompson HK Jr, Starmer CF, Whalen RE, et al. Indicator transit time considered as a gamma variate. Circ Res 1964;14:502–15.

20. Leiva-Salinas C, Provenzale JM, Kudo K, et al. The alphabet soup of perfusion CT and MR imaging: terminology revisited and clarified in five questions. Neuroradiology 2012;54:907–18.

21. Boxerman JL, Schmainda KM, Weisskoff RM. Relative cerebral blood volume maps corrected for contrast agent extravasation significantly correlate with glioma tumor grade, whereas uncorrected maps do not. AJNR Am J Neuroradiol 2006;27: 859–67.

22. Smith AM, Grandin CB, Duprez T, et al. Whole brain quantitative CBF, CBV, and MTT measurements using MRI bolus tracking: implementation and application to data acquired from hyperacute stroke patients. J Magn Reson Imaging 2000;12: 400–10.

23. Wintermark M, Sesay M, Barbier E, et al. Comparative overview of brain perfusion imaging techniques. Stroke 2005;36:e83–99.

24. Knutsson L, Stahlberg F, Wirestam R. Absolute quantification of perfusion using dynamic susceptibility contrast MRI: pitfalls and possibilities. MAGMA 2010;23:1–21.

25. Tofts PS, Brix G, Buckley DL, et al. Estimating kinetic parameters from dynamic contrast-enhanced T(1)-weighted MRI of a diffusable tracer: standardized quantities and symbols. J Magn Reson Imaging 1999;10:223–32.

26. Evelhoch JL. Key factors in the acquisition of contrast kinetic data for oncology. J Magn Reson Imaging 1999;10:254–9.

27. Gowland P, Mansfield P, Bullock P, et al. Dynamic studies of gadolinium uptake in brain tumors using inversion-recovery echo-planar imaging. Magn Reson Med 1992;26:241–58.

28. Parker GJ, Suckling J, Tanner SF, et al. Probing tumor microvascularity by measurement, analysis and display of contrast agent uptake kinetics. J Magn Reson Imaging 1997;7:564–74.

29. Brookes JA, Redpath TW, Gilbert FJ, et al. Accuracy of T1 measurement in dynamic contrast-enhanced breast MRI using two- and three-dimensional variable flip angle fast low-angle shot. J Magn Reson Imaging 1999;9:163–71.

30. Lebel R, Jones J, Ferré JC, et al. Highly accelerated dynamic contrast enhanced imaging with prospective undersampling. Annual meeting proceedings of the International Society for Magnetic Resonance in Medecine. 2012.

31. Smith DS, Welch EB, Li X, et al. Quantitative effects of using compressed sensing in dynamic contrast enhanced MRI. Phys Med Biol 2011;56: 4933–46.

32. Daniel BL, Yen YF, Glover GH, et al. Breast disease: dynamic spiral MR imaging. Radiology 1998;209: 499–509.

33. Patlak CS, Blasberg RG, Fenstermacher JD. Graphical evaluation of blood-to-brain transfer constants from multiple-time uptake data. J Cereb Blood Flow Metab 1983;3:1–7.

34. Larsson HB, Stubgaard M, Frederiksen JL, et al. Quantitation of blood-brain barrier defect by magnetic resonance imaging and gadolinium-DTPA in patients with multiple sclerosis and brain tumors. Magn Reson Med 1990;16:117–31.

35. Tofts PS, Kermode AG. Measurement of the blood-brain barrier permeability and leakage space using dynamic MR imaging. 1. Fundamental concepts. Magn Reson Med 1991;17:357–67.

36. Gaustad JV, Brurberg KG, Simonsen TG, et al. Tumor vascularity assessed by magnetic resonance imaging and intravital microscopy imaging. Neoplasia 2008;10:354–62.

37. Tofts PS. Modeling tracer kinetics in dynamic Gd-DTPA MR imaging. J Magn Reson Imaging 1997; 7:91–101.

38. St Lawrence KS, Lee TY. An adiabatic approximation to the tissue homogeneity model for water exchange in the brain: I. Theoretical derivation. J Cereb Blood Flow Metab 1998;18:1365–77.

39. Paldino MJ, Barboriak DP. Fundamentals of quantitative dynamic contrast-enhanced MR imaging. Magn Reson Imaging Clin N Am 2009;17:277–89.

40. Schabel MC, Fluckiger JU, DiBella EV. A model-constrained Monte Carlo method for blind arterial input function estimation in dynamic contrast-enhanced MRI: I. Simulations. Phys Med Biol 2010;55:4783–806.

41. Cha S, Knopp EA, Johnson G, et al. Intracranial mass lesions: dynamic contrast-enhanced susceptibility-weighted echo-planar perfusion MR imaging. Radiology 2002;223:11–29.

42. Kassner A, Annesley DJ, Zhu XP, et al. Abnormalities of the contrast re-circulation phase in cerebral tumors demonstrated using dynamic susceptibility contrast-enhanced imaging: a possible marker of vascular tortuosity. J Magn Reson Imaging 2000; 11:103–13.

43. Quarles CC, Schmainda KM. Assessment of the morphological and functional effects of the anti-angiogenic agent SU11657 on 9L gliosarcoma vasculature using dynamic susceptibility contrast MRI. Magn Reson Med 2007;57:680–7.

44. Copen WA, Schaefer PW, Wu O. MR perfusion imaging in acute ischemic stroke. Neuroimaging Clin N Am 2011;21:259–83, x.

45. Grigoryan M, Tung CE, Albers GW. Role of diffusion and perfusion MRI in selecting patients for reperfusion therapies. Neuroimaging Clin N Am 2011;21: 247–57, ix-x.

46. Shiroishi MS, Habibi M, Rajderkar D, et al. Perfusion and permeability MR imaging of gliomas. Technol Cancer Res Treat 2011;10:59–71.

47. Vajkoczy P, Menger MD. Vascular microenvironment in gliomas. J Neurooncol 2000;50:99–108.

48. Provenzale JM, Wang GR, Brenner T, et al. Comparison of permeability in high-grade and low-grade brain tumors using dynamic susceptibility contrast MR imaging. AJR Am J Roentgenol 2002;178:711–6.

49. Roberts HC, Roberts TP, Brasch RC, et al. Quantitative measurement of microvascular permeability in human brain tumors achieved using dynamic contrast-enhanced MR imaging: correlation with histologic grade. AJNR Am J Neuroradiol 2000; 21:891–9.

50. Wetzel SG, Cha S, Johnson G, et al. Relative cerebral blood volume measurements in intracranial mass lesions: interobserver and intraobserver reproducibility study. Radiology 2002;224: 797–803.

51. Camacho DL, Smith JK, Castillo M. Differentiation of toxoplasmosis and lymphoma in AIDS patients by using apparent diffusion coefficients. AJNR Am J Neuroradiol 2003;24:633–7.

52. Chiang IC, Hsieh TJ, Chiu ML, et al. Distinction between pyogenic brain abscess and necrotic brain tumour using 3-tesla MR spectroscopy, diffusion and perfusion imaging. Br J Radiol 2009;82: 813–20.

53. Holmes TM, Petrella JR, Provenzale JM. Distinction between cerebral abscesses and high-grade neoplasms by dynamic susceptibility contrast perfusion MRI. AJR Am J Roentgenol 2004;183: 1247–52.

54. Haris M, Gupta RK, Singh A, et al. Differentiation of infective from neoplastic brain lesions by dynamic contrast-enhanced MRI. Neuroradiology 2008;50: 531–40.

55. Cha S, Pierce S, Knopp EA, et al. Dynamic contrast-enhanced T2*-weighted MR imaging of tumefactive demyelinating lesions. AJNR Am J Neuroradiol 2001;22:1109–16.

56. Ge Y, Law M, Johnson G, et al. Dynamic susceptibility contrast perfusion MR imaging of multiple sclerosis lesions: characterizing hemodynamic impairment and inflammatory activity. AJNR Am J Neuroradiol 2005;26:1539–47.

57. Weber MA, Zoubaa S, Schlieter M, et al. Diagnostic performance of spectroscopic and perfusion MRI for distinction of brain tumors. Neurology 2006;66: 1899–906.

58. Mangla R, Kolar B, Zhu T, et al. Percentage signal recovery derived from MR dynamic susceptibility contrast imaging is useful to differentiate common enhancing malignant lesions of the brain. AJNR Am J Neuroradiol 2011;32:1004–10.

59. Law M, Yang S, Wang H, et al. Glioma grading: sensitivity, specificity, and predictive values of perfusion MR imaging and proton MR spectroscopic imaging compared with conventional MR imaging. AJNR Am J Neuroradiol 2003;24: 1989–98.

60. Aronen HJ, Perkio J. Dynamic susceptibility contrast MRI of gliomas. Neuroimaging Clin N Am 2002;12:501–23.

61. Law M, Teicher N, Zagzag D, et al. Dynamic contrast enhanced perfusion MRI in mycosis fungoides. J Magn Reson Imaging 2003;18:364–7.

62. Shin JH, Lee HK, Kwun BD, et al. Using relative cerebral blood flow and volume to evaluate the histopathologic grade of cerebral gliomas: preliminary results. Am J Roentgenol 2002;179:783–9.

63. Roberts HC, Roberts TP, Bollen AW, et al. Correlation of microvascular permeability derived from dynamic contrast-enhanced MR imaging with histologic grade and tumor labeling index: a study in human brain tumors. Acad Radiol 2001;8:384–91.

64. Law M, Yang S, Babb JS, et al. Comparison of cerebral blood volume and vascular permeability from dynamic susceptibility contrast-enhanced perfusion MR imaging with glioma grade. AJNR Am J Neuroradiol 2004;25:746–55.

65. Nguyen TB, Cron GO, Mercier JF, et al. Diagnostic accuracy of dynamic contrast-enhanced mr imaging using a phase-derived vascular input function in the preoperative grading of gliomas. AJNR Am J Neuroradiol 2012. http://dx.doi.org/10.3174/ajnr.A3012.

66. Patankar TF, Haroon HA, Mills SJ, et al. Is volume transfer coefficient (K(trans)) related to histologic grade in human gliomas? AJNR Am J Neuroradiol 2005;26:2455–65.

67. Lupo JM, Cha S, Chang SM, et al. Dynamic susceptibility-weighted perfusion imaging of high-grade gliomas: characterization of spatial heterogeneity. AJNR Am J Neuroradiol 2005;26:1446–54.

68. Bisdas S, Kirkpatrick M, Giglio P, et al. Cerebral blood volume measurements by perfusion-weighted MR imaging in gliomas: ready for prime time in predicting short-term outcome and recurrent disease? AJNR Am J Neuroradiol 2009;30:681–8.

69. Hirai T, Murakami R, Nakamura H, et al. Prognostic value of perfusion MR imaging of high-grade astrocytomas: long-term follow-up study. AJNR Am J Neuroradiol 2008;29:1505–10.

70. Cao Y, Nagesh V, Hamstra D, et al. The extent and severity of vascular leakage as evidence of tumor aggressiveness in high-grade gliomas. Cancer Res 2006;66:8912–7.

71. Law M, Young RJ, Babb JS, et al. Gliomas: predicting time to progression or survival with cerebral blood volume measurements at dynamic susceptibility-weighted contrast-enhanced perfusion MR imaging. Radiology 2008;247:490–8.

72. Kelly PJ, Daumas-Duport C, Kispert DB, et al. Imaging-based stereotaxic serial biopsies in untreated intracranial glial neoplasms. J Neurosurg 1987;66:865–74.

73. Danchaivijitr N, Waldman AD, Tozer DJ, et al. Low-grade gliomas: do changes in rCBV measurements at longitudinal perfusion-weighted MR imaging predict malignant transformation? Radiology 2008;247:170–8.

74. Clarke JL, Chang S. Pseudoprogression and pseudoresponse: challenges in brain tumor imaging. Curr Neurol Neurosci Rep 2009;9:241–6.

75. Hu LS, Baxter LC, Smith KA, et al. Relative cerebral blood volume values to differentiate high-grade glioma recurrence from posttreatment radiation effect: direct correlation between image-guided tissue histopathology and localized dynamic susceptibility-weighted contrast-enhanced perfusion MR imaging measurements. AJNR Am J Neuroradiol 2009;30:552–8.

76. Hazle JD, Jackson EF, Schomer DF, et al. Dynamic imaging of intracranial lesions using fast spin-echo imaging: differentiation of brain tumors and treatment effects. J Magn Reson Imaging 1997;7:1084–93.

77. Hygino da Cruz LC Jr, Rodriguez I, Domingues RC, et al. Pseudoprogression and pseudoresponse: imaging challenges in the assessment of posttreatment glioma. AJNR Am J Neuroradiol 2011;32:1978–85.

78. Gupta A, Shah A, Young R, et al. Pseudoprogression and the Macdonald response criteria in patients with glioblastoma. Proceedings of the Radiological Society of North America. 2009.

79. Young RJ, Gupta A, Shah AD, et al. Potential utility of conventional MRI signs in diagnosing pseudoprogression in glioblastoma. Neurology 2011;76:1918–24.

80. Law M, Lacerda S, Shiroishi MS, et al. Characterization of disease progression versus pseudoprogression after concomitant radiochemotherapy treatment using perfusion, permeability, and MR spectroscopy in high grade gliomas. Proceedings of the Radiological Society of North America. 2009.

81. Meyzer C, Dhermain F, Ducreux D, et al. A case report of pseudoprogression followed by complete remission after proton-beam irradiation for a low-grade glioma in a teenager: the value of dynamic contrast-enhanced MRI. Radiat Oncol 2010;5:9.

82. Norden AD, Drappatz J, Muzikansky A, et al. An exploratory survival analysis of anti-angiogenic therapy for recurrent malignant glioma. J Neurooncol 2009;92:149–55.

83. Batchelor TT, Sorensen AG, di Tomaso E, et al. AZD2171, a pan-VEGF receptor tyrosine kinase inhibitor, normalizes tumor vasculature and alleviates edema in glioblastoma patients. Cancer Cell 2007;11:83–95.

84. Sorensen AG, Batchelor TT, Zhang WT, et al. A "vascular normalization index" as potential mechanistic biomarker to predict survival after a single dose of cediranib in recurrent glioblastoma patients. Cancer Res 2009;69:5296–300.

85. Baird AE, Benfield A, Schlaug G, et al. Enlargement of human cerebral ischemic lesion volumes measured by diffusion-weighted magnetic resonance imaging. Ann Neurol 1997;41:581–9.

86. Barber PA, Darby DG, Desmond PM, et al. Prediction of stroke outcome with echoplanar

perfusion- and diffusion-weighted MRI. Neurology 1998;51:418–26.

87. Tong DC, Yenari MA, Albers GW, et al. Correlation of perfusion- and diffusion-weighted MRI with NIHSS score in acute (<6.5 hour) ischemic stroke. Neurology 1998;50:864–70.

88. Beaulieu C, de Crespigny A, Tong DC, et al. Longitudinal magnetic resonance imaging study of perfusion and diffusion in stroke: evolution of lesion volume and correlation with clinical outcome. Ann Neurol 1999;46:568–78.

89. Fink JN, Selim MH, Kumar S, et al. Is the association of National Institutes of Health Stroke Scale scores and acute magnetic resonance imaging stroke volume equal for patients with right- and left-hemisphere ischemic stroke? Stroke 2002;33:954–8.

90. Tissue plasminogen activator for acute ischemic stroke. The National Institute of Neurological Disorders and Stroke rt-PA Stroke Study Group. N Engl J Med 1995;333:1581–7.

91. Bluhmki E, Chamorro A, Davalos A, et al. Stroke treatment with alteplase given 3.0-4.5 h after onset of acute ischaemic stroke (ECASS III): additional outcomes and subgroup analysis of a randomised controlled trial. Lancet Neurol 2009;8:1095–102.

92. Albers GW, Thijs VN, Wechsler L, et al. Magnetic resonance imaging profiles predict clinical response to early reperfusion: the diffusion and perfusion imaging evaluation for understanding stroke evolution (DEFUSE) study. Ann Neurol 2006;60:508–17.

93. Davis SM, Donnan GA, Parsons MW, et al. Effects of alteplase beyond 3 h after stroke in the Echoplanar Imaging Thrombolytic Evaluation Trial (EPITHET): a placebo-controlled randomised trial. Lancet Neurol 2008;7:299–309.

94. Furlan AJ, Eyding D, Albers GW, et al. Dose Escalation of Desmoteplase for Acute Ischemic Stroke (DEDAS): evidence of safety and efficacy 3 to 9 hours after stroke onset. Stroke 2006;37:1227–31.

95. Hacke W, Albers G, Al-Rawi Y, et al. The Desmoteplase in Acute Ischemic Stroke Trial (DIAS): a phase II MRI-based 9-hour window acute stroke thrombolysis trial with intravenous desmoteplase. Stroke 2005;36:66–73.

96. Dani KA, Thomas RG, Chappell FM, et al. Systematic review of perfusion imaging with computed tomography and magnetic resonance in acute ischemic stroke: heterogeneity of acquisition and postprocessing parameters: a translational medicine research collaboration multicentre acute stroke imaging study. Stroke 2011;43:563–6.

97. Chalela JA, Kang DW, Luby M, et al. Early magnetic resonance imaging findings in patients receiving tissue plasminogen activator predict outcome: insights into the pathophysiology of acute stroke in the thrombolysis era. Ann Neurol 2004;55:105–12.

98. Kassner A, Roberts T, Taylor K, et al. Prediction of hemorrhage in acute ischemic stroke using permeability MR imaging. AJNR Am J Neuroradiol 2005; 26:2213–7.

99. Vidarsson L, Thornhill RE, Liu F, et al. Quantitative permeability magnetic resonance imaging in acute ischemic stroke: how long do we need to scan? Magn Reson Imaging 2009;27:1216–22.

100. Bang OY, Buck BH, Saver JL, et al. Prediction of hemorrhagic transformation after recanalization therapy using T2*-permeability magnetic resonance imaging. Ann Neurol 2007;62:170–6.

101. Zlokovic BV. Neurovascular pathways to neurodegeneration in Alzheimer's disease and other disorders. Nat Rev Neurosci 2011;12:723–38.

102. Farrall AJ, Wardlaw JM. Blood-brain barrier: ageing and microvascular disease–systematic review and meta-analysis. Neurobiol Aging 2009;30:337–52.

103. Starr JM, Farrall AJ, Armitage P, et al. Blood-brain barrier permeability in Alzheimer's disease: a case-control MRI study. Psychiatry Res 2009; 171:232–41.

104. Wang H, Golob EJ, Su MY. Vascular volume and blood-brain barrier permeability measured by dynamic contrast enhanced MRI in hippocampus and cerebellum of patients with MCI and normal controls. J Magn Reson Imaging 2006;24:695–700.

105. Anderson VC, Lenar DP, Quinn JF, et al. The blood-brain barrier and microvascular water exchange in Alzheimer's disease. Cardiovasc Psychiatry Neurol 2011;2011:615829.

106. Adhya S, Johnson G, Herbert J, et al. Pattern of hemodynamic impairment in multiple sclerosis: dynamic susceptibility contrast perfusion MR imaging at 3.0 T. Neuroimage 2006;33:1029–35.

107. Inglese M, Adhya S, Johnson G, et al. Perfusion magnetic resonance imaging correlates of neuropsychological impairment in multiple sclerosis. J Cereb Blood Flow Metab 2008;28:164–71.

108. Law M, Saindane AM, Ge Y, et al. Microvascular abnormality in relapsing-remitting multiple sclerosis: perfusion MR imaging findings in normal-appearing white matter. Radiology 2004;231:645–52.

109. Ingrisch M, Sourbron S, Morhard D, et al. Quantification of perfusion and permeability in multiple sclerosis: dynamic contrast-enhanced MRI in 3D at 3T. Invest Radiol 2012;47:252–8.

Use of Magnetic Resonance Imaging Contrast Agents in the Liver and Biliary Tract

Christina LeBedis, MD[a],*, Antonio Luna, MD[b,c], Jorge A. Soto, MD[a]

KEYWORDS

- Hepatobiliary-specific MRI contrast • Gadobenate dimeglumine • Multihance • Gadoxetic acid
- Eovist/Primovist • Gd-DTPA • Magnevist

KEY POINTS

- Hepatobiliary-specific contrast agents can distinguish between hepatocyte- and non–hepatocyte-containing lesions. One important example is the ability of gadobenate dimeglumine and gadoxetic acid to differentiate focal nodular hyperplasia from hepatic adenoma, 2 benign lesions with different follow-up and treatment strategies.
- Hepatobiliary-specific agent use is controversial in hepatocellular carcinoma detection and characterization because they do not provide increased sensitivity with respect to the extracellular agents, their uptake may be compromised in the setting of abnormal liver function, and well-differentiated hepatocellular carcinoma may accumulate hepatobiliary-specific agents on delayed hepatocyte imaging, making them indistinguishable from benign hepatocyte-containing lesions.
- Contrast-enhanced magnetic resonance cholangiography has exciting potential uses, including troubleshooting abnormalities encountered at T2-weighted magnetic resonance cholangiography, preoperative biliary anatomy assessment, postoperative biliary tree complications such as bile leaks, and functional biliary tree imaging to aid in the diagnosis of choledocholithiasis and cholecystitis.

INTRODUCTION

Contrast agents have been used in magnetic resonance (MR) imaging since 1986.[1,2] Since the clinical approval of gadolinium (Gd) deglumine in 1988, the daily use of MR contrast agents became widespread. MR imaging contrast improves detection and characterization of liver lesions by increasing lesion-to-liver contrast as a result of decreased T1 relaxation times of liver parenchyma and enhancing lesions.

The major classes of MR contrast agents currently used for liver imaging include extracellular Gd chelates, hepatobiliary-specific agents (including hepatocyte-selective and combined agents), reticuloendothelial agents, and blood pool agents. In this article, the extracellular and hepatobiliary-specific agents will be discussed in detail, highlighting clinical indications, mechanism of action, imaging pitfalls, current clinical applications, and potential future uses.

EXTRACELLULAR CONTRAST AGENTS

Extracellular contrast agents, which are composed of Gd chelated to an organic compound, have been

[a] Department of Radiology, Boston University Medical Center, 3rd Floor FGH Building, 820 Harrison Avenue, Boston, MA 02118, USA; [b] Clinica Las Nieves, Carmelo Torres 2, Jaén 23007, Spain; [c] Department of Radiology, Case Western Reserve University, Cleveland, OH, USA
* Corresponding author.
E-mail address: christina.lebedis@bmc.org

Magn Reson Imaging Clin N Am 20 (2012) 715–737
http://dx.doi.org/10.1016/j.mric.2012.07.006
1064-9689/12/$ – see front matter © 2012 Elsevier Inc. All rights reserved.

in clinical use the longest and remain the most frequently used MR contrast agents.[3,4] Several formulations of extracellular agents exist (Table 1); however, their pharmacologic and imaging characteristics are essentially identical.[4] Some of the benefits of the extracellular Gd chelates are that they are considered safe when given at clinically applicable doses in patients without renal failure, they demonstrate other abdominal organ lesions in addition to those of the liver, and they are the least expensive.

CLINICAL INDICATIONS

In the liver, indications for extracellular contrast agent use include lesion detection, lesion characterization, and liver vasculature assessment.[4] Furthermore, most of the "state-of-the-art" liver MR protocols include a dynamic series using an extracellular contrast agent.

MECHANISM OF ACTION

Extracellular contrast agents enter the liver via the hepatic artery and portal vein and freely redistribute from the intravascular to the interstitial space.[5] Liver lesion detection and characterization with extracellular agents rely on differential blood flow between the liver and the tumor.[6] Gd is highly paramagnetic and shortens the T1 (longitudinal) and T2 (transverse) relaxation times of adjacent water protons, causing T1-weighted signal enhancement and T2-weighted signal loss.[4,7] At clinical doses of the extracellular fluid agents, T1 shortening is observed in essentially all tissues.[4,5] Although iodinated contrast and Gd chelates have similar pharmacokinetics, Gd exhibits an amplification effect as a result of its paramagnetic properties, allowing for depiction of subtle areas of contrast accumulation that may not be seen on contrast-enhanced computed tomography (CT). Gd chelates offer better enhancement of the blood

pool on equilibrium-phase images than iodinated contrast agents, enabling better delineation of blood vessels than on contrast-enhanced CT.[5,8]

DOSAGE AND ELIMINATION

The recommended dose of extracellular fluid agents is 0.1 mmol/kg, rendering a dose of 20 mL effective in most adults for liver imaging. Renal elimination predominates with the extracellular agents.[9] In patients with normal renal function, documented adverse effects of the extracellular contrast agents are mild and include headache, nausea, and vomiting. Anaphylaxis is exceedingly rare.[10,11] Patients with renal failure are at risk for nephrogenic systemic fibrosis after the administration of any Gd-based contrast agent; however, these risks can be minimized by adhering to restrictive Gd-based contrast agent administration guidelines.[12]

All extracellular fluid agents are labeled class C drugs by the Food and Drug Administration (FDA) with a teratogenic effect demonstrated in animal studies; however, no controlled human studies have been performed. Therefore, Gd chelates are typically avoided in pregnancy, particularly in the first trimester.[13] The effect of Gd excreted in breast milk is unknown, but studies have shown that the expected absorbed dose by the infant from ingesting breast milk is less than 0.05% of the recommended pediatric dose.[14]

IMAGING PROTOCOL

Three- (or more) phase dynamic postcontrast imaging with T1-weighted 2- or 3-dimensional (3D) spoiled gradient echo sequences with chemically selective fat suppression is of paramount importance with the extracellular fluid agents because lesion detection and characterization hinge on differential blood flow between the liver parenchyma and the characteristic enhancement

Table 1
Extracellular contrast agents used for liver MR imaging

Generic Name	Abbreviated Name	Trade Name	Manufacturer
Gadopentetate dimeglumine	Gd-DTPA	Magnevist	Bayer, Wayne, NJ
Gadodiamide	Gd-DTPA-BMA	Omniscan	Nycomed Amersham, Princeton, NJ
Gadoteridol	Gd-HP-DO3A	ProHance	Bracco, Princeton, NJ
Gadoversetamide	Gd-DTPA-BMEA	Optimark	Mallinckrodt Imaging, Hazelwood, MO
Gadoterate meglumine[a]	Gd-DOTA	Dotarem	Guerbet, Villepinte, France
Gadobuterol[a]	Gd-BT-DO3A	Gadovist	Bayer, Wayne, NJ

[a] Not approved by the FDA for use in the United States.

patterns of lesions.[15] A sample contrast-enhanced liver MR protocol is listed in **Table 2**.

TIMING OF THE ARTERIAL PHASE OF DYNAMIC MR IMAGING

To accurately capture the arterial phase of enhancement, which is critical for vascular imaging and assessment of arterially enhancing masses, it is imperative to match the peak of the contrast bolus with the acquisition of the central lines of k-space, which encode tissue contrast. To achieve this, several different methods are available. The first uses a fixed scan delay that is constant from patient to patient. This method produces erratic contrast timing because of physiologic differences (especially cardiac output) between patients and is considered to be the least accurate. A second method uses MR "fluoroscopic" triggering, which involves administration of the entire volume of contrast and acquisition of multiple low-resolution MR images through a prescribed region, such as the aorta. Acquisition of a high-resolution breath-hold sequence begins immediately after a certain intensity threshold has been reached. This method is potentially problematic if the patient is unable to breath-hold once the threshold value has been reached because the entire contrast bolus has already been administered. The most reliable method for capturing the arterial phase involves the use of a small test bolus of Gd, usually 2 mL, followed by a 20- to 30-mL saline chaser. A low-resolution image, which repeats every second, is chosen through a specific anatomic region near the target organ. For liver imaging, the upper abdomen is customarily chosen. The technologist measures the time to peak enhancement after giving a 2-mL test bolus. Subsequently, determination of proper timing depends on the k-space acquisition strategy of the particular sequence. If the contrast-encoding center lines of k-space are acquired first (contrast-enhanced, centric reordered 3D MR angiography), the scan delay will then be equivalent to the time to peak enhancement as determined by the test bolus. If a linear k-space strategy is used, whereby the peripheral lines of k-space, which encode for detail, are acquired first, followed by acquisition of the center lines of k-space at the half-way point of the scan, then a timing run equation should be used to match the bolus peak with acquisition of the center lines of k-space:

$$\text{Delay} = \tfrac{1}{2}\,\text{IT} + \text{TTP} - \tfrac{1}{2}\,\text{AT}$$

where AT is acquisition time, IT is injection time, and TTP is time to peak aortic enhancement.[16]

EXTRACELLULAR CONTRAST AGENT PITFALLS

Malignant and benign liver lesions can demonstrate overlap in their enhancement patterns with the extracellular contrast agents given their nonspecific mechanism of action. In addition, timing of the dynamic phase postcontrast sequences can be challenging in patients who are unable to hold their breath. In situations in which a free breathing protocol is necessary, the arterial phase along with its diagnostic information is severely compromised.

HEPATOBILIARY AGENTS

To overcome some of the limitations of extracellular contrast agents, hepatobiliary agents were developed.[17] The hepatobiliary agents are paramagnetic compounds that are taken up to varying degrees by functioning hepatocytes and excreted in bile, causing T1 shortening and, thus, increased

Table 2
Contrast-enhanced liver MR protocol

Sequence	TR (ms)	TE (ms)	Flip Angle (°)
SSTSE coronal	∞	80	90
SSTSE axial	∞	140	90
T2 SPIR axial	1720	80	90
T1 GRE axial			
In phase	180	4.6	80
Out of phase	180	2.3	80
Diffusion axial b = 0 and b = 600			
ADC[d] map			
3D T1 GRE with SPIR	3.5	1.7	15
Precontrast			
Arterial phase – obtained using a test bolus			
Portal venous – acquired approximately 30 s after the arterial phase			
Equilibrium – acquired approximately 30 s after the portal venous phase			
Hepatocyte phase			
Gadobenate dimeglumine –acquired 60–240 min after initial administration			
Gadoxetic acid – acquired 10–20 min after initial administration			
Subtraction images of the arterial, portal venous, and equilibrium phases			

Abbreviations: ADC, apparent diffusion coefficient; GRE, gradient recalled echo; SPIR, spectral inversion recovery; SSTSE, single shot turbo spin echo.

signal intensity of the liver and biliary tree and hepatocyte-containing lesions. By extension, non–hepatocyte-containing lesions appear hypointense on T1-weighted images. There are 2 types of hepatobiliary-specific agents: hepatocyte-selective (mangafodipir trisodium) and combined (extracellular and hepatocyte-selective) agents (gadobenate dimeglumine and gadoxetic acid) (Table 3). Mangafodipir was removed from the US market in 2006; however, much of the experience with hepatobiliary-specific agents has been with this contrast agent and it shares delayed phase imaging characteristics with the other hepatobiliary-specific agents.[6] Hepatocyte-selective agents are more expensive that the nonspecific extracellular agents, but improved liver lesion detection and characterization can avoid additional imaging tests or even biopsy.[6]

INDICATIONS/USES

Hepatobiliary-specific agents allow for improved liver lesion detection in the hepatobiliary phase, characterization of lesions as hepatocellular or nonhepatocellular, and evaluation of biliary tree anatomy and function. Given their robust biliary excretion ($\geq$50%), mangafodipir and gadoxetic acid provide good delayed hepatic and biliary tree imaging, whereas gadobenate dimeglumine with its 5% biliary excretion can only depict the central biliary tree reliably.[6] Mangafodipir is taken up only by hepatocytes; thus, its major indications for use are to characterize lesions as hepatocellular or nonhepatocellular (Fig. 1) and for liver metastasis surveillance, particularly in patients with colorectal adenocarcinoma.[5] Mangafodipir only allows for delayed phase imaging. If an extracellular contrast is administered in conjunction with mangafodipir for the same MR examination, dynamic postcontrast imaging of the liver can also be performed.[5] Of note, the biliary applications of hepatobiliary-specific agents are not approved for clinical use in the United States.

MECHANISM OF ACTION
Hepatocyte-Selective Agents

Mangafodipir is a manganese chelate that is taken up by hepatocyte vitamin B6 receptors as a result of its chemical similarity to vitamin B6.[18] Extrahepatic uptake of mangafodipir is observed when some manganese dissociates from its ligand within the blood circulation. Mangafodipir shortens the T1 and T2 relaxation times of water protons, and at low concentrations, T1 shortening predominates, resulting in T1 high signal intensity.

Combined Agents

The combined agents, gadobenate dimeglumine and gadoxetic acid, have extracellular Gd chelate, hepatocyte-selective, and blood pool characteristics, allowing for dynamic phase imaging for liver lesion detection and characterization similar to the extracellular contrast agents. Their uptake into hepatocytes from the blood and excretion into the bile via the organic anion transport protein are analogous to bilirubin uptake. In their hepatocyte-selective phase, these agents provide prolonged opacification of liver parenchyma. At dynamic phase imaging, the Gd-based hepatobiliary-specific agents (gadobenate dimeglumine and gadoxetic acid) have been shown to be equivalent to the extracellular agents for liver lesion characterization.[19,20] Although the dynamic phases of the extracellular contrast agents and gadobenate dimeglumine are similar, gadoxetic acid does not demonstrate a pure arterial phase and its equilibrium and hepatobiliary phases overlap, altering the typical enhancement pattern of several lesions, including high-flow hemangiomas (Fig. 2).[21,22]

Dosage and Elimination

The recommended adult dosagee of mangafodipir is 0.5 µmol/kg injected slowly at a rate of 2 to 3 mL/min. Hepatic enhancement peaks at 15 minutes and persists for several hours.[15] More than 50%

Table 3			
Hepatobiliary contrast agents used for liver MR imaging			
Generic Name	**Abbreviated Name**	**Trade Name**	**Manufacturer**
Mangafodipir trisodium[a]	Mn-DPDP	Teslascan	GE Healthcare, Princeton, NJ
Gadobenate dimeglumine	Gd-BOPTA	MultiHance	Bracco, Princeton, NJ
Gadoxetic acid	Gadoxetic acid	Eovist[b]	Bayer, Wayne, NJ

Abbreviation: Gadolinium dimeglumine (Gd-DTPA) – Magnevist.
 [a] Taken off the US market in 2006.
 [b] Eovist is the trade name in the United States. Primovist is the trade name in the European Union, Australia, and Japan.

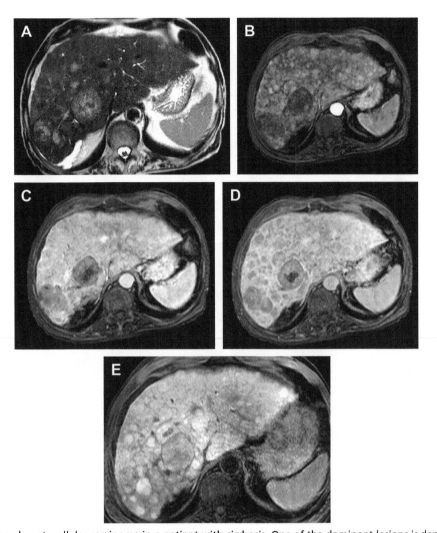

Fig. 1. Diffuse hepatocellular carcinoma in a patient with cirrhosis. One of the dominant lesions is denoted with an arrow. MR imaging demonstrates multiple focal liver lesions, which are moderately hyperintense on T2-weighted images (*A*), most of them enhancement of arterial phase (*B*), and show delayed washout (*C* and *D* on the dynamic series with extracellular contrast agent), although the largest ones shows little arterial enhancement. The enhancement of all nodules with mangafodipir rules out metastasis and confirms their hepatocellular origin (*E*). (*A*) T2-weighted image. (*B*) Arterial phase extracellular contrast agent. (*C*) Portal venous phase. (*D*) Equilibrium phase. (*E*) Mangafodipir. (*Courtesy of* Dr Enrique Ramón, Gregorio Marañón Hospital, Madrid, Spain.)

of the injected mangafodipir is eliminated through the biliary system, with the remainder eliminated by the kidneys. Mangafodipir is a class C drug and should not be administered to pregnant women. The effect of excreted mangafodipir in breast milk on nursing infants in not known.[15]

The recommended adult dosage of gadobenate dimeglumine is 0.1 mmol/kg administered in a bolus injection (2 mL/s). Dynamic imaging can be performed, and peak hepatic enhancement occurs at 1 to 2 hours with peak biliary excretion, which is necessary for functional biliary imaging

occurring at approximately 1 hour. Up to 5% of gadobenate dimeglumine is excreted via the biliary system with 95% being eliminated through the kidneys. The recommended adult dosage of gadoxetic acid is 0.025 mmol/kg administered in a bolus injection (1–2 mL/s). If gadoxetic acid is administered more rapidly, a ring artifact around the aorta may appear. As with gadobenate dimeglumine, dynamic imaging can be performed; however, hepatic enhancement peaks between 10 minutes to hours with peak biliary excretion, which is necessary for functional biliary imaging

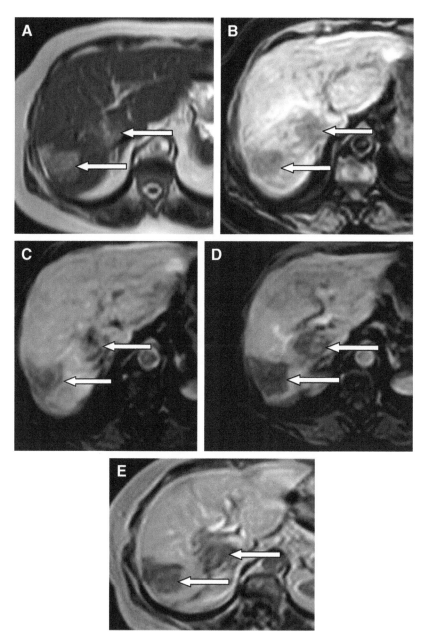

Fig. 2. High-flow hemangiomas. The hemangiomas are hyperintense on T2-weighted imaging (*A*) and hypointense on precontrast T1 fat-saturated imaging (*B*). Gadoxetic acid does not demonstrate a pure arterial phase (*C*) and its equilibrium (*D*) and hepatobiliary (*E*) phases overlap, altering the typical enhancement pattern of several lesions including high-flow hemangioma (*arrows*). (*A*) T2 single shot turbo spin echo (SSTSE). (*B*) T1 High resolution isotropic volume examination (THRIVE) precontrast. (*C*) THRIVE arterial. (*D*) THRIVE equilibrium. (*E*) Hepatobiliary phase.

occurring at approximately 10 minutes. Gadoxetic acid undergoes approximately 50% biliary excretion and 50% renal excretion.

Gadobenate dimeglumine and gadoxetic acid are labeled class C drugs by the FDA and should not be administered to pregnant women. The effect of excreted Gd in breast milk on nursing infants is unknown.[13]

Side effects of the hepatobiliary-selective agents are mild and include flushing, nausea, dizziness, raised blood pressure and heart rate, injection site pain, and taste perversion.[5,15]

Imaging Protocol

As mentioned previously, the combined agents have the same features as the nonspecific extracellular agents paired with the advantage of hepatocyte specificity. Given this, gadobenate dimeglumine and gadoxetic acid use the same imaging protocol as the extracellular agents with the addition of a delayed hepatobiliary sequence obtained at approximately 120 and 20 minutes, respectively. Because of the 120-minute delay between gadobenate dimeglumine injection and the hepatobiliary phase, the patient must be scanned twice. With gadoxetic acid, all of the imaging is performed at once with acquisition of the T2-weighted or diffusion-weighted images between the dynamic and hepatobiliary phases to shorten the examination time. Given the prolonged hepatobiliary phases of enhancement of both gadobenate dimeglumine and gadoxetic acid, additional imaging to assess for enhancement on the hepatobiliary phase. Gadobenate dimeglumine has applications in MR angiography because of its transient binding to serum albumin and resultant increased T1 relaxivity of gadobenate dimeglumine compared with other Gd chelates.

Hepatobiliary-Specific Agent Pitfalls

The T2 shortening effect of hepatobiliary/combined agents necessitates routine T2-weighted MR cholangiopancreatographic (MRCP) images to be obtained before contrast administration because the bile ducts become hypointense on T2-weighted images with these contrast agents. Hyperintense signal intensity on T1-weighted images of a hematoma or of iodine may mimic a bile leak on contrast-enhanced cholangiography. Hepatic insufficiency may require a delay in image acquisition.[15]

The attractive feature of gadoxetic acid is the ability to perform both dynamic and hepatocyte phase imaging in a reasonable time-frame in the same examination, which cannot be done with gadobenate dimeglumine.[6] The Gd-based contrast agents carry a risk of nephrogenic systemic fibrosis (NSF). To the best of our knowledge, gadoxetic acid has not been related to NSF. However, gadobenate dimeglumine has shown an association with several reported confounded NSF cases.[23] The hepatocyte phase can be performed as early as 10 minutes after gadoxetic acid injection in noncirrhotic patients. In cirrhotic

Table 4
Typical MR characteristics of common solid benign and malignant focal liver lesions

Lesion	T1-Weighted Images	T2-Weighted Images	Dynamic Contrast Enhancement	Hepatocyte Phase	Additional Features
FNH	Isointense to hypointense	Isointense to hyperintense	Intense arterial enhancement, isointense to hyperintense to liver in portal venous phase	Isointense to hyperintense to liver	Central scar in 80%, which is usually T2-weighted image hyperintense with delayed enhancement
HA	Isointense to hyperintense, heterogeneous	Variable	Intense arterial enhancement	No enhancement with gadobenate dimeglumine, variable enhancement with gadoxetic acid	T1- and T2-weighted image are variable if hemorrhage or fat are present
Metastasis	Variable (usually hypointense)	Variable	Variable	Hypointense	
HCC	Variable	Isointense to hyperintense	Intense arterial enhancement, washout in portal venous phase	Hypointense (isointense or hyperintense in well-differentiated lesions)	Hypovascular lesions may not demonstrate intense arterial enhancement

patients or in patients with elevated bilirubin levels, a longer delay (>20 minutes) is necessary.[24,25]

Liver Lesion Characterization

Benign liver lesions occur commonly in the general population, making accurate characterization of liver lesions important. At dynamic imaging, the hepatobiliary-specific agents have been shown to be equivalent to the nonspecific extracellular agents[20,26] at liver lesion characterization based on enhancement characteristics. As previously mentioned, gadoxetic acid does not have a pure arterial phase and the equilibrium and hepatobiliary phases overlap, altering the typical enhancement patterns of several lesions such as high-flow hemangiomas. Because the hepatobiliary agents are taken up by functioning hepatocytes in the delayed phase, they are useful in distinguishing between lesions that are of hepatocellular or non-hepatocellular origin and, thus, benign and malignant lesions because malignant lesions typically do not take up hepatocyte-specific contrast agents.[27] Furthermore, the addition of hepatobiliary phase imaging to the dynamic series increases the sensitivity and accuracy for detection of focal hepatic lesions.[28] **Table 4** is a summary of the typical MR appearance of common solid benign and malignant focal liver lesions.

Focal nodular hyperplasia (FNH) and hepatic adenoma (HAs) are encountered in similar patient populations and can share imaging features, leading to a diagnostic dilemma when nonspecific extracellular contrast agents are used. Research indicates that FNH can be diagnosed with use of the hepatobiliary-specific agents with a high

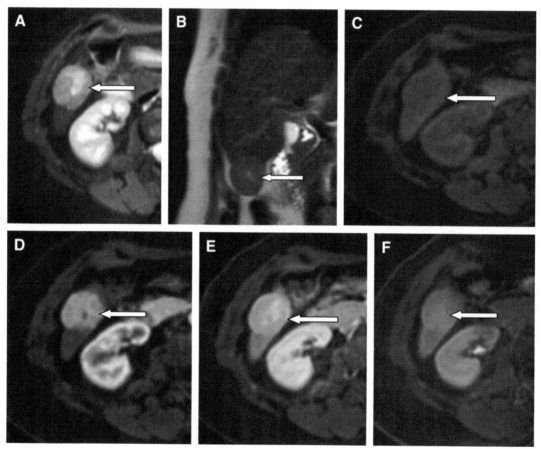

Fig. 3. A 44-year-old woman with FNH. The known FNH (*arrow*) demonstrates the typical T2 hyperintense scar (*A, B*) and classic enhancement pattern on T1 high resolution isotropic volume examination (THRIVE) precontrast (*C*), arterial phase (*D*), equilibrium phase (*E*), and hepatobiliary phase (*F*) with gadobenate dimeglumine. Notice that with gadobenate dimeglumine, the scar enhances on the hepatobiliary phase (*F*). (*A*) FNH T2 short tau inversion recovery (STIR). (*B*) FNH T2 single shot turbo spin echo (SSTSE) coronal. (*C*) THRIVE precontrast. (*D*) THRIVE arterial phase with gadobenate dimeglumine. (*E*) THRIVE equilibrium phase with gadobenate dimeglumine. (*F*) THRIVE hepatocyte phase (1 hour) with gadobenate dimeglumine.

degree of confidence,[26,29,30] allowing for conservative management. HAs, on the other hand, may require close monitoring, surgical excision, or possible transarterial embolization because of the risk of hemorrhage and malignant transformation into hepatocellular carcinoma (HCC).[31,32]

FNH is composed of functional hepatocytes and abnormal blind-ending biliary ductules, which do not communicate with the biliary tree.[33] FNH accumulates hepatobiliary-specific agents at delayed phase imaging because of slow biliary excretion and a high density of hepatocytes.[26,34] Atypical

enhancement of FNH on the hepatobiliary phase is usually related to a large central scar or fat component.[30] Usually, the central scar of FNH enhances on the hepatobiliary phase with gadobenate dimeglumine and not with gadoxetic acid (**Figs. 3** and **4**).[35]

HAs contain glycogen and lipid-rich hepatocytes arranged in sheaths separated by fibrous septae containing sinusoidal arteries but lacking bile ductules.[32] At least 4 subtypes of HAs have been characterized by cytogenetics, with the β-catenin–activated HAs being at greater risk for

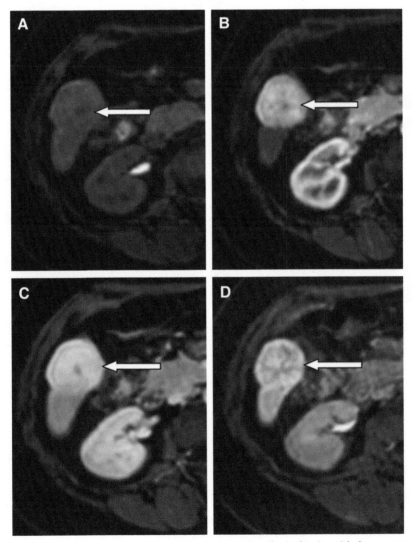

Fig. 4. A 44-year-old woman with FNH (same patient as in **Fig. 3**). Gadxetic acid demonstrates the typical enhancement pattern of an FNH (*arrow*) on the dynamic series. (*A*) Precontrast. (*B*) Arterial phase. (*C*) Equilibrium phase. (*D*) Hepatobiliary phase. However, the central scar does not enhance on the hepatobiliary phase (*D*). This difference has been reported between gadobenate dimeglumine and gadoxetic acid recently. (*A*) T1 High resolution isotropic volume examination (THRIVE) precontrast. (*B*) THRIVE arterial phase with gadoxetic acid. (*C*) T1 High resolution isotropic volume examination (THRIVE) equilibrium phase with gadoxetic acid. (*D*) THRIVE hepatobiliary phase (20 minutes) with gadoxetic acid.

malignant transformation.[36] Although HAs are composed of hepatocytes, they have decreased or absent accumulation of hepatobiliary-specific agent in the hepatocyte phase (**Figs. 5** and **6**).[20] Recent cytogenetic classification of HAs helps to explain the differences in hepatobiliary phase enhancement among HAs. The inflammatory subtype of HA usually demonstrates absence of enhancement on the hepatobiliary phase, although this is variable (**Fig. 7**). HNF1α–mutated HAs demonstrate an absence of enhancement of hepatobiliary phase, whereas β-catenin–mutated

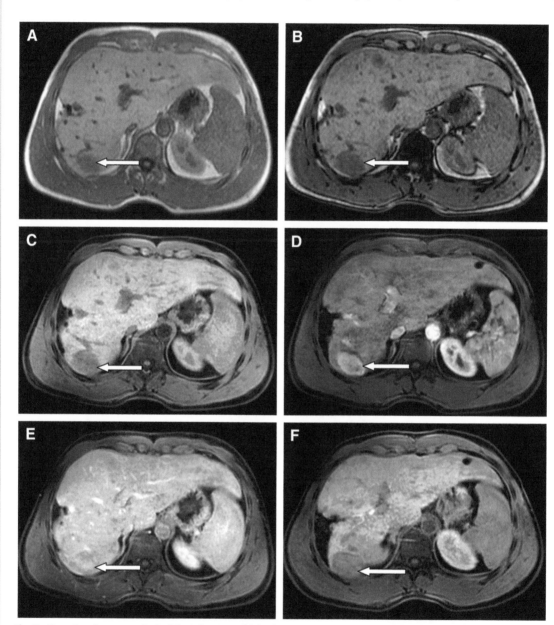

Fig. 5. Hepatic adenomatosis. In (*A*) and opposed (*B*), phase T1 gradient-echo (GRE) images demonstrate multiple liver lesions that show signal loss on the opposed phase, consistent with lesions that contain intravoxel fat. Dynamic contrast-enhanced imaging [(*C*) precontrast, (*D*) arterial phase, (*E*) equilibrium phase, (*F*) hepatobiliary phase] with gadobenate dimeglumine demonstrates that these lesions are arterially enhancing with washout that is most conspicuous on the equilibrium phase. Absence of lesion enhancement on hepatobiliary phase is consistent with multiple hepatocellular adenomas. The largest lesion is denoted with an arrow. (*A*) T1 GRE in phase. (*B*) T1 GRE opposed phase. (*C*) T1 High resolution isotropic volume examination (THRIVE) precontrast. (*D*) THRIVE arterial phase gadobenate dimeglumine. (*E*) THRIVE equilibrium gadobenate dimeglumine. (*F*) THRIVE hepatobiliary phase (1 hour) with gadobenate dimeglumine.

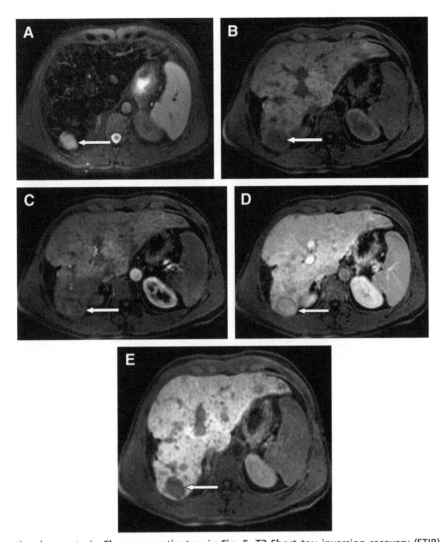

Fig. 6. Hepatic adenomatosis. The same patient as in **Fig. 5.** T2 Short tau inversion recovery (STIR) image (*A*) demonstrates that several of the known HAs are T2 hyperintense. Dynamic contrast-enhanced imaging [(*B*) precontrast, (*C*) arterial phase, (*D*) equilibrium phase, (*E*) hepatobiliary phase] with gadoxetic acid demonstrates that these lesions are less avidly enhancing on the arterial phase than with gadobenate dimeglumine, and they show lack of enhancement of washout in the equilibrium phase because of the overlap of equilibrium and early hepatospecific phase with gadoxetic acid. However, in the hepatobiliary phase, the absence of enhancement of all of the lesions is more evident than with gadobenate dimeglumine. Note that on the gadoxetic acid equilibrium phase, the HAs continue to demonstrate enhancement, whereas they heterogeneously wash out on the equilibrium phase with gadobenate dimeglumine (**Fig. 5E**). The largest lesion is denoted with an arrow. (*A*) T2 STIR. (*B*) T1 High resolution isotropic volume examination (THRIVE) precontrast. (*C*) THRIVE arterial phase gadoxetic acid. (*D*) THRIVE equilibrium phase gadoxetic acid. (*E*) THRIVE hepatobiliary phase (20 minutes) with gadoxetic acid.

HAs usually show enhancement.[37,38] Differentiation of FNH from HAs is similar when imaged with gadoxetic acid and gadobenate dimeglumine; however, gadobenate dimeglumine achieves better results with a higher sensitivity and specificity than gadoxetic acid.[29,30] In summary, all hepatobiliary-specific agents can be used to diagnose FNH with a high degree of accuracy.[29,30] Gadobenate dimeglumine and gadoxetic acid are particularly useful in distinguishing FNH from HAs

because HAs typically do not take up these agents in the hepatobiliary phase.[29,30] Occasionally, HAs can accumulate hepatobiliary-specific contrast agents on the hepatobiliary phase, leading to a potential pitfall (**Fig. 8**).

HCC

In North America, the incidence of HCC is rising.[39] Cirrhosis is the strongest predisposing factor for

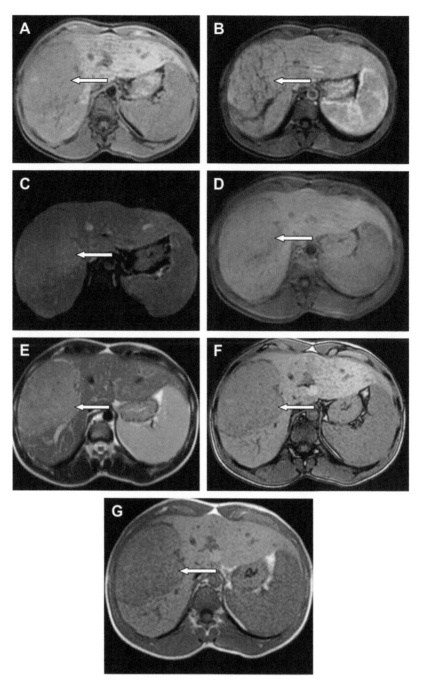

Fig. 7. Inflammatory HA (*arrow*) demonstrating classic dynamic phase enhancement [(*A*) precontrast, (*B*) arterial phase, (*C*) equilibrium phase, (*D*) hepatobiliary phase] with gadobenate dimeglumine with intense arterial enhancement (*B*) that persists on delayed phase imaging (*C, D*). Inflammatory HAs are typically hyperintense on T2-weighted imaging (*E*) and do not demonstrate signal loss on T1 gradient-echo (GRE) opposed phase (*F*) compared with T1 GRE in phase (*G*) imaging. (*A*) T1 High resolution isotropic volume examination (THRIVE) precontrast. (*B*) THRIVE arterial. (*C*) THRIVE equilibrium phase. (*D*) THRIVE hepatobiliary phase. (*E*) T2 single shot turbo spin echo (SSTSE). (*F*) T1 GRE opposed phase. (*G*) T1 GRE in phase.

HCC with common causes including hepatitis C virus, hepatitis B virus, alcohol consumption, and nonalcoholic steatohepatitis. Viral hepatitis (chronic hepatitis B and C) is the main risk factor for cirrhosis and is associated with most cases of HCC (approximately 80%).[39,40] Early detection of small HCC (<2 cm) is important because the efficacy of treatments and survival of patients with

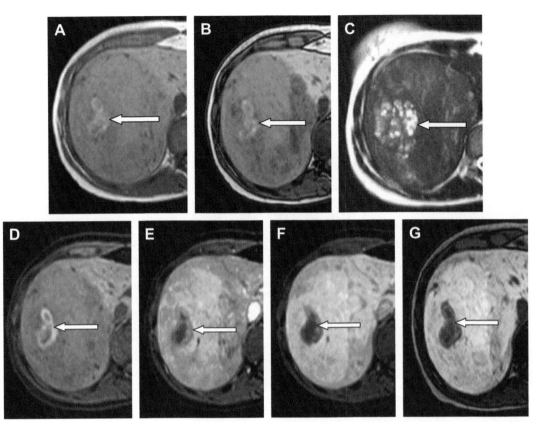

Fig. 8. HA with hepatobiliary phase enhancement – a potential pitfall. This biopsy-proved HA (*small arrows*) demonstrated heterogeneous signal loss on opposed (*A*) compared with in-phase T1 gradient-echo (GRE) imaging (*B*) and was heterogeneously hyperintense on T2-weighted imaging (*C*), likely because of the known central regions of fat (*star*) and hemorrhage (*arrowhead*). Dynamic postcontrast imaging [(*D*) precontrast, (*E*) arterial, (*F*) equilibrium, (*G*) hepatobiliary] illustrates a potential pitfall with the hepatocyte-specific agents in that occasionally HAs can enhance on the hepatobiliary phase (*G*). (*A*) Opposed phase T1 GRE. (*B*) In-phase T1 GRE. (*C*) T2 single shot turbo spin echo (SSTSE). (*D*) T1 precontrast. (*E*) T1 arterial phase. (*F*) T1 equilibrium. (*G*) T1 hepatobiliary. (*Courtesy of* Dr Enrique Ramón, Gregorio Marañón Hospital, Madrid, Spain.)

early-stage HCC, as defined by the Milan criteria, are significantly better than those of patients with advanced disease. Liver MR imaging is being increasingly used for screening high-risk individuals[40,41,42] because although the detection of HCC with ultrasound and CT is specific (pooled estimates of 97% and 93%, respectively), they are insufficiently sensitive (pooled estimates of 60% and 68%, respectively) to support an effective HCC surveillance program.[43]

Small HCCs pose a diagnostic challenge because of decreased sensitivity and increased frequency of atypical features on imaging. In addition, the inhomogeneity of cirrhotic livers as a result of fibrosis and heterogeneous enhancement complicates lesion detection and characterization.[6] Differentiating early HCC from benign regenerative or premalignant dysplastic nodules is of paramount importance because there are

implications for lesion management and patient survival (**Fig. 9**).[42]

There is limited experience using hepatobiliary-specific agents in the evaluation of HCC but interest is growing. The overall sensitivity of the hepatobiliary-specific agents for lesion detection is similar to that of the extracellular agents (**Table 5**). In addition, the rate of detection for HCC is similar for gadoxetic acid and gadobenate dimeglumine.[45]

Recent data have shown that gadoxetic acid is taken up by hepatocytes via the organic anion transporting peptide-8 (OATP8) and exits to bile through the canalicular transporter multidrug resistance–associated protein 3 (MRP3).[46] The immunohistochemical expression of OATP8 significantly decreases during multistep hepato-carcinogenesis, which may explain the decrease in enhancement ratio on gadoxetic acid–enhanced MR imaging.[47] In severe liver disease, gadobenate

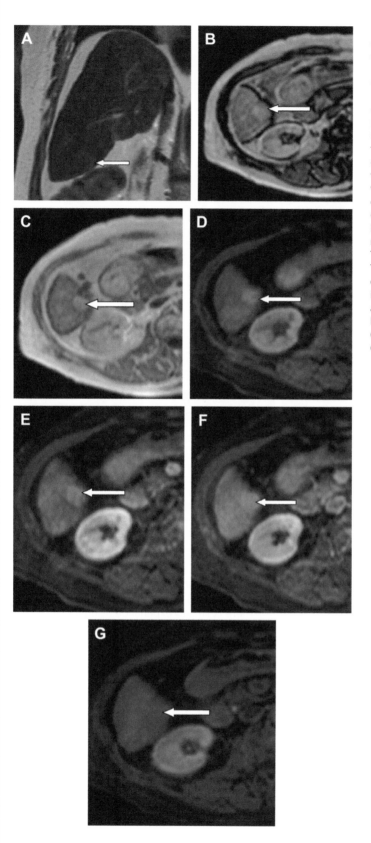

Fig. 9. Dysplastic nodule in a 68-year-old man with known cirrhosis. This segment 6 nodule (*arrow*) is slightly hyperintense on T2-weighted imaging (A) and does not demonstrate signal loss on opposed phase T1 gradient echo images (B) compared with in-phase T1 gradient-echo images (C). On precontrast T1-weighted imaging, this nodule is hyperintense (D) and enhanced on the arterial (E) and portal venous (F) phases with gadoxetic acid when subtraction images were created. On the hepatobiliary phase (G), this nodule was isointense to the liver parenchyma, favoring a dysplastic nodule or well-differentiated HCC. This nodule was stable for 1 year. (A) T2 single shot turbo spin echo (SSTSE) coronal. (B) T1 opposed phase. (C) T1 in-phase. (D) T1 precontrast. (E) T1 arterial phase Eovist. (F) T1 High resolution isotropic volume examination (THRIVE) equilibrium phase Eovist. (G) T1 THRIVE 20 minutes post Eovist.

Table 5
HCC detection sensitivities of liver MR contrast agents

Extracellular Agents	Gadobenate Dimeglumine	Gadoxetic Acid
81% (pooled estimate[43])	80%–85%[44,45]	80%[45]

dimeglumine functions as an extracellular agent because of the low level of OATPs expression. In addition, gadobenate dimeglumide remains trapped within hepatocytes in rats lacking the MRP2 canilicular transporter because it cannot reflux back to the sinusoids through other basolateral transporters such as MRP3.[47] These differences in hepatocyte transporters may explain why there are better preliminary results with gadoxetic acid than with gadobenate dimeglumine in the differentiation of dysplastic nodules from early HCC.[48]

Most HCCs are hypointense on hepatobiliary phase; however, different degrees of enhancement are possible and are related to residual hepatobiliary function. The combined interpretation of dynamic and hepatobiliary phase MR images improves the diagnostic accuracy of gadobenate dimeglumine–enhanced MR imaging for the detection of HCC compared with either dynamic MR or multiphasic multidetector CT images alone.[49] For characterizing small (1- to 2-cm) hepatic nodules in patients at high risk for HCC with gadobenate dimeglumine, improved sensitivity with a small reduction of specificity was achieved by adding lesion hyperintensity on T2-weighted images and lesion hypointensity on the hepatobiliary phase as

diagnostic criteria for HCC to nodules fitting the American Association for the Study of Liver Diseases' practice guideline (arterial phase hyperintensity and washout) (**Fig. 10**).[50]

There is overlap in the degree of enhancement during the hepatobiliary phase of dysplastic nodules and HCC, and well-differentiated and poorly differentiated HCC, with both gadobenate dimeglumine and gadoxetic acid; however, most of the hyperintense HCCs on the hepatobiliary phase are hypervascular on the arterial phase, and hyperintense dysplastic nodules on the hepatobiliary phase are isointense on the arterial phase.[51] Nodules suspicious for HCC on precontrast MR imaging that are hypointense on the hepatobiliary phase and hypovascular on the arterial phase likely represent HCC.

To summarize, although there is insufficient evidence to include the hepatobiliary phase in the MR imaging protocol for HCC, there is a trend toward an increased sensitivity in the differentiation of dysplastic nodules and early HCC, using hepatobiliary contrast agents in combination with the information of dynamic series and other ancillary MR findings, especially with gadoxetic acid, as a result of different mechanisms at the level of hepatic transporter expression in HCC.

Liver Metastases

The identification and resection of curable liver metastases improve the survival of patients with several types of cancer, most notably colorectal cancer.[52] Dynamic contrast-enhanced liver MR imaging with the nonspecific extracellular agents is as or more sensitive as fluorine 18 fluorodeoxyglucose positron emission tomography (PET) and

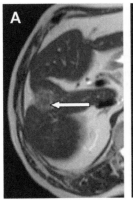 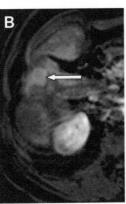 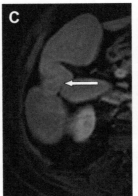 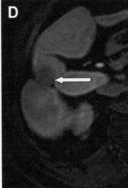

Fig. 10. A 63-year-old man with cirrhosis secondary to hemochromatosis and HCC. Axial T2-weighted (A) image demonstrates a hyperintense lesion in segment 6 that demonstrates arterial enhancement (B) with heterogeneous washout on equilibrium phase imaging (C) with gadoxetic acid (denoted by arrows). Note the lack of enhancement of this HCC on the hepatobiliary phase (D) (arrow). (A) T2 single shot turbo spin echo (SSTSE). (B) Arterial phase. (C) Equilibrium phase. (D) Hepatobiliary phase.

contrast-enhanced CT, respectively, in delineating colorectal liver metastases and more specific than both at liver lesion characterization.[53,54] Liver MR imaging performed with hepatobiliary-specific agents depicts more colorectal liver metastases with improved diagnostic confidence compared with the nonspecific extracellular agents, because metastases, which can have variable enhancement on the dynamic phases, typically appear hypointense on delayed phase imaging given their nonhepatocellular nature[15] (Figs. 11 and 12). The hepatobiliary-specific agents, such as gadoxetic acid, are more accurate than contrast-enhanced PET-CT, especially for the detection of small (<1-cm) lesions.[55] Atypical patterns of enhancement on hepatobiliary phase have been reported, such as ringlike peripheral enhancement. Rarely, diffuse enhancement of metastases in ischemic regions of the liver is also possible.

Cholangiocarcinoma

Differentiation of cirrhous HCC and cholangiocarcinoma is significantly improved using hepatospecific phase compared with dynamic enhancement pattern and unenhanced MR features.[56] Intrahepatic cholangiocarcinoma usually shows a

target-like enhancement because of the absence of hepatocytes. Central enhancement of cholangiocarcinomas in the hepatospecific phase has been described, related not to true enhancement, but due to contrast pooling in the fibrous areas (Fig. 13).

Biliary Tree Imaging with Hepatobiliary-Specific Contrast Agents

Contrast-enhanced T1-weighted MR cholangiography is possible with all of the hepatobiliary-specific agents because they are all excreted into the biliary tree to varying degrees, causing T1 shortening of bile. Contrast-enhanced MR cholangiography has the potential to be a powerful adjunctive or even primary tool in the evaluation of the biliary tree in patients with normal liver function. However, as noted previously, hepatobiliary-specific contrast agents are not approved for evaluation of the biliary tree by the FDA.

Troubleshooting Abnormalities on T2-Weighted MR Cholangiography

One important role that contrast-enhanced MR cholangiography can play is that of a problem-solving modality for T2-weighted MR cholangiography when the distinction between a filling defect

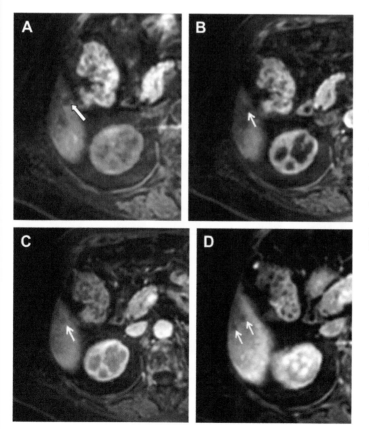

Fig. 11. Breast cancer liver metastases. Delayed phase with gadoxetic acid demonstrates more hepatic metastases (arrows) than on the dynamic series [(A) precontrast, (B) arterial phase, (C) portal venous phase, (E) hepatobiliary phase]. For example, in segment 5, only 1 hepatic metastasis was visible on the arterial (B) and portal venous (C) phases, whereas the hepatobiliary phase demonstrates 2 hepatic metastases (D). (A) T1 High resolution isotropic volume examination (THRIVE) precontrast. (B) THRIVE arterial phase Eovist. (C) THRIVE portal venous phase Eovist. (D) THRIVE 20 minutes post Eovist.

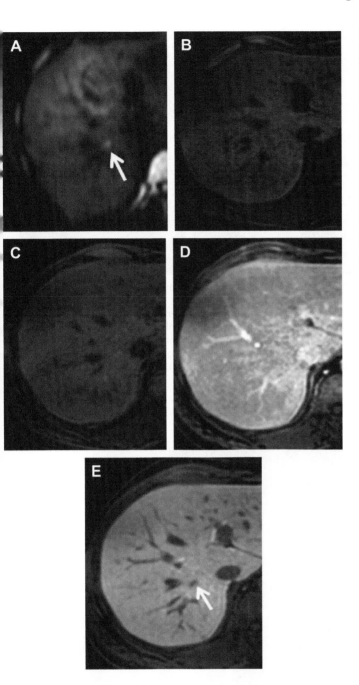

Fig. 12. A 45-year-old man with chronic myelogenous lymphoma (CLL) involving the liver. Several nodular lesions were detected and best depicted on diffusion-weighted images (DWI b = 1000, *A*, *arrow*). The largest of these is marked with an arrow. These lesions were isointense to the liver parenchyma on T1-weighted, T2-weighted, and all of the phases of the dynamic postcontrast series [(*B*) precontrast, (*C*) arterial phase, (*D*) equilibrium phase] with the exception of the hepatobiliary phase (*arrow*, *E*). (*A*) B1000. (*B*) T1 High resolution isotrpic volume examination (THRIVE) precontrast. (*C*) THRIVE arterial phase. (*D*) THRIVE portal phase. (*E*) THRIVE 20 minutes post gadoxetic acid.

within the biliary tree such as choledocholithiasis or tumor and flow artifact can be difficult.[57] If a flow artifact is confirmed, the patient may be spared endoscopic retrograde cholangiopancreatography.

Biliary Tree Anatomy

Assessment of the biliary tree for anatomic variant is of paramount importance preoperatively

because a detailed understanding of bile ducts can prevent surgical complications such as unintended bile ligation or transsection. Contrast-enhanced MRCP using 3D gradient echo can offer better assessment with higher-resolution images and reconstructions compared with T2-weighted MRCP, which uses T2-weighted fast spin echo sequences. Because the 3D gradient echo contrast-enhanced MRCP sequence is acquired

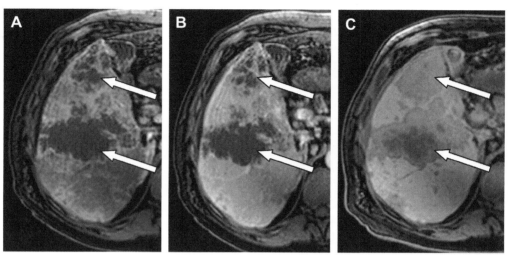

Fig. 13. An 81-year-old man with recurrent intrahepatic cholangiocarcinoma. There is progressive peripheral enhancement of the nodules on dynamic postcontrast imaging [(A) arterial, (B) equilibrium, (C) hepatobiliary]. On the hepatobiliary phase with gadobenate dimeglumine (C), there is enhancement of all of the nodules (arrows); peripheral enhancement in the largest nodule and homogeneous enhancement in the remainder. These regions of delayed enhancement represent contrast pooling in the fibrous components of these tumors, as cholangiocarcinomas lack hepatocytes. (A) Arterial phase with gadobenate dimeglumine. (B) Equilibrium phase with gadobenate dimeglumine. (C) Hepatobiliary phase with gadobenate dimeglumine.

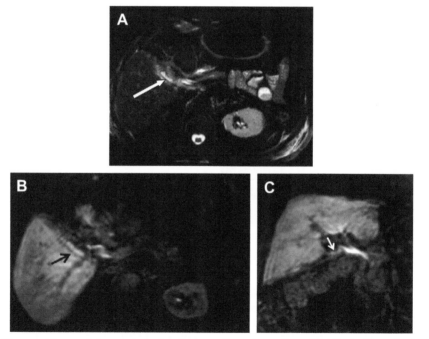

Fig. 14. An 80-year-old man status post cholecystectomy 2 weeks earlier with bile leaking via the subhepatic percutaneous drain. T2-weighted imaging demonstrates a small collection in operative bed (A) that shows delayed enhancement with gadoxetic acid on T1-weighted imaging (B), consistent with a biliary leak. The point of bile leak was detected at proximal cystic duct on T1 coronal contrast-enhanced MR cholangiography (C). (A) Single-shot spectral selection attenuated inversion recovery (SPAIR). (B) Axial gadoxetic acid. (C) Coronal gadoxetic acid.

in a shorter amount of time than the T2-weighted MRCP, there is potential for improved breath-hold compliance on the part of the patient.[6]

Dynamic Assessment of the Biliary Tree

Hepatobiliary scintigraphy is widely used for its functional assessment of the biliary tree[58]; however, it lacks the spatial resolution or anatomic detail provided by CT and MR imaging. The introduction of the hepatobiliary-specific agents and contrast-enhanced MRCP adds a new dimension to biliary tree evaluation because they combine both anatomic and functional biliary assessment in patients with normal liver function as off-label indications.[59] Potential future applications include acute and chronic cholecystitis,[60,61] distinction between biliary and extrabiliary lesions including choledocholithiasis, biliary leak (**Fig. 14**) and stricture delineation (**Fig. 15**), sphincter of Oddi dysfunction, and biliary enteric anastomoses.[62,63]

Postoperative and Traumatic Biliary Tree Injuries

At the time of surgery or trauma, the biliary tree can sustain injuries that are difficult to detect on CT or

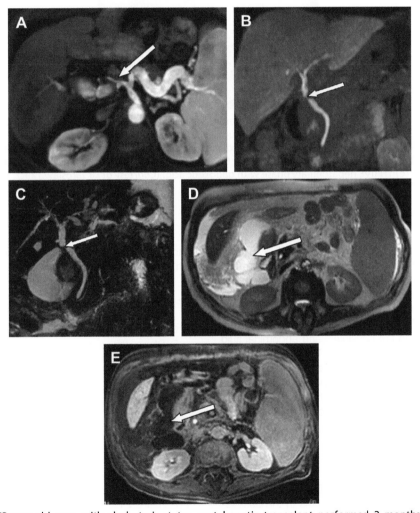

Fig. 15. A 53-year-old man with cholestasis status post hepatic transplant performed 3 months earlier. MR imaging is performed to assess the hepatic artery and biliary anastomosis. The hepatic artery was thinned, but patent as demonstrated in axial maximum intensity projection (MIP) of arterial phase (*A*). MR cholangiography and functional cholangiography with gadoxetic acid show stenosis of biliary anastomosis (*B, C*) and absence of biliary leak. A postsurgical collection of nonbiliary origin was identified (*D*), as it did not show delayed enhancement with gadoxetic acid (*E*). Of note, the MIP images (*B, C*) demonstrate common bile duct stenosis and not an artifact from the hepatic artery (images not shown). (*A*) "Hepatic artery." (*B*) MIP gadoxetic acid excretory phase. (*C*) MIP 3D gadoxetic acid cholangiography. (*D*) Axial T2 single shot turbo spin echo (SSTSE). (*E*) Axial collection post gadoxetic acid.

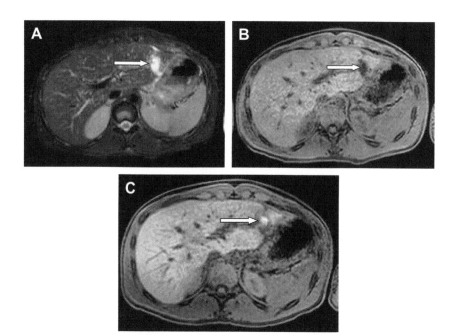

Fig. 16. A 30-year-old man with a grade II liver laceration status post motor vehicle accident. Axial T2-weighted image demonstrates a grade II liver laceration through segments 2/3 (*A*). Precontrast (*B*) and hepatobiliary phase (*C*) images demonstrate gadoxetic acid contrast extravasation from the liver laceration, consistent with a bile leak. (*A*) Axial T2 spectral inversion recovery (SPIR). (*B*) Precontrast T1 high resolution isotropic volume examination (THRIVE). (*C*) THRIVE hepatobiliary phase with gadoxetic acid. (*Courtesy of* Dr Jaroslaw Tkacz, Boston University Medical Center, Boston, MA.)

extracellular agent contrast-enhanced liver MR imaging such as in the setting of liver laceration (**Fig. 16**). The presence of bile leaks or bile duct ligations warrants rapid diagnosis and treatment because they portend a higher morbidity and mortality. On T2-weighted MRCP, identification of the site of biliary leakage is often not possible[64] and abdominal fluid collections further obscure T2-weighted biliary imaging findings.[6] Biliary strictures are also important to recognize and consider for possible intervention. The combination of functional and anatomic evaluation provided by contrast-enhanced MRCP optimizes identification of these entities.

SUMMARY

Extracellular and hepatobiliary-specific MR contrast agents are powerful tools in the assessment of liver lesions. In particular, the hepatocyte-specific agents provide unique opportunities to improve the detection and characterization of liver lesions not afforded by other modalities such as contrast-enhanced CT or contrast-enhanced PET/CT. Potential future applications of the hepatobiliary-specific agents lie in their ability to generate contrast-enhanced MRCP

examinations, combining functional information with exquisite anatomic detail.

REFERENCES

1. Carr DH, Graif M, Niendorf HP, et al. Gadolinium-DTPA in the assessment of liver tumours by magnetic resonance imaging. Clin Radiol 1986;37: 347–53.
2. Hamm B, Wolf KJ, Felix R. Conventional and rapid MR imaging of the liver with Gd-DTPA. Radiology 1987;2:313–20.
3. Edelman RR, Siegel JB, Singer A, et al. Dynamic MR imaging of the liver with Gd-DTPA: initial clinical results. AJR Am J Roentgenol 1989;153:1213–9.
4. Semelka RC, Helmberger TK. Contrast agents for MR imaging of the liver. Radiology 2001;218:27–38.
5. Gandhi SN, Brown MA, Wong JG, et al. MR contrast agents for liver imaging: what, when, how. Radiographics 2006;26:1621–36.
6. Seale MK, Catalano OA, Saini S, et al. Hepatobiliary-specific MR contrast agents: role in imaging the liver and biliary tree. Radiographics 2009;29: 1725–48.
7. Wood ML, Hardy PA. Proton relaxation enhancement. J Magn Reson Imaging 1993;3:149–56.

8. Balci NC, Semelka RC. Contrast agents for MR imaging of the liver. Radiol Clin North Am 2005;43: 887–98.

9. Weinmann HJ, Brasch RC, Press WR, et al. Characteristics of gadolinium-DTPA complex: a potential NMR contrast agent. AJR Am J Roentgenol 1984; 142:619–24.

10. Shellock FG, Kanal E. Safety of magnetic resonance imaging contrast agents. J Magn Reson Imaging 1999;10:477–84.

11. Niendorf HP, Alhassan A, Geens VR, et al. Safety review of gadopentetate dimeglumine: experience after more than five million applications. Invest Radiol 1994;29(Suppl 2):S179–82.

12. Wang Y, Alkasab TK, Narin O, et al. Incidence of nephrogenic systemic fibrosis after adoption of restrictive gadolinium-based contrast agent guidelines. Radiology 2011;260(1):105–11.

13. Wang PI, Chong ST, Kielar AZ, et al. Imaging of pregnant and lactating patients: part 1, evidence-based review and recommendations. AJR Am J Roentgenol 2012;198:778–84.

14. American College of Radiology (ACR) Website. ACR manual on contrast media, version 7. 2010. Available at: http://www.acr.org/Quality-Safety/Resources/Contrast-Manual. Accessed May 28, 2012.

15. Reimer P, Schneider G, Schima W. Hepatobiliary contrast agents for contrast-enhanced MRI of the liver: properties, clinical development and applications. Eur Radiol 2004;14:559–78.

16. Hussain HK, Londy FJ, Francis IR, et al. Hepatic arterial phase MR imaging with automated bolus-detection three-dimensional fast gradient-recalled-echo sequence: comparison with test-bolus method. Radiology 2003;226:558–66.

17. Bellini MF, Vasile M, Morel-Precetti S. Currently used non-specific extracellular MR contrast media. Eur Radiol 2003;13:2688–98.

18. Rofsky NM, Earls JP. Magnafodipir trisodium injection (Mn-DPDP): a contrast agent for abdominal MR imaging. Magn Reson Imaging Clin N Am 1996;4:73–85.

19. Schneider G, Maas R, Schultze Kool L, et al. Low-dose gadobenate dimeglumine versus standard dose gadopentetate dimeglumine for contrast-enhanced magnetic resonance imaging of the liver: an individual crossover comparison. Invest Radiol 2003;38:85–94.

20. Purysko AS, Remer EM, Veniero JC. Focal liver lesion detection and characterization with Gd-EOB-DTPA. Clin Radiol 2011;66(7):673–84.

21. Tamada T, Ito K, Yamamoto A, et al. Hepatic hemangiomas: evaluation of enhancement patterns at dynamic MRI with gadoxetate disodium. AJR Am J Roentgenol 2011;196(4):824–30.

22. Doo KW, Lee CH, Choi JW, et al. "Pseudo washout"-sign in high-flow hepatic hemangioma on gadoxetic acid contrast-enhanced MRI mimicking hypervascular tumor. AJR Am J Roentgenol 2009;193(6): W490–6.

23. Sadowski EA, Bennett LK, Chan MR, et al. Nephrogenic systemic fibrosis: risk factores and incidence estimation. Radiology 2007;243(1):148–57.

24. Tschirch FT, Struwe A, Petrowsky H, et al. Contrast-enhanced MR cholangiography with Gd-EOB-DTPA in patients with liver cirrhosis: visualization of the biliary ducts in comparison with patients with normal liver parenchyma. Eur Radiol 2008;18:1577–86.

25. Kanki A, Tamada T, Higaki A, et al. Hepatic parenchymal enhancement at Gd-EOB-DTPA-enhanced MR imaging: correlation with morphological grading of severity in cirrhosis and chronic hepatitis. Magn Reson Imaging 2012;30:356–60.

26. Huppertz A, Balzer T, Blakeborough A. Improved detection of focal liver lesions at MR imaging: multicenter comparison of gadoxetic acid-enhanced MR images with intraoperative findings. Radiology 2004; 230:226–75.

27. Morana G, Grazioli L, Kirchin MA, et al. Solid hypervascular liver lesions: accurate identification of true benign lesions on enhanced dynamic and hepatobiliary phase magnetic resonance imaging after gadobenate dimeglumine administration. Invest Radiol 2011;46(4):225–39.

28. Fu GL, Zee CS, Yang HF, et al. Gadobenate dimeglumine-enhanced liver magnetic resonance imaging: value of hepatobiliary phase for the detection of focal liver lesions. J Comput Assist Tomogr 2012;36(1):14–9.

29. Grazioli L, Morana G, Kirchin MA, et al. Accurate differentiation of focal nodular hyperplasia from hepatic adenoma at gadobenate dimeglumine-enhanced MR imaging: prospective study. Radiology 2005;236:166–77.

30. Grazioli L, Bondioni MP, Haradome H, et al. Hepatocellular adenoma and focal nodular hyperplasia: value of gadoxetic acid-enhanced MR imaging in differential diagnosis. Radiology 2012; 262:520–9.

31. Huurman VA, Schaapherder AF. Management of ruptured hepatocellular adenoma. Dig Surg 2010; 27:56–60.

32. Bunchorntavakul C, Bahirwani R, Drazek D, et al. Clinial features and natural history of hepatocellular adenomas: the impact of obesity. Aliment Pharmacol Ther 2011;34(6):664–74.

33. Marin D, Brancatelli G, Federle MP, et al. Focal nodular hyperplasia: typical and atypical MRI findings with emphasis on the use of contrast media. Clin Radiol 2008;63:577–85.

34. Grazioli L, Morana G, Federle MP, et al. Focal nodular hyperplasia: morphologic and functional information from MR imaging with gadobenate dimeglumine. Radiology 2001;221:731–9.

35. Karam AR, Shankar S, Surapaneni P, et al. Focal nodular hyperplasia: central scar enhancement pattern using gadoxetate disodium. J Magn Reson Imaging 2010;32(2):341–4.

36. Bioulac-Sage P, Balabaud C, Zucman-Rossi J. Subtype classification of hepatocellular adenoma. Dig Surg 2010;27:39–45.

37. Katabathina VS, Menias CO, Shanbhogue AK, et al. Genetics and imaging of hepatocellular adenomas: 2011 update. Radiographics 2011;31(6):1529–43.

38. Shanbhogue AK, Prasad SR, Takahashi N, et al. Recent advances in cytogenetics and molecular biology of adult hepatocellular tumors: implications for imaging and management. Radiology 2011; 258(3):673–93.

39. El-Serag HB. Epidemiology of viral hepatitis and hepatocellular carcinoma. Gastroenterology 2012; 142(6):1264–73.

40. Lee JM, Choi BI. Hepatocellular nodules in liver cirrhosis: MR evaluation. Abdom Imaging 2011; 36(3):282–9.

41. Willatt JM, Hussain HK, Adusumilli S, et al. MR imaging of hepatocellular carcinoma in the cirrhotic liver: challenges and controversies. Radiology 2008;247:311–30.

42. Chanyputhipong J, Low SC, Chow PK. Gadoxetate acid-enhanced MR imaging for HCC: a review for clinicians. Int J Hepatol 2011;2011:489342.

43. Colli A, Fraquelli M, Casazza G, et al. Accuracy of ultrasonography, spiral CT magnetic resonance and alpha-fetoprotein in diagnosing hepatocellular carcinoma: a systematic review. Am J Gastroenterol 2006;101:513–23.

44. Choi SH, Lee JM, Yu NC, et al. Hepatocellular carcinoma in liver transplantation candidates: detection with gadobenate dimeglumine-enhanced MRI. AJR Am J Roentgenol 2008;191(2):529–36.

45. Park Y, Kim SH, Kim SH, et al. Gadoxetic acid (Gd-EOB-DTPA)-enhanced MRI versus gadobenate dimeglumine (Gd-BOPTA)-enhanced MRI for preoperatively detecting hepatocellular carcinoma: an initial experience. Korean J Radiol 2010;11(4): 433–40.

46. Kitao A, Matsui O, Yoneda N, et al. The uptake transporter OATP8 expression decreases during multistep hepatocarcinogenesis: correlation with gadoxetic acid enhanced MR imaging. Eur Radiol 2011; 21(10):2056–66.

47. Pastor CM. Gadoxetic acid-enhanced hepatobiliary phase MR imaging: cellular insight. Radiology 2010;257(2):589.

48. Sano K, Ichikawa T, Motosugi U, et al. Imaging study of early hepatocellular carcinoma: usefulness of gadoxetic acid-enhanced MR imaging. Radiology 2011;261(3):834–44.

49. Marin D, Di Martino M, Guerrisi A, et al. Hepatocellular carcinoma in patients with cirrhosis: qualitative comparison of gadobenate dimeglumine-enhanced MR imaging and multiphasic 64-section CT. Radiology 2009;251(1):85–95.

50. Kim TK, Lee KH, Jang HJ, et al. Analysis of gadobenate dimeglumine-enhanced MR findings for characterizing small (1-2-cm) hepatic nodules in patients at high risk for hepatocellular carcinoma. Radiology 2011;259(3):730–8.

51. Goodwin MD, Dobson JE, Sirlin CB, et al. Diagnostic challenges and pitfalls in MR imaging with hepatocyte-specific contrast agents. Radiographics 2011;31(6):1547–68.

52. Vigano L, Ferrero A, Lo Tesoriere R, et al. Liver surgery for colorectal mestastases: results after 10 years of follow-up. Long-term sruvivors, late recurrences, and prognostic role of morbidity. Ann Surg Oncol 2008;15(9):2458–64.

53. Cantwell CP, Setty BN, Holalkere N, et al. Liver lesion detection and characterization in patients with colorectal cancer: a comparison of low radiation dose non-enhanced PET/CT, contrast-enhanced PET/CT, and liver MRI. J Comput Assist Tomogr 2008;32(5): 738–44.

54. Niekel MC, Bipat S, Stoker J. Diagnostic imaging of colorectal liver metastases with CT, MR imaging, FDG PET, and/or FDG PET/CT: a meta-analysis of prospective studies including patients who have not previously undergone treatment. Radiology 2010;257(3):674–84.

55. Seo HJ, Kim MJ, Lee JD, et al. Gadoxetate disodium-enhanced magnetic resonance imaging versus contrast-enhanced 18F-fluorodeoxyglucose positron emission tomography/computed tomography for the detection of colorectal liver metastases. Invest Radiol 2011;46(9):548–55.

56. Jeon TY, Kim SH, Lee WJ, et al. The value of gadobenate dimeglumine-enhanced hepatobiliary-phase MR imaging for the differentiation of scirrhous hepatocellular carcinoma and cholangiocarcinoma with or without hepatocellular carcinoma. Abdom Imaging 2010;35(3):337–45.

57. Irie H, Honda H, Kuroiwa T, et al. Pitfalls in MR cholangiopancreatographic interpretation. Radiographics 2001;21(1):23–37.

58. Ziessman HA. Nuclear medicine hepatobiliary imaging. Clin Gastroenterol Hepatol 2010;8(2):111–6.

59. Gupta RT, Brady CM, Lotz J, et al. Dynamic MR imaging of the biliary system using hepatocyte-specific contrast agents. AJR Am J Roentgenol 2010;195: 405–13.

60. Akpinar E, Turkbey B, Karcaaltincaba M, et al. Initial experience on utility of Gadobenate dimeglumine (Gd-BOPTA) enhanced T1-weighted MR cholangiography in diagnosis of acute cholecystitis. J Magn Reson Imaging 2009;30:578–85.

61. Krishnan P, Gupta RT, Boll DT, et al. Functional evaluation of cystic duct patency with Gd-EOB-DTPA MR imaging: an alternative to hepatobiliary

scintigraphy for diagnosis of acute cholecystitis? Abdom Imaging 2012;37:457–64.

62. Lee NK, Kim S, Lee JW, et al. Biliary MR imaging with Gd-EOB-DTPA and its clinical applications. Radiographics 2009;29:1707–24.

63. Marin D, Bova V, Agnello F, et al. Gadoxetate disodium-enhanced magnetic resonance cholangiography for the noninvasive detection of an active bile leak after laparoscopic cholecystectomy. J Comput Assist Tomogr 2010;34:213–6.

64. Hoeffel C, Azizi L, Lewin M. Normal and pathologic features of the postoperative biliary tract at 3D MR cholangiopancreatography and MR imaging. Radiographics 2006;26:1603–20.

Contrast-Enhanced Cardiac Magnetic Resonance Imaging

Carlos S. Restrepo, MD[a],*, Sina Tavakoli, MD[a],
Alejandro Marmol-Velez, MD[b]

KEYWORDS

- Cardiac magnetic resonance imaging • Contrast-enhanced magnetic resonance imaging
- Delayed myocardial enhancement • Myocardial perfusion imaging • Coronary MR angiography
- Myocardial viability

KEY POINTS

- Clinical assessment of myocardial perfusion remains critical in determining the diagnosis, management, and prognosis of patients with suspected or known coronary artery disease (CAD).
- Multiparametric cardiac magnetic resonance (CMR) (stress perfusion, rest perfusion, and late gadolinium enhancement) has better sensitivity and negative predictive value (NPV) than single-photon emission CT (SPECT) for the diagnosis of CAD.
- Current guidelines and appropriate use criteria indicate that coronary artery magnetic resonance (MR) angiography is useful for identifying coronary artery anomalies, in particular in younger individuals, without exposure to ionizing radiation or iodinated contrast medium.
- Delayed enhancement CMR, one of the most common examinations for tissue characterization both in ischemic and nonischemic myocardial diseases, has become the gold standard for visualization and quantification of infarcted myocardium and scar tissues as well as for the detection of infiltrative diseases of the heart.

INTRODUCTION

Despite a significant decline in the death rate attributable to cardiovascular diseases in recent years, they are still responsible for 1 in every 3 deaths (32.8%) in the United States. More than 2200 Americans die each day from cardiovascular diseases (1 every 39 seconds). CAD causes 1 of every 6 deaths, with more than 400,000 deaths annually. An estimate of 785,000 Americans have a new coronary artery attack and 470,000 have a recurrent coronary artery attack each year. Additionally, approximately 195,000 silent first myocardial infarctions (MIs) occur annually. All this together means a coronary event every 25 seconds with a death rate of 1 every minute.[1]

MYOCARDIAL PERFUSION IMAGING

Clinical assessment of myocardial perfusion remains critical in determining the diagnosis, management, and prognosis of patients with suspected or known CAD. Even though catheter angiography and cardiac-gated CT angiography are excellent modalities to demonstrate the patency of coronary arteries, they tell little about the downstream microvascular flow within the myocardium. Myocardial ischemia is detected in fewer than half of patients with obstructive CAD; and 10% of patients with normal angiogram and low to intermediate probability of CAD have abnormal myocardial perfusion.[2] Because perfusion abnormalities proceed systolic dysfunction, there is no surprise

[a] Department of Radiology, The University of Texas Health Science Center at San Antonio, 7703 Floyd Curl Drive, San Antonio, TX 78229, USA; [b] Division of Cardiology, Department of Medicine, The University of Texas Health Science Center at San Antonio, 7703 Floyd Curl Drive, San Antonio, TX 78229, USA
* Corresponding author.
E-mail address: crestr@gmail.com

Magn Reson Imaging Clin N Am 20 (2012) 739–760
http://dx.doi.org/10.1016/j.mric.2012.07.005
1064-9689/12/$ – see front matter © 2012 Elsevier Inc. All rights reserved.

that direct perfusion imaging has higher sensitivity than indirect imaging (eg, wall motion dysfunction) for detection of ischemia, a concept described as "ischemic cascade" (**Fig. 1**).[3]

Stress Echocardiography and Perfusion Scintigraphy

Stress echocardiography can evaluate myocardial perfusion by detecting wall motion abnormalities in response to physical (exercise) or pharmacologic (mainly dobutamine or dipyridamole) stress. The sensitivity and specificity of exercise echocardiography range from 74% to 97% and 64% to 86%, respectively. For dobutamine stress echocardiogram, the sensitivity and specificity are 61% to 95% and 51% to 95%. Dipyridamole stress echocardiogram has sensitivity and specificity in the range of 61% to 81% and 90% to 94%, respectively.[4] Like perfusion scintigraphy, the diagnostic performance of stress echocardiography is decreased in multivessel disease. Although stress echocardiography is a versatile tool that does not involve radiation exposure, interpretation is mainly qualitative and based on the visual assessment of wall motion (thickening). Diagnostic performance is operator dependent with moderate interobserver agreement of 73% and κ value of 0.37.[4,5] Additionally, finding of an appropriate acoustic window can be challenging in some cases. Sympathomimetic effect of dobutamine may induce hypotension, headache, anxiety, and arrhythmias. Contraindications of dobutamine administration include several conditions that are common in patients with cardiovascular disease (eg, severe arterial hypertension, unstable angina, significant aortic stenosis, complex cardiac arrhythmias, hypertrophic obstructive cardiomyopathy, myocarditis, uncontrolled heart failure, and history of hypersensitivity

to the medication). Dobutamine stress CMR has also been extensively used for detection of inducible ischemia with good sensitivity (79%–96%) and specificity (70%–90%); but many of the limitations (discussed previously) for stress echocardiography (eg, subjective visual assessment and contraindication to the use of dobutamine) also apply to this technique. This imaging modality is also limited in patients with moderate to severe reduction in ejection fraction and in those with left ventricular hypertrophy.[6] More recently, real-time contrast echocardiography using encapsulated microbubbles has been introduced for evaluation of myocardial perfusion. Limitations include low spatial resolution with inadequate endocardial border definition, limited acoustic windows, and concerns related to potential mechanical obstruction of the coronary vasculature by microbubbles. Contraindications to the use of microbubbles include intra-arterial injection, intracardiac shunt, unstable heart failure, acute MI or coronary syndrome, ventricular arrhythmias, respiratory failure, pulmonary hypertension and hypersensitivity to perflutren, blood products, or albumin.[7]

Nuclear cardiac imaging with SPECT using ^{201}Tl-labeled or ^{99m}Tc-labeled agents is probably the most widely used noninvasive imaging technique for evaluation of myocardial perfusion. Cardiac nuclear imaging, however, exposes patients to a significant dose of ionizing radiation and has important limitations, including poor spatial resolution, inability to perform quantitative measurements, and susceptibility to attenuation artifacts. In addition, the acquisition time for stress-induced myocardial ischemia is lengthy, and it usually requires the stress and rest portions of the study to be performed in separate sessions. More recently, positron emission tomography (PET) with different tracers (ammonia N 13, water O 15, or rubidium chloride Rb 82) has proved useful for the quantitative measurement of myocardial blood flow and coronary flow reserve.[8] PET also has significant shortcomings, however: it is not widely available, it is expensive, and, because of the short half-life of the radiotracers used for perfusion imaging (ammonia N 13, 9.8 minutes; water O 15, 2.4 minutes; and rubidium chloride Rb 82, 78 seconds), it requires a cyclotron on site.[8]

The NPV of exercise myocardial perfusion scintigraphy or echocardiography is high. Several different meta-analysis, including many studies with thousands of patients, have demonstrated the value, cost-effectiveness, and safety of myocardial perfusion scintigraphy and stress echocardiography for the diagnosis of CAD. A meta-analysis that included 17 nuclear medicine perfusion studies (8008 patients) and 4 exercise

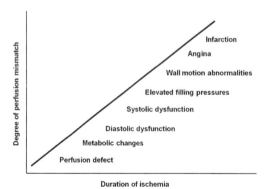

Fig. 1. The ischemic cascade refers to the temporal sequence of events that develop over time when there is a progressive imbalance between myocardial oxygen demand and supply with abnormal myocardial perfusion being the first detectable event.

echocardiography studies (3021 patients) reported greater than 98% NPV for MI and cardiac death over a 36-month follow up.[9] In a different meta-analysis, the pooled annualized event rate for cardiac death and MI are substantially (5-fold) higher in patients with abnormal stress perfusion imaging.[10] A more recent meta-analysis in hypertensive patients found sensitivity of 90% and 77% and specificity of 63% and 89% for myocardial perfusion scintigraphy and stress echocardiography, respectively, in this population at risk for CAD.[11]

Magnetic Resonance Myocardial Perfusion Imaging

CMR imaging is a multiparametric study, given its ability to assess multiple aspects of cardiovascular pathology in a single examination, including myocardial and coronary artery anatomy, ventricular function, myocardial perfusion, and viability. First-pass contrast-enhanced MR imaging has emerged as an excellent alternative imaging modality for the assessment of myocardial perfusion. The higher contrast and spatial/temporal resolution of CMR imaging compared with other techniques not only allow a more accurate detection of ischemia and CAD but also provide detailed anatomic and functional information.

CMR has evolved significantly in the past decade and has finally established its place in the menu of imaging technologies available in the evaluation of CAD. In the European Cardiovascular Magnetic Resonance Registry pilot study, conducted in 20 German centers, in which a total of 11,400 patients were included, 88% of patients received a gadolinium-based contrast and 21% underwent adenosine stress perfusion. Image quality was considered good (90%) or moderate (8%) in the vast majority of studies performed. Severe complications were rare (0.05%), with no death during CMR examinations. In two-thirds of patients, the findings of CMR imaging had an impact on clinical management; the final diagnosis was entirely different in 16% of cases, which resulted in a complete change in management. And finally, in more than 86% of cases, CMR alone satisfied all imaging needs for patient care, so that no additional imaging was required.[12] The American College of Cardiology, American College of Radiology, American Heart Association, North American Society for Cardiovascular Imaging, and Society for Cardiovascular Magnetic Resonance Imaging Expert Consensus Document on Cardiovascular Magnetic Resonance indicates that the use of CMR stress testing (vasodilator or dobutamine) is appropriate in individuals with intermediate pretest probability of CAD, patients with an uninterpretable EEG, or those unable to exercise. CMR stress testing is also appropriate for cardiac risk assessment in patients with prior coronary angiography or stenosis of unclear clinical significance.[13]

Clinical Validation of MR Perfusion Imaging

Many single-center studies have demonstrated excellent performance of CMR for the detection of CAD compared with other imaging modalities.[14–19] The few multicenter studies that have been performed, which probably better reflect the real world than specialized single-center studies, have similarly demonstrated the superiority of CMR over other imaging techniques.[20–22] In a large prospective trial, including 752 patients, in which CMR and SPECT were compared with x-ray coronary angiography as the reference standard, multiparametric CMR (stress perfusion, rest perfusion, and late gadolinium enhancement) had better sensitivity than SPECT (86.5% vs 66.5%) and NPV (90.5% vs 79.1%) for diagnosis of CAD. When considered alone, the stress perfusion part of the examination also out-performed SPECT both in the single-vessel and the multivessel disease groups.[23] Stress myocardial perfusion MR also helps with risk stratification of patients with known coronary artery stenosis of intermediate angiographic severity and may help identification of patients at risk of major adverse cardiovascular event (ie, death, stroke, and MI). Patients with coronary lesions of intermediate severity (50%–75% diameter stenosis) with myocardial perfusion defect have significantly higher incidence of adverse outcome (4%–20%) than those with equivalent coronary artery stenosis without perfusion abnormality.[24,25] In addition, a normal stress test is associated with low event rate. In a series of 513 patients with known or suspected CAD, those with normal CMR stress test (adenosine stress perfusion and dobutamine stress wall motion) had a 3-year event-free survival rate greater than 99%.[26]

Two different recent meta-analyses have reported CMR perfusion imaging to have sensitivity of 89% to 91% and specificity of 80% to 81% for the detection of CAD.[27,28] The exact role of myocardial perfusion MR imaging in patients with acute chest pain and acute coronary syndrome presenting to the emergency department is still to be defined. Some studies have demonstrated, however, that CMR perfusion imaging is feasible in these patients and has high diagnostic accuracy for detection of true acute coronary syndromes, particularly when adenosine vasodilator stress is used (sensitivity: 77%–100%, specificity: 83%–93%, and accuracy: 87%). Follow-up after normal perfusion CMR examinations has demonstrated an excellent NPV of 94% to 100% for adverse outcome or subsequent diagnosis of CAD after hospital discharge.[29–32] An imaging strategy involving perfusion CMR may also reduce cost in patient care by reducing unnecessary admissions and cardiac catheterizations without missing true positive acute coronary syndromes.[33] It remains unclear how versatile and cost-effective CMR would be compared with other imaging modalities (ie, SPECT) used for early detection of acute coronary syndrome in the emergency department.

Imaging Technique

First-pass perfusion CMR examination is based on dynamic rapid imaging of the heart during the circulation of a gadolinium-based contrast agent from the cardiac cambers into the myocardium. CMR perfusion imaging can be performed as a stand-alone technique or more commonly as part of a comprehensive CMR protocol (multiparametric examination), which includes noncontrast acquisition for morphologic and functional assessment as well as delayed enhancement (DE) images. Different protocols exist for comprehensive examination of the heart, but all contain morphologic and functional sequences; a stress dynamic first-pass perfusion after contrast administration, which is compared with a similar acquisition at rest; and finally delayed images for the detection of late gadolinium enhancement. Many variations exist depending on the type of magnet, coils, clinical question at hand, stressor agent used, and personal preferences.[34]

A typical MR protocol begins with localizers that are used to determine the true left ventricular short and long axes. These localizers are usually obtained as single-shot technique either as half-Fourier acquisition single-shot turbo spin-echo (HASTE) or as steady-state free precession (SSFP). Subsequently, functional images with white blood techniques are obtained in the short axis from the mitral valve through the apex, in vertical long axis, and in horizontal long axis views. Next, perfusion MR is obtained during the first pass of a gadolinium-based contrast agent after intravenous injection during pharmacologic vasodilation with adenosine or dipyridamole. Approximately 10 to 15 minutes later, allowing for contrast media elimination from the circulation, rest imaging is performed in the same plane and with an identical sequence (short-axis saturation recovery). Finally myocardial viability and infarction are evaluated with DE technique in which a heavily T1-weighted segmented gradient-recalled echo (GRE) sequence is acquired

in at least 2 planes, usually short axis and vertical long axis.[35] Some investigators prefer to perform the stress myocardial perfusion study first, followed by MR coronary angiography and resting myocardial perfusion study. Subsequently, additional intravenous injection of gadolinium is administered in preparation for delayed images. In the meantime, resting wall images are obtained, with DE images acquired at the end.[36] Other investigators prefer to perform the resting perfusion examination first, followed by cine images, MR angiography, and subsequently the stress perfusion and viability examination performed at the end of the exam.[32] A stress-only protocol has been proposed based on the high diagnostic performance of the hyperemia data from different studies.[22,37] Adding T2-weighted imaging for depiction of edema has also been proposed for better detection of patients with acute coronary syndrome.[31] The order in which stress and rest perfusion are performed may also be influenced by whether adenosine or dipyridamole is used as the stressor agent. Because adenosine has a short half-life (<10 seconds), it may be better to perform the stress study first so that the rest perfusion examination is not influenced by residual gadolinium injected at rest, which may accumulate in areas of scar tissue. If dipyridamole is used, it may be better to perform the rest study first, and then the stress study, because it has a significant longer half-life (30 minutes) and may delay the completion of the study (**Fig. 2**).

Stress Agents

Adenosine is a naturally occurring substance that activates A_2 cell-surface receptors of vascular smooth muscle cells causing relaxation and hence vasodilation. Unlike normal vessels or mildly abnormal arteries, the more diseased coronary arteries have a reduced blood flow reserve and cannot further dilate in response to adenosine, which creates a heterogeneous flow pattern across the myocardium. The vasodilatory effect may create mild to moderate reduction in systolic and diastolic blood pressure and reflex tachycardia. Significant advantages of adenosine over other stress agents used in cardiovascular imaging are its short half-life and excellent safety profile, with rare serious complications.[38] Contraindications of adenosine include second-degree and third-degree atrioventricular block, sick sinus syndrome, symptomatic bradycardia, severe asthma, and chronic obstructive pulmonary disease.

Dipyridamole is an indirect coronary vasodilator that inhibits intracellular reuptake and deamination of adenosine, increasing intravascular adenosine levels. Regadenoson, a selective A_{2A} adenosine

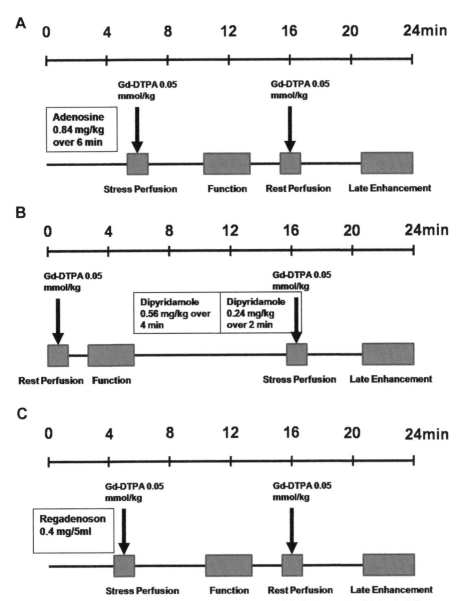

Fig. 2. (*A*) Typical first-pass perfusion protocol for adenosine stress perfusion CMR. (*B*) Typical first-pass perfusion protocol for dipyridamole stress perfusion CMR. (*C*) Typical first-pass perfusion protocol for regadenoson stress perfusion CMR. (*Modified from* Gerber BL, Raman SV, Nayak K, et al. Myocardial first-pass perfusion cardiovascular magnetic resonance: history, theory, and current state of the art. J Cardiovasc Magn Reson 2008;10:18.)

receptor agonist, is a newly introduced stressor agent that induces functional and perfusion results similar to nonselective adenosine and is used for stress perfusion imaging examinations.[39,40] Regadenoson has several advantages over adenosine: it is administered as an intravenous bolus fixed dose (400 µg independent of the patient weight); has fewer adverse effects, including atrioventricular block and bronchospasm; can be used in patients with mild to moderate reactive airway disease; and is cheaper.[41] Patients should be advised to restrain from smoking, drinking tea, coffee, or any caffeine-containing substance at least for 12 hours (some prefer up to 48 hours) previous to the examination due to the competitive interaction between caffeine and adenosine or regadenoson, which may attenuate the coronary hyperemic response by competitive blockade of A_{2A} receptors. For stress perfusion imaging, intravenous adenosine is administered at a dose of 140 µg/kg/min. Approximately 4 minutes into the adenosine infusion, an intravenous bolus injection of

0.05 mmol/kg to 0.01 mmol/kg of gadolinium-based contrast at 3 mL/min to 4 mL/min is administered, followed by 15 mL of saline flush at 5 mL/s, during end-expiratory breath hold.

The majority of clinical trials published so far have been done with 1.5-T magnets but the 3-T magnets are being used more and more in the clinical arena. Imaging at 3 T differs significantly from 1.5 T because it suffers from increased susceptibility artifacts, difference in tissue relaxation, and radiofrequency homogeneity problems. At the same time, higher field strength increases the signal-to-noise ratio, which theoretically improves image quality and may reduce imaging time. Only a few studies of myocardial perfusion performed by 3-T magnets have been published, but so far they tend to demonstrate a better contrast and spatial resolution, with improved accuracy in diagnosis of myocardial perfusion defects, with sensitivity as high as of 90%.[42,43]

Image Interpretation

Qualitative interpretation of perfusion CMR imaging is the most common approach in clinical practice. Image interpretation usually begins with review of delayed images for the presence of scar from previous MI. In absence of scar, the nonischemic myocardium exhibits uniform enhancement during first-pass perfusion at rest and with vasodilator stress. Ischemic but noninfarcted myocardium shows perfusion abnormality at stress that normalizes at rest (**Fig. 3**). Matched stress and rest perfusion defects in the absence of DE in the same region are considered artifactual.[44] Quantitative analysis of CMR perfusion examination is possible but complex. It can be significantly affected by several artifacts and variables (timing of saturation pulse, concentration of the contrast agent, magnetic field strength, phase of the cardiac cycle, and so forth) and has not been entirely validated or standardized. Therefore, quantitative analysis is more commonly used in research than in clinical practice.[34,45]

A common artifact that is seen in as many as 1 in every 4 studies is the endocardial dark rim artifact, which can be seen in dynamic sequences when the bolus of gadolinium first enters into the left ventricle and mimics a perfusion defect (**Fig. 4**). This dark rim is considered an artifact from susceptibility effect from gadolinium itself, from motion, or from resolution effect, because the artifact is perpendicular to the direction with the lowest spatial resolution (typically the phase-encoding direction). The most common location is at the interventricular septum in the left anterior descending artery vascular territory between the right and left ventricular cavities (>50%). Unlike true perfusion defects, this artifact is transient and does not remain after the bolus of contrast, a feature that helps in their differentiation.[43,46]

Limitations and Contraindications

Contraindications of perfusion CMR can be related to the high magnetic field, contrast agent, or pharmacologic stressor used. Contraindications related to the magnetic field are the same as those for other MR examination, including patients with electronic devices, such as most pacemakers and defibrillators, neurostimulators, ear implants, and cerebral aneurysm clips. These are usually considered absolute contraindications. Currently, the use of gadolinium contrast agents for cardiac imaging is off-label in the United States. Severe anaphylactic reaction to gadolinium is rare. A contraindication to the use of intravascular gadolinium is renal insufficiency because of the risk of nephrogenic systemic fibrosis, especially with the use of linear gadolinium chelates. Finally, contraindication for the use of adenosine or dipyridamole include asthma, severe chronic obstructive pulmonary disease, unstable angina, severely high or low blood pressure, heart block or sick sinus syndrome, and severe heart

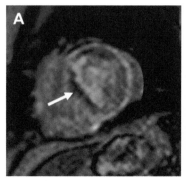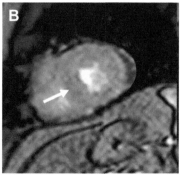

Fig. 3. Stress perfusion CMR. (*A*) Stress image shows subendocardial hypoperfusion of the interventricular septum (*arrow*). (*B*) Corresponding rest image reveals normal enhancement of the ischemic zone (*arrow*).

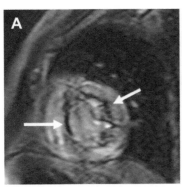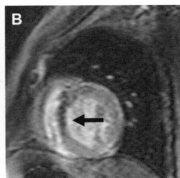

Fig. 4. Dark rim artifact versus perfusion defect. (*A*) The dark rim artifact is seen as a thin endocardial low signal region (*white arrows*). (*B*) Perfusion defect in the interventricular septum (*black arrow*). The dark rim artifact is usually transient whereas real perfusion defect persist longer during the first pass of the bolus of contrast.

failure. Claustrophobia, seen in approximately 5% of patients, is a relative contraindication that can be modified with the use of superficial sedatives or tranquilizers.

CORONARY ARTERY MR ANGIOGRAPHY

Despite impressive advances in cross-sectional imaging in recent years, coronary artery MR angiography remains an unconquered territory. Many obstacles (eg, cardiac and respiratory motions, tortuous anatomy, vessel size, and high signal from epicardial fat) have technically complicated this imaging modality. MR angiography is currently accepted as the imaging modality of choice for many vascular territories, including head, neck, abdomen, pelvis, and the extremities, but for coronary arteries it has remained challenging.

Current guidelines and appropriate use criteria indicate that coronary artery MR angiography is useful for identifying coronary artery anomalies, in particular in younger individuals, to determine the patency of coronary arteries, and to identify patients with multivessel CAD without exposure to ionizing radiation or iodinated contrast medium. It is also excellent in the detection and follow-up of coronary artery aneurysms in patients with Kawasaki disease and in those with ectatic coronary arteries and fistulas who may require serial imaging surveillance and follow-up.[13]

Many imaging techniques have been proposed and technical refinements developed with important advances in overcoming these challenges. The introduction of EEG triggering, faster pulse sequences, and navigator echoes have worked well in reducing motion artifacts. Prepulse sequences that enhance contrast-to-noise ratio and 3-D acquisition that allows significant postprocessing manipulation are additional useful tools. Two types of sequences can be used for coronary artery

MR angiography: noncontrast flow-sensitive sequences and contrast-enhanced sequences. Free-breathing, navigator-gated 3-D segmented GRE sequence has shown promising results, especially for evaluation of the proximal coronary arteries (**Figs. 5** and **6**). Single-center and multicenter studies have reported sensitivities of 74% to 100% and specificities of 50% to 98%.[47–50] In a prospective study comparing MR and CT angiography for coronary artery stenosis, both techniques showed similar diagnostic accuracy (83% vs 87%), sensitivity (87% vs 90%), and specificity (77% vs 83%); and both techniques were similar in their ability to identify patients who would subsequently need revascularization.[51] Similar numbers have been obtained more recently in a national

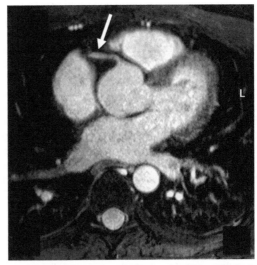

Fig. 5. MR coronary angiography. Free-breathing 3-D noncontrast turbo field-echo image demonstrates normal morphology and origin of the proximal right coronary artery (*arrow*).

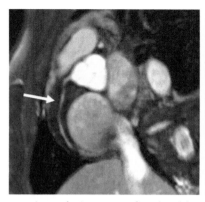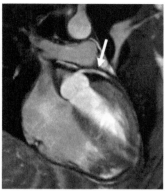

Fig. 6. MR coronary angiography in a young female athlete with exercise-induced chest pain. Free breathing 3-D noncontrast turbo field-echo images demonstrate normal origin and course of the proximal right and left coronary arteries (*arrows*).

multicenter trial in Japan, which revealed a high sensitivity and NPV (87% and 88%, respectively) and moderate specificity and positive predictive value (72% and 71%, respectively) for detection of significant coronary artery stenosis, suggesting that MR angiography could be used to rule out CAD given its high NPV.[52] A meta-analysis comprising 20 studies with 989 patients revealed sensitivity and specificity of 87.1% and 70.3% for the detection of coronary artery stenosis of 50% or greater, using catheter angiography as the reference standard.[53]

Coronary MR angiography can also be performed after intravenous injection of gadolinium-based contrast agents to shorten the T1 relaxation time of blood and increase the contrast-to-noise ratio. The currently available extravascular contrast agents, however, rapidly extravasate from the intravascular compartment, requiring rapid breath-hold first-pass imaging, which is technically challenging. Contrast-enhanced coronary artery MR angiography, with 3-T magnet during slow infusion of a gadolinium-based contrast agent using a 3-D spoiled GRE technique, has shown good results with sensitivity, specificity, and accuracy of 91.6%, 83.1%, and 84.1% on a per-segment analysis and 94.1%, 82.1%, and 88.7% on a per-patient analysis.[54] For prolonging the T1 shortening of the blood during the acquisition of the images, this technique requires a higher dose of gadolinium-based contrast (0.2 mmol/kg body weight), slowly infused (0.3 mL/s) using a power injector, followed by 20 mL of saline at the same rate.

New intravascular (blood pool) MR imaging contrast agents are being developed and evaluated for coronary MR angiography. These intravascular agents (based on gadolinium or ultrasmall superparamagnetic iron oxide particles) remain longer in the vasculature, allowing longer scan time with free breathing or repeated breath-holding technique. Experience with these new agents is limited, and even though initial reports are promising with good sensitivity, specificity, and accuracy for detection of coronary artery abnormalities, further studies are needed to better define their role in the clinical arena.[55–60]

DE-CMR IMAGING

DE-CMR imaging is one of the most common examinations for tissue characterization both in ischemic and nonischemic myocardial diseases. This technique has become the gold standard for visualization and quantification of infarcted myocardium and scar tissues as well as detection of infiltrative diseases of the heart. Differential myocardial enhancement in infarcted myocardium was initially described in the 1970s with CT after iodine contrast injection and demonstrated also as corresponding to areas of increased uptake of technetium pyrophosphate, an infarct-avid radiotracer, and to areas of decreased perfusion with [201]Tl.[61] Later, in the early 1980s, preferential and persistent enhancement of infarcted myocardium was also recognized with MR after gadolinium injection.[62,63] Significant refinement in MR technology with EEG-gated sequences, faster image acquisition, improved spatial and temporal resolution, and specialized imaging sequences, including use of an inversion pulse to null the signal of the normal myocardium, enables more reliable results and more consistent tissue characterization for routine clinical practice.[64] Today, DE-CMR is considered an appropriate imaging technique for determination of the location and extent of myocardial necrosis, assessment of post-acute MI patients, assessment of viability before revascularization, establishing the likelihood of functional recovery with coronary artery revascularization, and evaluation of nonischemic cardiomyopathy and myocarditis.[65]

Imaging Technique

Inversion-recovery T1-weighted or GRE (spoiled GRE or SSFP) sequences are typically acquired 10 to 30 minutes after intravenous administration of the contrast agent (0.1–0.2 mmol/kg of gadolinium chelates [eg, gadolinium-diethylenetriamine pentaacetic acid]).[66–68] A 180° inversion radiofrequency pulse is applied before 90° pulse to suppress, or null, the signal from the healthy myocardium.[67] This myocardial nulling technique accentuates the contrast between the normal myocardium, which appears dark, and abnormal enhancing myocardium.[67] The optimum inversion time (TI) varies among the individuals. Therefore, myocardial nulling is optimized for individual patients by acquiring TI scout images after applying progressively longer TIs (typically from 200 to 350 ms) and visual evaluation of the images for maximal signal suppression of the normal myocardium (**Fig. 7**).[67]

DE-CMR IN ISCHEMIC HEART DISEASE
Mechanisms of Myocardial DE

Gadolinium chelates are unable to diffuse through the intact cell membranes. Therefore, DE reflects the distribution of the contrast agents in the extracellular myocardial compartment.[69] Intracellular volume constitutes approximately 70% to 80% of the tissue volume in the normal myocardium.[69,70] The loss of cell membrane integrity in acute ischemia and necrosis, however, allows free passage of the gadolinium chelates to the intracellular space. Distribution of the contrast agent in both extracellular space and within the necrotic cells results in a higher concentration of the contrast agent, thus tissue hyperenhancement.[69,71] Using MR-derived partition coefficients in a rat model, fractional distribution volume of gadopentetate dimeglumine was measured as 0.23 in normal and 0.90 in infarcted myocardium. These values correspond well to the fractional volume of the extracellular space only and combined intracellular plus extracellular spaces, respectively.[72] Alteration in functional capillary density, capillary permeability, and washin/washout kinetics of the contrast agents are other factors that contribute to DE in acute MI.[73] In the chronic phase of myocardial ischemia/infarction, the necrotic tissue is replaced by fibrosis (ie, collagenous scar). Fibrotic tissues contain markedly larger extracellular volume and, therefore, enhance more compared with normal myocardium, which is densely packed with cardiomyocytes.[69,71]

Despite having different mechanisms of DE, acute and chronic MI cannot be readily distinguished by the use of extracellular gadolinium agents. This distinction is of high clinical significance in patients with known history of MI in whom superimposed acute MI is suspected. Combination of DE pattern with other CMR findings (eg, myocardial thinning and increased T2 signal[74]) and blood oxygen level–dependent imaging[75] may help establish the diagnosis. Recently, the combined use of high molecular weight contrast agents that remain exclusively in

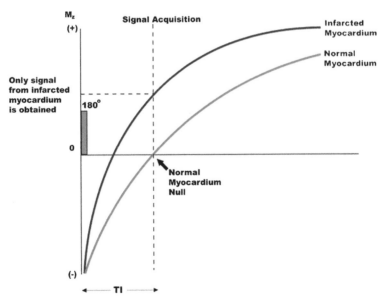

Fig. 7. Diagram illustrates how signal from a specific type of tissue is nulled. At signal acquisition in this diagram normal myocardium is giving zero signal and thus appears dark in the image. This can be applied between multiple tissues or substances as long as they have different T1 relaxation times.

the intravascular space (eg, gadomeritol) and standard extracellular contrast agents have been reported to help the distinction of acute and chronic MI in a pig model.[76] Microvascular integrity is only breached in acutely infarcted, but not chronically, scarred myocardium. Thereby, DE is only observed in acute MI after intravascular contrast administration, allowing the distinction from chronic MI.[76] This method, however, is not yet in routine clinical practice.

Myocardial Infarction

Myocardial ischemic injury, and therefore, DE most often begins at the subendocardium and extends to variable degrees toward the subepicardium.[77] Several mechanisms contribute to the susceptibility of the subendocardial myocardium to ischemic insult, including systolic compression of the subendocardial vessels and backflow to epicardial vessels as well as accelerated energy use by subendocardial myocardium.[77,78] In MI, DE follows a vascular distribution, which distinguishes it from other causes of subendocardial and transmural enhancement. DE-CMR after gadolinium-based contrast injection (with a 0.3 mmol/kg contrast dose) is highly sensitive in diagnosis of acute MI and chronic MI, reaching 99% and 94%, respectively, compared with the sensitivity of 11% of non–contrast-enhanced CMR imaging.[79] DE has been reported superior in identification of small subendocardial infarcts, which are not recognizable on SPECT,[80] and is also particularly helpful in diagnosis of non–Q-wave silent MI.[69]

In addition to DE caused by myocardial necrosis and scarring, aggregation of atheromatous debris, inflammatory cells, and platelets may occlude the microvascular and produce a core of no flow on first-pass perfusion imaging in acute MI.[81,82] This microvascular obstruction may persist even after

restoration of perfusion to the epicardial coronary artery.[69,81,82] Contrast-enhanced CMR imaging can identify microvascular obstruction through the no-flow phenomenon, which is associated with adverse ventricular remodeling and predicts a poor clinical outcome.[69,81,82]

Myocardial Viability

In addition to the irreversible myocardial damage (ie, necrosis), there are 2 distinct but related states of reversible myocardial contractile dysfunction (ie, stunning and hibernation). Stunning refers to a prolonged, but temporary, contractile dysfunction that occurs after brief episode(s) of acute nonlethal ischemia.[83] There is no pathologic evidence of irreversible myocardial damage,[84] and functional recovery occurs within hours, days, or weeks after restoration of blood flow.[83] Cumulative stunning as a result of repetitive episodes of acute ischemia seems an important contributor to development of contractile dysfunction in patients with CAD.[83] Alternatively, hibernation is a state of reversible suppressed contractility and energy demands in "chronically" ischemic myocardium and may protect against development of irreversible injury.[85]

Several studies have reported the presence of substantial amount of viable myocardium in more than 50% of patients with chronic ischemic heart disease.[86,87] Many retrospective studies have suggested that the presence of viable myocardium is predictive of improved left ventricular contractility and overall outcome on revascularization.[86–94] A cutoff of 50% transmural extension of DE has been considered to distinguish patients who experience significant recovery of myocardial contractility after revascularization (Figs. 8–10).[95,96] A large recent multicenter randomized clinical trial (Surgical Treatment for Ischemic Heart Failure [STICH])

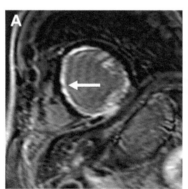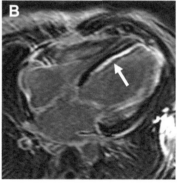

Fig. 8. MI in a 50-year-old man. Viability study in short axis (A) and horizontal long axis (B) demonstrates subendocardial enhancement of the interventricular septum with some focal areas of transmural infarction. Based on the MRI findings, surgical revascularization was performed with significant improvement of the left ventricular function.

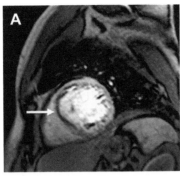

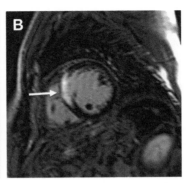

Fig. 9. Rest ischemia. A 61-year-old man with history of recent MI. (*A*) First-pass perfusion demonstrates hypoperfusion of the interventricular septum (*arrow*). (*B*) DE MR reveals nearly transmural DE of the midseptum, matching the ischemic zone (*arrow*).

demonstrated that patients with significant viable myocardium have an overall better outcome.[97] Viability, however, as assessed by dobutamine stress echocardiography and SPECT, did not influence the likelihood of survival benefit from combined medical therapy and coronary artery bypass graft compared with medical therapy alone.[97] The findings of this trial have been debated, considering the controversy with the bulk of other retrospective studies.[98] Additionally, this trial has been criticized for its randomization methodology.[98] Whether viability assessment by DE-CMR imaging improves the identification of patients who benefit most from revascularization versus medical therapy has not been addressed in this trial and needs to be further studied in randomized trials.

DE-CMR IN NONISCHEMIC HEART DISEASE

DE has been described in a variety of nonischemic heart diseases. These diseases are less common than myocardial ischemia. The pattern and distribution of DE often allows radiologists to make a distinction between these entities. The most common nonischemic conditions associated with DE are reviewed.

Dilated Cardiomyopathy

Dilated cardiomyopathy is the most common cause of nonischemic cardiomyopathy. It is characterized by myocardial contractile dysfunction that causes progressive dilation of the ventricular chambers with normal wall thickness.[99] The majority of cases are sporadic and may be idiopathic in etiology or result from a wide range of pathologic insults, including myocarditis (viral, bacterial, fungal, rickettsial, and parasitic), autoimmune disease, vasculitis, alcoholism, chemotherapeutic drugs (eg, anthracyclines), and toxins (eg, lead, mercury, and arsenic).[99] In 20% to 35% of cases, dilated cardiomyopathy is familial; the predominant pattern of inheritance is autosomal dominant with incomplete penetrance and variable expression, but X-linked inheritance and mitochondrial inheritance are well described.[99]

DE helps distinguish ischemic and nonischemic forms of dilated cardiomyopathy.[100–103] Although

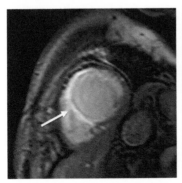

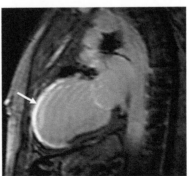

Fig. 10. Viability MR in a 55-year-old male patient with history of CAD and percutaneous intervention considered for revascularization surgery. Contrast-enhanced MR demonstrates extensive DE (*arrows*) and left ventricular dilation consistent with transmural infarction with true left ventricular aneurysm.

DE is almost invariably present in patients with ischemic cardiomyopathy, it is identified in only approximately 30% to 40% of patients with nonischemic causes.[103,104] Additionally, the most common pattern of DE in nonischemic dilated cardiomyopathy is focal or diffuse midwall myocardial enhancement, sparing the subendocardium (**Fig. 11**).[100,101] Subendocardial or transmural enhancement, however, may be seen in a minority of cases and may represent an underlying or concomitant CAD.[103] DE is associated with increased left ventricular remodeling, wall stress, and systolic dysfunction and may be of prognostic significance in predicting development of heart failure and arrhythmias in patients with dilated cardiomyopathy.[104,105]

Hypertrophic Cardiomyopathy

Hypertrophic cardiomyopathy is a genetic disease that affects approximately 0.2% of the population.[106,107] The most common pattern of inheritance is autosomal dominant with incomplete penetrance and variable expression.[106] It is the leading cause of sudden cardiac death in young people, including athletes.[107] Patients may be asymptomatic or present with exertional chest pain and dyspnea. Pathologically, hypertrophic cardiomyopathy is characterized by focal or diffuse left ventricular hypertrophy, most prominent in the subaortic basal anterior septum.[108] Commonly, the papillary muscle anomalously inserts into the body, instead of the tip, of the mitral valve. Mitral valve leaflet length is also increased. These anomalies allow systolic anterior motion of the distal portion of the mitral valve.[108] The combined effect of subaortic septal hypertrophy and anterior motion of the mitral valve produces left ventricular outflow stenosis during systole.[108] At the microscopic level,

cardiomyocyte hypertrophy, sarcomere disarray and interstitial fibrosis are present.[108]

Transthoracic echocardiography is generally the first-line imaging diagnostic tool. CMR examination, however, complements the diagnostic workup and provides unique information about the mitral valve and left ventricle morphology and function and fibrosis burden. Myocardial hypertrophy is often diffuse (affecting >50% of the left ventricular wall) but may be focal.[106,109–113] MR imaging, in particular, is superior to echocardiogram in identification of focal hypertrophy of the anterolateral free wall, posterior septum, and apex, areas where echocardiography is technically limited.[106,109–113] CMR imaging may also identify papillary muscle and mitral valve abnormalities and apical aneurysms and demonstrate the degree of left ventricular outflow tract obstruction.[109]

DE has been reported in approximately 60% of patients[114] and represents areas of myocardial ischemia and replacement fibrosis from subclinical ischemia caused by poor blood supply to hypertrophied myocardium by intramural coronary arteries and dysfunctional microvasculature.[109,115] Expansion of the extracellular space as a result of cardiomyocyte disorganization allows further accumulation of the contrast agents and may contribute to DE.[109] Abnormal enhancement is typically subepicardial or midmyocardial and almost always spares the subendocardium (**Fig. 12**).[96] In more than 30% of patients, both the left ventricular free wall and septum are affected.[109] In the remaining patients, focal enhancement, often in regions of myocardial hypertrophy, may be seen involving the left ventricular free wall, septum (particularly at the insertion site of the right ventricle), apex, or even right ventricular wall and papillary muscles.[109] DE does not follow a vascular distribution in these patients (**Fig. 13**).[109]

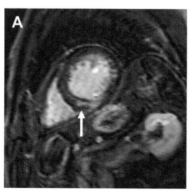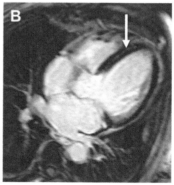

Fig. 11. Dilated cardiomyopathy in a 60-year-old man. Delayed images after contrast injection in short axis (*A*) and horizontal long axis (*B*) demonstrate abnormal late gadolinium enhancement in the midventricular wall, with a nonvascular distribution (*arrows*).

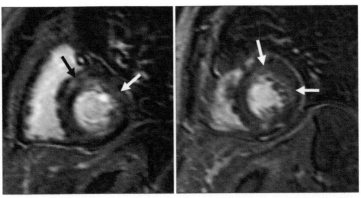

Fig. 12. Hypertrophic cardiomyopathy in a 53-year-old male. Irregular areas of contrast enhancement are appreciated in this short axis delayed images after contrast injection (*arrows*).

Extensive DE is associated with heart failure in patients with hypertrophic cardiomyopathy.[109] It is also strongly associated with the risk of ventricular arrhythmias[109,116] and predicts future cardiac complications.[114] A recent meta-analysis with 1063 patients demonstrated that DE is associated with cardiovascular, heart failure, and all-cause mortality in patients with this condition.[114] DE may also be appreciated in areas of scar tissue formation after alcohol ablation (**Fig. 14**).

Myocarditis

Myocarditis is caused by a variety of insults, including infectious agents, autoimmune diseases, and toxins.[117] In developed countries, viral infections (eg, coxsackieviruses A, B3 and B4, adenovirus, parvovirus B19, and human herpesvirus 6) account for the majority of cases. Autoimmune disease (eg, rheumatic heart disease) and parasitic infections (eg, Chagas disease) remained important causes of myocarditis in developing countries.[117] The clinical presentation is often nonspecific and includes fatigue, chest pain, arrhythmias, heart

block, EEG changes, elevation of cardiac enzymes, and acute heart failure.[117,118] Considering the nonspecificity of the clinical findings, diagnosis of myocarditis is challenging and generally made by exclusion of other cardiac pathologies, in particular MI.[117] Sampling errors and interobserver variability weaken the diagnostic value of endomyocardial biopsy.[119,120]

CMR imaging is of great value in diagnosis of acute myocarditis and may guide endomyocardial biopsy or even circumvent its need. Diffusion of contrast agents into necrotic cells seems the mechanism of DE in acute myocarditis.[121] In an appropriate clinical setting, myocardial contractile abnormality, increased T2 signal, and late gadolinium enhancement in a nonvascular distribution are highly suggestive.[96,122] T2 signal abnormality and DE may be patchy or diffuse and, unlike MI, typically originate from the subepicardial or midwall regions and spare the subendocardium.[123] In severe cases, transmural DE may be present.[123] It does not, however, follow a vascular distribution (**Figs. 15** and **16**).[124] Additionally, DE is often milder in myocarditis compared with MI,[123] likely due

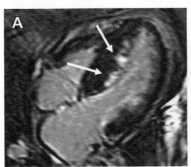
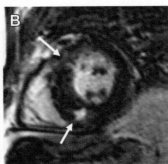

Fig. 13. Hypertrophic cardiomyopathy. A 50-year-old woman with history of syncope and chest pain. Viability study, horizontal long axis (*A*), and short-axis (*B*) images depict abnormal thickening of the interventricular septum, with irregular areas of DE (*arrows*).

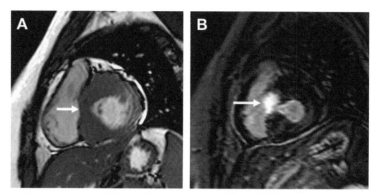

Fig. 14. Postalcohol ablation scar in a 36-year-old woman with history of hypertrophic cardiomyopathy. (*A*) White blood short axis view (balanced fast field echo [FFE]) shows focal thinning (*arrow*) between 2 areas of thick left ventricular myocardium. (*B*) DE short-axis image shows significant contrast retention in the area of thinning (*arrow*) consistent with postablation changes.

to patchy distribution of cardiomyocyte necrosis in the former compared with a homogeneous and extensive necrosis in the latter.[121,123] Some viral causes are reported to demonstrate a preferential distribution of DE (eg, human herpesvirus and parvovirus predominantly affect the midwall interventricular septum and subepicardial lateral wall).[124]

DE tends to decrease in size and intensity within weeks to months during the recovery.[66] It may eventually resolve or appear as a vague diffuse enhancement in the chronic phase. Areas of residual midwall or subepicardial DE persist, however, in approximately 70% of patients,[96] corresponding to foci of fibrosis.[66,121] Myocardial DE with a pattern compatible with myocarditis has a high specificity (up to 100%).[96] Its sensitivity, however, has been variable among different reports, ranging from 27% to 95%.[96] Early CMR imaging (ie, within 2 weeks of onset of symptoms) markedly improves the sensitivity of DE in acute myocarditis.[122]

The kinetics of gadolinium washout has been reported different in acute myocarditis compared with MI. Unlike the stable enhancement in patients with MI, significant contrast washout has been identified in patients with acute myocarditis 5 to 15 minutes post contrast injection. This finding suggests that an earlier image acquisition may improve the sensitivity of DE and provide a better delineation of myocardial involvement.[125] Prognostically, DE is a strong predictor of development of heart failure[126] and mortality in patients with viral myocarditis.[127]

Sarcoidosis

Sarcoidosis is a multisystem granulomatous disease of unknown cause. Multiple genetic and environmental factors, including immunologic and infectious, have been suggested as contributing to its pathogenesis.[128] Autopsy and advanced imaging techniques, including CMR and PET, demonstrate myocardial involvement in up to 40%

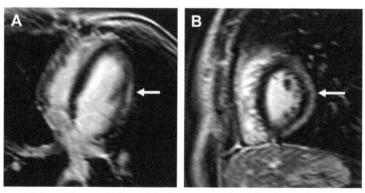

Fig. 15. Acute myocarditis in a 15-year-old boy with chest pain and mildly elevated troponins. (*A*) DE axial image shows abnormal late gadolinium enhancement on the lateral wall of the left ventricle (*arrow*). (*B*) Short-axis view shows the characteristic epicardial pattern of enhancement associated with acute myocarditis (*arrow*).

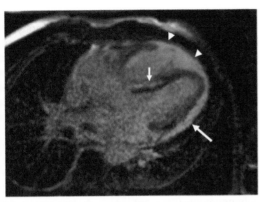

Fig. 16. Giant cell myocarditis in a 45-year-old man with arrhythmia and heart failure. CMR delayed images after contrast injection reveal abnormal late gadolinium enhancement of the right ventricle (*arrowheads*), left ventricle (*large arrow*), and basal interventricular septum (*small arrow*).

of cases. Clinically evident cardiac disease, however, is seen in only 5% of patients.[128,129] The myocardium, in particular septum and left ventricular free wall, is most commonly involved.[128] Any cardiac structure, however (eg, conduction system, pericardium, and endocardium), may be involved. Clinical manifestations vary depending on the affected organs. Cardiac involvement often occurs along other manifestations of sarcoidosis, although the heart rarely is the initial organ involved. Patients may develop dilated cardiomyopathy, arrhythmias and heart block, pericardial effusion, pericarditis, and even sudden death.[130]

Diagnosis of cardiac sarcoidosis may be difficult, in particular if cardiac disease precedes other manifestations. Most diagnostic tests are not highly sensitive and specific. Therefore, often a combination of diagnostic tests (eg, serum markers, EEG, echocardiogram, perfusion myocardial scintigraphy, and fludeoxyglucose F 18 PET) is

required for diagnosis.[129,131] The patchy distribution of noncaseating granulomas in sarcoidosis complicates the diagnosis, reducing the sensitivity of endomyocardial biopsy to approximately 20%.[129]

CMR imaging markedly improves the diagnostic sensitivity[131] and helps guide endomyocardial biopsy. In the acute phase, CMR imaging demonstrates wall motion abnormalities, focal myocardial thickening, T2 hyperintensity (due to edema), and both early and late gadolinium enhancement.[66,128] In the chronic phase, areas of fibrosis develop that result in focal or diffuse myocardial thinning and DE.[66,128] DE is typically subepicardial or midmyocardial but can also be transmural, does not follow a vascular distribution, and primarily affects the basal segments of left ventricle and midventricular septum.[131,132] Although regions of DE with a pattern similar to CAD may be observed in approximately half of the patients, the majority of patients (86%) have at least one area of DE with a nonvascular pattern (**Fig. 17**).[131] Myocardial DE may less commonly be identified in other regions of heart, including the right ventricular side of the interventricular septum, right ventricular free wall, outflow tract, anterobasal segments of the right ventricle, and papillary muscles.[131]

Extensive DE is associated with left ventricular dysfunction.[96,131,133,134] It also predicts the risk of future complications, including ventricular tachyarrhythmia, atrioventricular block, and cardiac death.[131] Additionally, corticosteroid therapy improves myocardial DE and increased T2 signal, suggesting a role for contrast-enhanced CMR imaging in monitoring the response to therapy.[135]

Amyloidosis

Systemic amyloidosis is a heterogeneous group of diseases in which there is abnormal extracellular

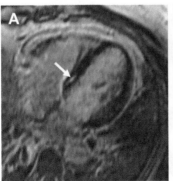
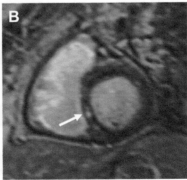

Fig. 17. Cardiac sarcoidosis. A 54-year-old man with history of pulmonary sarcoidosis who presents with cardiac arrhythmia. Viability imaging in horizontal long axis (*A*) and short axis (*B*) reveals abnormal focal areas of late gadolinium enhancement within the interventricular septum (*arrows*).

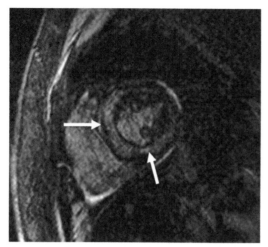

Fig. 18. Cardiac amyloidosis in a 63-year-old man with refractory congestive heart failure. Short axis inversion recovery delayed image 12 minutes after contrast injection shows diffuse late gadolinium enhancement of the left ventricular myocardium (*arrows*).

deposition of amyloid protein. Every year, several new cases (10 per million) of acquired amyloidosis are identified in the United States.[136] Amyloid light chain and transthyretin deposition constitutes the majority of cases.[137,138] The heart, which is after the kidney the second most commonly affected organ, develops endomyocardial deposition of amyloid, which causes progressive wall thickening and diastolic dysfunction.[137] The extent of cardiac involvement is one of the major prognostic factors in systemic amyloidosis. Unfortunately, the clinical symptoms are nonspecific until late in the course of the disease.[139]

The most commonly used modality to assess the cardiac involvement is echocardiography. It is not sensitive in early stages of the disease and cannot differentiate different patterns of amyloid deposition. Endomyocardial biopsy is the gold standard for diagnosis but it is invasive and prone to sampling errors. Recently, contrast-enhanced CMR imaging with DE has been used to assess cardiac involvement.[139]

Several patterns of myocardial DE have been described.[123,139–141] The 2 most common patterns are global subendocardial enhancement and global homogenous or heterogeneous transmural enhancement (Fig. 18).[123,139] A less common pattern is patchy focal enhancement. Finally, suboptimal nulling has also has been described, in which no proper TI can be found despite multiple cine-inversion recovery sequences. In this latter group, the endomyocardium has a darker appearance as opposed to global hyperenhancement, the blood appears darker than usual, and images have lower signal-to-noise ratio.[139] In a series of 34 pathologically proven cases of cardiac amyloidosis, Syed and colleagues[139] demonstrated global transmural or subendocardial enhancement in 83%, patchy focal enhancement in 6%, and suboptimal nulling in 3% of patients. Global transmural or subendocardial enhancement was associated with greater degrees of amyloid deposition on pathology examination.

Other Rare Nonischemic Causes of Myocardial DE

DE has been described in other uncommon cardiac pathologies, including Churg-Strauss syndrome,

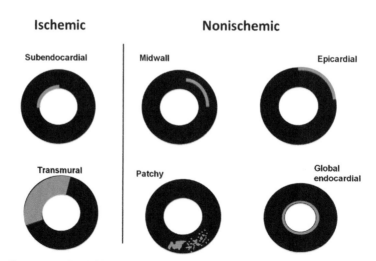

Fig. 19. Diagram illustrating the difference between the DE observed in ischemic and nonischemic diseases. Ischemic disease presents a vascular territory distribution and characteristically involves the endocardium. In nonischemic conditions, the abnormal DE may be midwall, patchy, epicardial, or global subendocardial.

endomyocardial fibrosis, myocardial noncompaction, arrhythmogenic right ventricular dysplasia, Takotsubo cardiomyopathy, and Anderson-Fabry disease. The pattern of myocardial DE in these diseases is reviewed elsewhere.[66,96,123]

SUMMARY

During the past 2 decades, there have been substantial technologic advances in CMR imaging, allowing better evaluation of cardiac physiology, anatomy, and pathology. Concurrent with these advances, there has been a steady growth in applications of CMR in clinical and research settings. Comprehensive multiparametric CMR, which includes perfusion, DE, and noncontrast imaging, is now considered an accurate and reliable diagnostic tool for identification of myocardial ischemia and is the study of choice for evaluation of myocardial viability. Identification of specific patterns of myocardial DE that occur in a variety of nonischemic diseases, such as myocarditis, sarcoidosis, hypertrophic cardiomyopathy, and amyloidosis, has further extended the clinical applications of contrast-enhanced CMR imaging (Fig. 19).

CMR imaging remains an active area of research. Ongoing and future studies are needed to better define the role of CMR in answering important clinical questions, such as patient prognosis, risk stratification, and patient response to therapeutic interventions, and to better define its role in clinical decision making in acute and chronic cardiovascular diseases.

REFERENCES

1. Roger VL, Go AS, Lloyd-Jones DM, et al. Heart disease and stroke statistics—2012 update: a report from the American Heart Association. Circulation 2012;125(1):e2–e220.
2. Groothuis JG, Beek AM, Brinckman SL, et al. Low to intermediate probability of coronary artery disease: comparison of coronary CT angiography with first-pass MR myocardial perfusion imaging. Radiology 2010;254(2):384–92.
3. Schinkel AF, Bax JJ, Geleijnse ML, et al. Noninvasive evaluation of ischaemic heart disease: myocardial perfusion imaging or stress echocardiography? Eur Heart J 2003;24(9):789–800.
4. Marwick TH. Stress echocardiography. Heart 2003; 89(1):113–8.
5. Hoffmann R, Lethen H, Marwick T, et al. Analysis of interinstitutional observer agreement in interpretation of dobutamine stress echocardiograms. J Am Coll Cardiol 1996;27(2):330–6.
6. Charoenpanichkit C, Hundley WG. The 20 year evolution of dobutamine stress cardiovascular magnetic resonance. J Cardiovasc Magn Reson 2010;12:59.
7. Modonesi E, Balbi M, Bezante GP. Limitations and potential clinical application on contrast echocardiography. Curr Cardiol Rev 2010;6(1):24–30.
8. Schindler TH, Schelbert HR, Quercioli A, et al. Cardiac PET imaging for the detection and monitoring of coronary artery disease and microvascular health. JACC Cardiovasc Imaging 2010; 3(6):623–40.
9. Metz LD, Beattie M, Hom R, et al. The prognostic value of normal exercise myocardial perfusion imaging and exercise echocardiography: a meta-analysis. J Am Coll Cardiol 2007;49(2):227–37.
10. Navare SM, Mather JF, Shaw LJ, et al. Comparison of risk stratification with pharmacologic and exercise stress myocardial perfusion imaging: a meta-analysis. J Nucl Cardiol 2004;11(5):551–61.
11. Gargiulo P, Petretta M, Bruzzese D, et al. Myocardial perfusion scintigraphy and echocardiography for detecting coronary artery disease in hypertensive patients: a meta-analysis. Eur J Nucl Med Mol Imaging 2011;38(11):2040–9.
12. Bruder O, Schneider S, Nothnagel D, et al. EuroCMR (European Cardiovascular Magnetic Resonance) registry: results of the German pilot phase. J Am Coll Cardiol 2009;54(15):1457–66.
13. Hundley WG, Bluemke DA, Finn JP, et al. ACCF/ACR/AHA/NASCI/SCMR 2010 expert consensus document on cardiovascular magnetic resonance: a report of the American College of Cardiology Foundation Task Force on Expert Consensus Documents. J Am Coll Cardiol 2010;55(23): 2614–62.
14. Al-Saadi N, Nagel E, Gross M, et al. Noninvasive detection of myocardial ischemia from perfusion reserve based on cardiovascular magnetic resonance. Circulation 2000;101(12):1379–83.
15. Schwitter J, Nanz D, Kneifel S, et al. Assessment of myocardial perfusion in coronary artery disease by magnetic resonance: a comparison with positron emission tomography and coronary angiography. Circulation 2001;103(18):2230–5.
16. Panting JR, Gatehouse PD, Yang GZ, et al. Echoplanar magnetic resonance myocardial perfusion imaging: parametric map analysis and comparison with thallium SPECT. J Magn Reson Imaging 2001; 13(2):192–200.
17. Paetsch I, Jahnke C, Wahl A, et al. Comparison of dobutamine stress magnetic resonance, adenosine stress magnetic resonance, and adenosine stress magnetic resonance perfusion. Circulation 2004;110(7):835–42.
18. Klem I, Heitner JF, Shah DJ, et al. Improved detection of coronary artery disease by stress perfusion

cardiovascular magnetic resonance with the use of delayed enhancement infarction imaging. J Am Coll Cardiol 2006;47(8):1630–8.

19. Ishida N, Sakuma H, Motoyasu M, et al. Non-infarcted myocardium: correlation between dynamic first-pass contrast-enhanced myocardial MR imaging and quantitative coronary angiography. Radiology 2003;229(1):209–16.

20. Wolff SD, Schwitter J, Coulden R, et al. Myocardial first-pass perfusion magnetic resonance imaging: a multicenter dose-ranging study. Circulation 2004;110(6):732–7.

21. Giang TH, Nanz D, Coulden R, et al. Detection of coronary artery disease by magnetic resonance myocardial perfusion imaging with various contrast medium doses: first European multi-centre experience. Eur Heart J 2004;25(18):1657–65.

22. Schwitter J, Wacker CM, van Rossum AC, et al. MR-IMPACT: comparison of perfusion-cardiac magnetic resonance with single-photon emission computed tomography for the detection of coronary artery disease in a multicentre, multivendor, randomized trial. Eur Heart J 2008;29(4):480–9.

23. Greenwood JP, Maredia N, Younger JF, et al. Cardiovascular magnetic resonance and single-photon emission computed tomography for diagnosis of coronary heart disease (CE-MARC): a prospective trial. Lancet 2012;379(9814):453–60.

24. Doesch C, Seeger A, Doering J, et al. Risk stratification by adenosine stress cardiac magnetic resonance in patients with coronary artery stenoses of intermediate angiographic severity. JACC Cardiovasc Imaging 2009;2(4):424–33.

25. Bodi V, Husser O, Sanchis J, et al. Prognostic implications of dipyridamole cardiac MR imaging: a prospective multicenter registry. Radiology 2012;262(1):91–100.

26. Jahnke C, Nagel E, Gebker R, et al. Prognostic value of cardiac magnetic resonance stress tests: adenosine stress perfusion and dobutamine stress wall motion imaging. Circulation 2007;115(13):1769–76.

27. Nandalur KR, Dwamena BA, Choudhri AF, et al. Diagnostic performance of stress cardiac magnetic resonance imaging in the detection of coronary artery disease: a meta-analysis. J Am Coll Cardiol 2007;50(14):1343–53.

28. Hamon M, Fau G, Nee G, et al. Meta-analysis of the diagnostic performance of stress perfusion cardiovascular magnetic resonance for detection of coronary artery disease. J Cardiovasc Magn Reson 2010;12(1):29.

29. Kwong RY, Schussheim AE, Rekhraj S, et al. Detecting acute coronary syndrome in the emergency department with cardiac magnetic resonance imaging. Circulation 2003;107(4):531–7.

30. Ingkanisorn WP, Kwong RY, Bohme NS, et al. Prognosis of negative adenosine stress magnetic resonance in patients presenting to an emergency department with chest pain. J Am Coll Cardiol 2006;47(7):1427–32.

31. Cury RC, Shash K, Nagurney JT, et al. Cardiac magnetic resonance with T2-weighted imaging improves detection of patients with acute coronary syndrome in the emergency department. Circulation 2008;118(8):837–44.

32. Plein S, Greenwood JP, Ridgway JP, et al. Assessment of non-ST-segment elevation acute coronary syndromes with cardiac magnetic resonance imaging. J Am Coll Cardiol 2004;44(11):2173–81.

33. Miller CD, Hwang W, Hoekstra JW, et al. Stress cardiac magnetic resonance imaging with observation unit care reduces cost for patients with emergent chest pain: a randomized trial. Ann Emerg Med 2010;56(3):209–219.e202.

34. Gerber BL, Raman SV, Nayak K, et al. Myocardial first-pass perfusion cardiovascular magnetic resonance: history, theory, and current state of the art. J Cardiovasc Magn Reson 2008;10:18.

35. Kim HW, Crowley AL, Kim RJ. A clinical cardiovascular magnetic resonance service: operational considerations and the basic examination. Magn Reson Imaging Clin N Am 2007;15(4):473–85, v.

36. Greenwood JP, Maredia N, Radjenovic A, et al. Clinical evaluation of magnetic resonance imaging in coronary heart disease: the CE-MARC study. Trial 2009;10:62.

37. Schwitter J, Arai AE. Assessment of cardiac ischaemia and viability: role of cardiovascular magnetic resonance. Eur Heart J 2011;32(7): 799–809.

38. Cerqueira MD, Verani MS, Schwaiger M, et al. Safety profile of adenosine stress perfusion imaging: results from the Adenoscan Multicenter Trial Registry. J Am Coll Cardiol 1994; 23(2):384–9.

39. Mahmarian JJ, Cerqueira MD, Iskandrian AE, et al. Regadenoson induces comparable left ventricular perfusion defects as adenosine: a quantitative analysis from the ADVANCE MPI 2 trial. JACC Cardiovasc Imaging 2009;2(8):959–68.

40. Lyons M, Javidan-Nejad C, Saeed IM, et al. Feasibility of detecting myocardial ischemia using first-pass contrast MRI and regadenoson. J Cardiovasc Magn Reson 2012;14(Suppl 1):P11.

41. Al Jaroudi W, Iskandrian AE. Regadenoson: a new myocardial stress agent. J Am Coll Cardiol 2009; 54(13):1123–30.

42. Araoz PA, Glockner JF, McGee KP, et al. 3 Tesla MR imaging provides improved contrast in first-pass myocardial perfusion imaging over a range of gadolinium doses. J Cardiovasc Magn Reson 2005; 7(3):559–64.

43. Gebker R, Jahnke C, Paetsch I, et al. Diagnostic performance of myocardial perfusion MR at 3 T in

patients with coronary artery disease. Radiology 2008;247(1):57–63.

44. Kim HW, Klem I, Kim RJ. Detection of myocardial ischemia by stress perfusion cardiovascular magnetic resonance. Cardiol Clin 2007;25(1): 57–70, vi.

45. Motwani M, Fairbairn TA, Larghat A, et al. Systolic versus diastolic acquisition in myocardial perfusion MR imaging. Radiology 2012;262(3):816–23.

46. Di Bella EV, Parker DL, Sinusas AJ. On the dark rim artifact in dynamic contrast-enhanced MRI myocardial perfusion studies. Magn Reson Med 2005; 54(5):1295–9.

47. Kim WY, Danias PG, Stuber M, et al. Coronary magnetic resonance angiography for the detection of coronary stenoses. N Engl J Med 2001;345(26): 1863–9.

48. Sommer T, Hofer U, Hackenbroch M, et al. Submillimeter 3D coronary MR angiography with real-time navigator correction in 107 patients with suspected coronary artery disease. Rofo 2002;174(4):459–66 [in German].

49. Sakuma H, Ichikawa Y, Chino S, et al. Detection of coronary artery stenosis with whole-heart coronary magnetic resonance angiography. J Am Coll Cardiol 2006;48(10):1946–50.

50. Dewey M, Teige F, Schnapauff D, et al. Noninvasive detection of coronary artery stenoses with multislice computed tomography or magnetic resonance imaging. Ann Intern Med 2006;145(6):407–15.

51. Hamdan A, Asbach P, Wellnhofer E, et al. A prospective study for comparison of MR and CT imaging for detection of coronary artery stenosis. JACC Cardiovasc Imaging 2011;4(1):50–61.

52. Kato S, Kitagawa K, Ishida N, et al. Assessment of coronary artery disease using magnetic resonance coronary angiography: a national multicenter trial. J Am Coll Cardiol 2010;56(12):983–91.

53. Schuetz GM, Zacharopoulou NM, Schlattmann P, et al. Meta-analysis: noninvasive coronary angiography using computed tomography versus magnetic resonance imaging. Ann Intern Med 2010;152(3): 167–77.

54. Yang Q, Li K, Liu X, et al. Contrast-enhanced whole-heart coronary magnetic resonance angiography at 3.0-T: a comparative study with X-ray angiography in a single center. J Am Coll Cardiol 2009; 54(1):69–76.

55. Herborn CU, Barkhausen J, Paetsch I, et al. Coronary arteries: contrast-enhanced MR imaging with SH L 643A–experience in 12 volunteers. Radiology 2003;229(1):217–23.

56. Huber ME, Paetsch I, Schnackenburg B, et al. Performance of a new gadolinium-based intravascular contrast agent in free-breathing inversion-recovery 3D coronary MRA. Magn Reson Med 2003;49(1):115–21.

57. Paetsch I, Jahnke C, Barkhausen J, et al. Detection of coronary stenoses with contrast enhanced, three-dimensional free breathing coronary MR angiography using the gadolinium-based intravascular contrast agent gadocoletic acid (B-22956). J Cardiovasc Magn Reson 2006;8(3):509–16.

58. Zheng J, Li D, Maggioni F, et al. Single-session magnetic resonance coronary angiography and myocardial perfusion imaging using the new blood pool compound B-22956 (gadocoletic acid): initial experience in a porcine model of coronary artery disease. Invest Radiol 2005;40(9):604–13.

59. Prompona M, Cyran C, Nikolaou K, et al. Contrast-enhanced whole-heart MR coronary angiography at 3.0 T using the intravascular contrast agent gadofosveset. Invest Radiol 2009;44(7):369–74.

60. Herborn CU, Schmidt M, Bruder O, et al. MR coronary angiography with SH L 643 A: initial experience in patients with coronary artery disease. Radiology 2004;233(2):567–73.

61. Siemers PT, Higgins CB, Schmidt W, et al. Detection, quantitation and contrast enhancement of myocardial infarction utilizing computerized axial tomography: comparison with histochemical staining and 99mTc-pyrophosphate imaging. Invest Radiol 1978;13(2):103–9.

62. McNamara MT, Higgins CB, Ehman RL, et al. Acute myocardial ischemia: magnetic resonance contrast enhancement with gadolinium-DTPA. Radiology 1984;153(1):157–63.

63. Wesbey GE, Higgins CB, Lipton MJ, et al. Enhancement of myocardial infarctions with nuclear magnetic resonance contrast media. Invest Radiol 1984;19(4):S151.

64. Simonetti OP, Kim RJ, Fieno DS, et al. An improved MR imaging technique for the visualization of myocardial infarction. Radiology 2001; 218(1):215–23.

65. Hundley WG, Bluemke DA, Finn JP, et al. ACCF/ACR/AHA/NASCI/SCMR 2010 expert consensus document on cardiovascular magnetic resonance: a report of the American College of Cardiology Foundation Task Force on Expert Consensus Documents. Circulation 2010;121(22):2462–508.

66. Vogel-Claussen J, Rochitte CE, Wu KC, et al. Delayed enhancement MR imaging: utility in myocardial assessment. Radiographics 2006; 26(3):795–810.

67. Gupta A, Lee VS, Chung YC, et al. Myocardial infarction: optimization of inversion times at delayed contrast-enhanced MR imaging. Radiology 2004;233(3):921–6.

68. Lim RP, Srichai MB, Lee VS. Non-ischemic causes of delayed myocardial hyperenhancement on MRI. AJR Am J Roentgenol 2007;188(6):1675–81.

69. Kim HW, Farzaneh-Far A, Kim RJ. Cardiovascular magnetic resonance in patients with myocardial

infarction: current and emerging applications. J Am Coll Cardiol 2009;55(1):1–16.

70. Dobson GP, Cieslar JH. Intracellular, interstitial and plasma spaces in the rat myocardium in vivo. J Mol Cell Cardiol 1997;29(12):3357–63.

71. Rehwald WG, Fieno DS, Chen EL, et al. Myocardial magnetic resonance imaging contrast agent concentrations after reversible and irreversible ischemic injury. Circulation 2002;105(2):224–9.

72. Arheden H, Saeed M, Higgins CB, et al. Measurement of the distribution volume of gadopentetate dimeglumine at echo-planar MR imaging to quantify myocardial infarction: comparison with 99mTc-DTPA autoradiography in rats. Radiology 1999; 211(3):698–708.

73. Kim RJ, Chen EL, Lima JA, et al. Myocardial Gd-DTPA kinetics determine MRI contrast enhancement and reflect the extent and severity of myocardial injury after acute reperfused infarction. Circulation 1996;94(12):3318–26.

74. Abdel-Aty H, Zagrosek A, Schulz-Menger J, et al. Delayed enhancement and T2-weighted cardiovascular magnetic resonance imaging differentiate acute from chronic myocardial infarction. Circulation 2004;109(20):2411–6.

75. Egred M, Al-Mohammad A, Waiter GD, et al. Detection of scarred and viable myocardium using a new magnetic resonance imaging technique: blood oxygen level dependent (BOLD) MRI. Heart 2003;89(7):738–44.

76. Saeed M, Weber O, Lee R, et al. Discrimination of myocardial acute and chronic (scar) infarctions on delayed contrast enhanced magnetic resonance imaging with intravascular magnetic resonance contrast media. J Am Coll Cardiol 2006; 48(10):1961–8.

77. Lowe JE, Cummings RG, Adams DH, et al. Evidence that ischemic cell death begins in the subendocardium independent of variations in collateral flow or wall tension. Circulation 1983;68(1):190–202.

78. Algranati D, Kassab GS, Lanir Y. Why is the subendocardium more vulnerable to ischemia? A new paradigm. Am J Physiol Heart Circ Physiol 2011; 300(3):H1090–100.

79. Kim RJ, Albert TS, Wible JH, et al. Performance of delayed-enhancement magnetic resonance imaging with gadoversetamide contrast for the detection and assessment of myocardial infarction: an international, multicenter, double-blinded, randomized trial. Circulation 2008;117(5):629–37.

80. Wagner A, Mahrholdt H, Holly TA, et al. Contrast-enhanced MRI and routine single photon emission computed tomography (SPECT) perfusion imaging for detection of subendocardial myocardial infarcts: an imaging study. Lancet 2003;361(9355):374–9.

81. Shapiro MD, Guarraia DL, Moloo J, et al. Evaluation of acute coronary syndromes by cardiac magnetic resonance imaging. Top Magn Reson Imaging 2008;19(1):25–32.

82. Strzelczyk J, Attili A. Cardiac magnetic resonance evaluation of myocardial viability and ischemia. Semin Roentgenol 2008;43(3):193–203.

83. Camici PG, Prasad SK, Rimoldi OE. Stunning hibernation, and assessment of myocardial viability. Circulation 2008;117(1):103–14.

84. Pomblum VJ, Korbmacher B, Cleveland S, et al. Cardiac stunning in the clinic: the full picture. Interact Cardiovasc Thorac Surg 2010;10(1): 86–91.

85. Vanoverschelde JL, Pasquet A, Gerber B, et al. Pathophysiology of myocardial hibernation. Implications for the use of dobutamine echocardiography to identify myocardial viability. Heart 1999; 82(Suppl 3):III1–7.

86. Auerbach MA, Schoder H, Hoh C, et al. Prevalence of myocardial viability as detected by positron emission tomography in patients with ischemic cardiomyopathy. Circulation 1999;99(22):2921–6.

87. Schinkel AF, Bax JJ, Boersma E, et al. How many patients with ischemic cardiomyopathy exhibit viable myocardium? Am J Cardiol 2001;88(5):561–4.

88. Gioia G, Powers J, Heo J, et al. Prognostic value of rest-redistribution tomographic thallium-201 imaging in ischemic cardiomyopathy. Am J Cardiol 1995; 75(12):759–62.

89. Gioia G, Milan E, Giubbini R, et al. Prognostic value of tomographic rest-redistribution thallium 201 imaging in medically treated patients with coronary artery disease and left ventricular dysfunction. J Nucl Cardiol 1996;3(2):150–6.

90. Williams MJ, Odabashian J, Lauer MS, et al. Prognostic value of dobutamine echocardiography in patients with left ventricular dysfunction. J Am Coll Cardiol 1996;27(1):132–9.

91. Petretta M, Cuocolo A, Bonaduce D, et al. Incremental prognostic value of thallium reinjection after stress-redistribution imaging in patients with previous myocardial infarction and left ventricular dysfunction. J Nucl Med 1997;38(2):195–200.

92. Afridi I, Grayburn PA, Panza JA, et al. Myocardial viability during dobutamine echocardiography predicts survival in patients with coronary artery disease and severe left ventricular systolic dysfunction. J Am Coll Cardiol 1998;32(4):921–6.

93. Pasquet A, Robert A, D'Hondt AM, et al. Prognostic value of myocardial ischemia and viability in patients with chronic left ventricular ischemic dysfunction. Circulation 1999;100(2):141–8.

94. Hage FG, Venkataraman R, Aljaroudi W, et al. The impact of viability assessment using myocardial perfusion imaging on patient management and outcome. J Nucl Cardiol 2010;17(3):378–89.

95. Kim RJ, Wu E, Rafael A, et al. The use of contrast-enhanced magnetic resonance imaging to identify

reversible myocardial dysfunction. N Engl J Med 2000;343(20):1445–53.

96. Ordovas KG, Higgins CB. Delayed contrast enhancement on MR images of myocardium: past, present, future. Radiology 2011;261(2):358–74.

97. Bonow RO, Maurer G, Lee KL, et al. Myocardial viability and survival in ischemic left ventricular dysfunction. N Engl J Med 2011;364(17):1617–25.

98. Grover S, Srinivasan G, Selvanayagam JB. Evaluation of myocardial viability with cardiac magnetic resonance imaging. Prog Cardiovasc Dis 2011; 54(3):204–14.

99. Maron BJ, Towbin JA, Thiene G, et al. Contemporary definitions and classification of the cardiomyopathies: an American Heart Association Scientific Statement from the Council on Clinical Cardiology, Heart Failure and Transplantation Committee; Quality of Care and Outcomes Research and Functional Genomics and Translational Biology Interdisciplinary Working Groups; and Council on Epidemiology and Prevention. Circulation 2006; 113(14):1807–16.

100. Bohl S, Wassmuth R, Abdel-Aty H, et al. Delayed enhancement cardiac magnetic resonance imaging reveals typical patterns of myocardial injury in patients with various forms of non-ischemic heart disease. Int J Cardiovasc Imaging 2008;24(6):597–607.

101. Calore C, Cacciavillani L, Boffa GM, et al. Contrast-enhanced cardiovascular magnetic resonance in primary and ischemic dilated cardiomyopathy. J Cardiovasc Med (Hagerstown) 2007;8(10):821–9.

102. Soriano CJ, Ridocci F, Estornell J, et al. Noninvasive diagnosis of coronary artery disease in patients with heart failure and systolic dysfunction of uncertain etiology, using late gadolinium-enhanced cardiovascular magnetic resonance. J Am Coll Cardiol 2005;45(5):743–8.

103. McCrohon JA, Moon JC, Prasad SK, et al. Differentiation of heart failure related to dilated cardiomyopathy and coronary artery disease using gadolinium-enhanced cardiovascular magnetic resonance. Circulation 2003;108(1):54–9.

104. Alter P, Rupp H, Adams P, et al. Occurrence of late gadolinium enhancement is associated with increased left ventricular wall stress and mass in patients with non-ischaemic dilated cardiomyopathy. Eur J Heart Fail 2011;13(9):937–44.

105. Lehrke S, Lossnitzer D, Schob M, et al. Use of cardiovascular magnetic resonance for risk stratification in chronic heart failure: prognostic value of late gadolinium enhancement in patients with non-ischaemic dilated cardiomyopathy. Heart 2011;97(9):727–32.

106. Desai MY, Ommen SR, McKenna WJ, et al. Imaging phenotype versus genotype in hypertrophic cardiomyopathy. Circ Cardiovasc Imaging 2011; 4(2):156–68.

107. Maron BJ. Contemporary insights and strategies for risk stratification and prevention of sudden death in hypertrophic cardiomyopathy. Circulation 2010;121(3):445–56.

108. Hughes SE. The pathology of hypertrophic cardiomyopathy. Histopathology 2004;44(5):412–27.

109. Maron MS. Clinical utility of cardiovascular magnetic resonance in hypertrophic cardiomyopathy. J Cardiovasc Magn Reson 2012;14:13.

110. Rickers C, Wilke NM, Jerosch-Herold M, et al. Utility of cardiac magnetic resonance imaging in the diagnosis of hypertrophic cardiomyopathy. Circulation 2005;112(6):855–61.

111. Maron MS, Lesser JR, Maron BJ. Management implications of massive left ventricular hypertrophy in hypertrophic cardiomyopathy significantly underestimated by echocardiography but identified by cardiovascular magnetic resonance. Am J Cardiol 2010;105(12):1842–3.

112. Moon JC, Fisher NG, McKenna WJ, et al. Detection of apical hypertrophic cardiomyopathy by cardiovascular magnetic resonance in patients with non-diagnostic echocardiography. Heart 2004; 90(6):645–9.

113. Fattori R, Biagini E, Lorenzini M, et al. Significance of magnetic resonance imaging in apical hypertrophic cardiomyopathy. Am J Cardiol 2010;105(11): 1592–6.

114. Green JJ, Berger JS, Kramer CM, et al. Prognostic value of late gadolinium enhancement in clinical outcomes for hypertrophic cardiomyopathy. JACC Cardiovasc Imaging 2012;5(4):370–7.

115. Maron MS, Olivotto I, Maron BJ, et al. The case for myocardial ischemia in hypertrophic cardiomyopathy. J Am Coll Cardiol 2009;54(9):866–75.

116. Fluechter S, Kuschyk J, Wolpert C, et al. Extent of late gadolinium enhancement detected by cardiovascular magnetic resonance correlates with the inducibility of ventricular tachyarrhythmia in hypertrophic cardiomyopathy. J Cardiovasc Magn Reson 2010;12:30.

117. Sagar S, Liu PP, Cooper LT Jr. Myocarditis. Lancet 2012;379(9817):738–47.

118. Childs H, Friedrich MG. Cardiovascular magnetic resonance imaging in myocarditis. Prog Cardiovasc Dis 2011;54(3):266–75.

119. Baughman KL. Diagnosis of myocarditis: death of Dallas criteria. Circulation 2006;113(4):593–5.

120. Cooper LT, Baughman KL, Feldman AM, et al. The role of endomyocardial biopsy in the management of cardiovascular disease: a scientific statement from the American Heart Association, the American College of Cardiology, and the European Society of Cardiology. Circulation 2007;116(19):2216–33.

121. Mahrholdt H, Goedecke C, Wagner A, et al. Cardiovascular magnetic resonance assessment of human myocarditis: a comparison to histology

and molecular pathology. Circulation 2004;109(10): 1250–8.

122. Monney PA, Sekhri N, Burchell T, et al. Acute myocarditis presenting as acute coronary syndrome: role of early cardiac magnetic resonance in its diagnosis. Heart 2011;97(16):1312–8.

123. Cummings KW, Bhalla S, Javidan-Nejad C, et al. A pattern-based approach to assessment of delayed enhancement in nonischemic cardiomyopathy at MR imaging. Radiographics 2009;29(1):89–103.

124. Cassone VM. Effects of melatonin on vertebrate circadian systems. Trends Neurosci 1990;13(11): 457–64.

125. Jacquier A, Prost C, Amabile N, et al. Gadolinium chelate kinetics in cardiac MR imaging of myocarditis: comparison to acute myocardial infarction and impact on late gadolinium enhancement. Invest Radiol 2011;46(11):705–10.

126. Mavrogeni S, Spargias C, Bratis C, et al. Myocarditis as a precipitating factor for heart failure: evaluation and 1-year follow-up using cardiovascular magnetic resonance and endomyocardial biopsy. Eur J Heart Fail 2011;13(8):830–7.

127. Grun S, Schumm J, Greulich S, et al. Long-term follow-up of biopsy-proven viral myocarditis: predictors of mortality and incomplete recovery. J Am Coll Cardiol 2012;59(18):1604–15.

128. Youssef G, Beanlands RS, Birnie DH, et al. Cardiac sarcoidosis: applications of imaging in diagnosis and directing treatment. Heart 2011;97(24):2078–87.

129. Yeboah J, Lee C, Sharma OP. Cardiac sarcoidosis: a review 2011. Curr Opin Pulm Med 2011;17(5): 308–15.

130. Sekhri V, Sanal S, Delorenzo LJ, et al. Cardiac sarcoidosis: a comprehensive review. Arch Med Sci 2011;7(4):546–54.

131. Patel MR, Cawley PJ, Heitner JF, et al. Detection of myocardial damage in patients with sarcoidosis. Circulation 2009;120(20):1969–77.

132. Smedema JP, Snoep G, van Kroonenburgh MP, et al. Cardiac involvement in patients with

pulmonary sarcoidosis assessed at two university medical centers in the Netherlands. Chest 2005; 128(1):30–5.

133. Ichinose A, Otani H, Oikawa M, et al. MRI of cardiac sarcoidosis: basal and subepicardial localization of myocardial lesions and their effect on left ventricular function. AJR Am J Roentgenol 2008; 191(3):862–9.

134. Smedema JP, Snoep G, van Kroonenburgh MP, et al. The additional value of gadolinium-enhanced MRI to standard assessment for cardiac involvement in patients with pulmonary sarcoidosis. Chest 2005; 128(3):1629–37.

135. Shimada T, Shimada K, Sakane T, et al. Diagnosis of cardiac sarcoidosis and evaluation of the effects of steroid therapy by gadolinium-DTPA-enhanced magnetic resonance imaging. Am J Med 2001; 110(7):520–7.

136. Selvanayagam JB, Leong DP. MR imaging and cardiac amyloidosis where to go from here? JACC Cardiovasc Imaging 2010;3(2):165–7.

137. Dubrey SW, Hawkins PN, Falk RH. Amyloid diseases of the heart: assessment, diagnosis, and referral. Heart 2011;97(1):75–84.

138. Kapoor P, Thenappan T, Singh E, et al. Cardiac amyloidosis: a practical approach to diagnosis and management. Am J Med 2011;124(11): 1006–15.

139. Syed IS, Glockner JF, Feng D, et al. Role of cardiac magnetic resonance imaging in the detection of cardiac amyloidosis. JACC Cardiovasc Imaging 2010;3(2):155–64.

140. Vogelsberg H, Mahrholdt H, Deluigi CC, et al. Cardiovascular magnetic resonance in clinically suspected cardiac amyloidosis: noninvasive imaging compared to endomyocardial biopsy. J Am Coll Cardiol 2008;51(10):1022–30.

141. Perugini E, Rapezzi C, Piva T, et al. Non-invasive evaluation of the myocardial substrate of cardiac amyloidosis by gadolinium cardiac magnetic resonance. Heart 2006;92(3):343–9.

Peripheral MR Angiography

J. Harald Kramer, MD[a,b,*], Thomas M. Grist, MD[a]

KEYWORDS

- Contrast-enhanced MRA • Peripheral arteries • Cardiovascular disease
- Magnetic Resonance Imaging

KEY POINTS

- Since the introduction of contrast-enhanced MR angiography (MRA), several different techniques for imaging of the peripheral arteries have evolved. All provide good diagnostic image quality, whereas some older techniques suffer from drawbacks, such as long acquisition time, impaired image quality from venous enhancement, or limited spatial resolution.
- Other techniques, such as CT angiography, digital subtraction angiography, and ultrasound, are superior to MRA in terms of spatial and/or temporal resolution. However, this superiority is only in certain anatomic areas or under certain circumstances.
- MRA provides the most comprehensive modality allowing the examination to be tailored to the patient and the specific question to be answered.

INTRODUCTION

Cardiovascular disease, with its major manifestations of coronary heart disease, cerebrovascular disease/stroke, and peripheral artery disease (PAD), still represents the leading cause of death in the United States.[1] Approximately 83 million American adults have one or more types of cardiovascular disease; 50% of these are older than 60 years of age. The prevalence of asymptomatic PAD lies between 3% and 10% in the general population, increasing to 15% to 20% in persons older than 70 years. Additionally, the prevalence of symptomatic PAD is approximately 3% in patients aged 40 years and 6% at 60 years.[2] However, these data might underestimate the total prevalence of cardiovascular disease, because screening studies showed that between 10% and 50% of all patients with intermittent claudication never consult a doctor about their symptoms. Besides family history of PAD, smoking is the most severe risk factor. Smokers are 3 times more often affected than nonsmokers. Furthermore, PAD is directly associated with arterial hypertension and diabetes mellitus,[3] and is the most common cause of nontraumatic limb amputation in the industrialized world, and thus an important economic factor in health care in the western world.[4]

The first clinical test performed to evaluate the presence or absence of PAD is calculation of the ankle brachial index (ABI), which is the ratio of the systolic pressure in the posterior tibial or dorsalis pedis artery divided by the systolic blood pressure in the brachial artery. A resting ABI of 0.90 or less correlates with a hemodynamically significant arterial stenosis, and therefore the ABI is often used to determine if suspected PAD is hemodynamically relevant. In symptomatic individuals, an ABI 0.90 or less is approximately 95% sensitive in detecting arteriogram-positive PAD and almost 100% specific in identifying healthy individuals.[5] Thus, this test is well suited for identifying individuals with PAD but is nonspecific for the exact localization of pathologic vascular lesions. Hence an

a Department of Radiology, University of Wisconsin–Madison, 600 Highland Avenue, Madison, WI 53792–3252, USA; b Institute for Clinical Radiology, Ludwig-Maximilians-University Hospital Munich, Marchioninistr. 15, 81377 Munich, Germany
* Corresponding author. Department of Radiology, University of Wisconsin–Madison, School of Medicine and Public Health, E1/372 Clinical Science Center, 600 Highland Avenue, Madison, WI 53792–3252.
E-mail address: hkramer3@wisc.edu

Magn Reson Imaging Clin N Am 20 (2012) 761–776
http://dx.doi.org/10.1016/j.mric.2012.08.002
1064-9689/12/$ – see front matter © 2012 Elsevier Inc. All rights reserved.

imaging modality that provides detailed information about the location and extent of vascular disease is of great interest.

Because digital subtraction angiography (DSA) has the highest spatial and temporal resolution compared with other imaging modalities and is the only technique that provides both diagnostic imaging and the opportunity of interventional procedures, it is still regarded as the standard of reference. However, the well-known disadvantages of DSA, including risks associated with the invasive procedure itself, ionizing radiation, and potentially nephrotoxic contrast agents, have led to a substantial change in the radiologic approach to the diagnosis of PAD in the past few years. CT angiography (CTA), MR angiography (MRA), and ultrasound, including Doppler techniques, can serve as noninvasive substitutes. The latter can provide high spatial resolution and dynamic information and vessel wall imaging in certain anatomic regions. However, other vascular territories are not accessible with ultrasound because of surrounding structures that impair imaging. Additionally, ultrasound in general suffers from its dependency on experienced examiners and patient preparation. CTA and MRA both feature user-independent noninvasive cross-sectional imaging of the entire arterial vasculature from head to toe. However, CTA suffers from the drawback of ionizing radiation and the need for potentially nephrotoxic contrast agents, and in some cases the influence of dense vessel wall calcifications on image analysis and rendering.

MRA, compared with other techniques, features the lowest spatial resolution but can provide dynamic information and vessel wall imaging with high soft tissue contrast without the definite need for contrast agents. However, the MR contrast agents are in general regarded as safe for the kidneys in patients with sufficient renal function (glomerular filtration rate >30 mL/min per 1.73 m^2) and are thus used in most MRA applications. Recently, some MRA contrast agents have been implicated in the development of nephrogenic systemic fibrosis in patients with significant renal insufficiency.[6,7] Therefore, new noncontrast MRA techniques have been developed to provide MRA images without the need for contrast agents. Recent technical developments, including the introduction of new image reconstruction algorithms and dedicated contrast agents, have pushed the limits of MRA toward higher spatial resolution and image quality and have enabled time-resolved imaging. The combination of multichannel MR systems, high field strength, multielement receiver coils for angiography and dedicated contrast agents has helped to substantially minimize most of the traditional drawbacks of MRA.[8]

CONTRAST AGENTS FOR MRA

Today, all contrast agents approved for MRA, or at least used for MRA, are gadolinium-based. However, these agents can be differentiated in several ways; besides relaxivity, the 2 most important ways depend on their molecular structure and their interaction with blood components. Diagnostic MRA examinations can be created with every gadolinium-based contrast agent (GBCA); however, the molecular structure, and therefore the characteristics of a GBCA, are of clinical importance in terms of resulting image quality. In addition, the molecular structure may be of significance in terms of molecular stability and the risk of releasing free gadolinium, which is highly toxic and seems to be the trigger for development of nephrogenic systemic fibrosis. The 2 structures present today are linear and cyclic molecules, although cyclic agents seem to be more stable than linear agents. The latter again can be divided into ionic and nonionic agents, although the ionic agents are regarded as more stable than the nonionic agents. In terms of interaction with blood components, most agents do not show any binding to blood components, specifically proteins (human serum albumin [HSA]). However, some agents feature at least a temporary linkage to blood proteins, which leads to a prolonged presence of contrast agent within the blood vessels because of a restricted transfer of contrast agent from the vessels to the surrounding tissue (**Table 1**).[9,10]

The current standard contrast agent for imaging of the entire body and vasculature is a 0.5-mol/L extracellular gadolinium chelate without any protein binding. This type of contrast agent provides reasonable image quality for nearly all clinical indications of MRA. The advent of innovative new contrast agents with properties distinct from those of the traditional extracellular gadolinium agents promises to further expand the clinical application of contrast-enhanced MRA (CE-MRA). For some anatomic regions or indications, high-relaxivity contrast agents with higher concentrations of gadolinium chelates and/or an at least transient binding to proteins seem to be beneficial. These indications include imaging of the carotid or renal arteries or time-resolved applications.[11–14]

Gadolinium chelates with protein binding feature a delayed passage or do not pass the vessel walls at all because of their size when bound to human serum proteins such as HSA. This effect helps make MRA more independent of the short-duration arterial first-pass imaging and allows for

Table 1
Ways to differentiate between contrast agents depending on their biochemical properties

	Linear		Cyclic	
	Ionic	**Nonionic**	**Ionic**	**Nonionic**
No protein binding	Gadopentetate dimeglumine (Magnevist)	Gadodiamide (Omniscan) Gadoversetamide (OptiMark)	Gadoterate meglumine (Dotarem)	Gadobutrol (Gadavist/Gadovist) Gadoteridol (ProHance)
Weak protein binding	Gadobenate dimeglumine (MultiHance) Gadoxetate disodium (Eovist/ Primovist)			
Strong protein binding	Gadofosveset trisodium (Ablavar)			

high spatial resolution at "steady state" (equilibrium state) with potentially prolonged acquisition times of up to several minutes.[15–18]

TECHNICAL CONCEPTS FOR PERIPHERAL MRA

The main prerequisite for any diagnostic imaging modality of the arterial vasculature is to get high enough spatial resolution for reliable stenosis grading in combination with sufficient vessel contrast. In addition, dynamic information can be of great value for comprehensive imaging of diseased vasculature. Detailed vessel wall evaluation also potentially helps to further increase the image quality and specificity of an examination. An MRA dataset of high image quality features excellent signal-to-noise ratio and is free of venous enhancement. To reach this goal with MRA, several technical concepts evolved over time. Of all available methods, CE-MRA has evolved as the preferred technique for MR imaging of the arterial vasculature.[8,19–21] CE-MRA can be performed in several different ways, and the contrast agent application scheme must be tailored to every CE-MRA technique (**Table 2**).

CE-MRA

The basic principle of CE-MRA is to image gadolinium-enhanced blood. Thus, gadolinium arterial first pass must be synchronized with the acquisition of at least central k-space information to acquire an angiogram of the arterial lumen during the arterial phase.[22,23] Peripheral parts of k-space are sampled not necessarily during peak arterial enhancement but rather should be while the injected contrast agent is present in the imaged field

of view (FOV) to avoid artifacts (eg, edge blurring). However, injection of GBCA only leads to transient T1 shortening of the blood pool. Generally, enough contrast must be injected to decrease the T1 of blood to values smaller than those of stationary background tissues. After having briefly enhanced the arterial vasculature, most GBCAs rapidly diffuse into the extravascular extracellular space. Relative to peak arterial concentration, the intravascular half-life of commercially approved standard GBCA is approximately 90 seconds. Some dedicated GBCAs feature a longer intravascular half-life because of interaction with proteins in the blood pool. The major challenge in CE-MRA is balancing arterial first pass, spatial resolution, anatomic coverage, and data acquisition time.

Depending on the clinical question, imaging at one or multiple phases is recommended. Before GBCA is injected, a nonenhanced acquisition with exactly the same sequence settings as the contrast-enhanced scans should be acquired for later subtraction. Many of the primary clinical questions can be answered with only one postcontrast acquisition during the arterial first pass, especially for the larger proximal vessels. However, sometimes additional phases are needed, such as in the case of imbalanced filling of the arterial vasculature of both legs or to detect low flow collaterals. To get best results for peripheral MRA in terms of image quality, several different acquisition schemes were developed and are still used.

STEP-BY-STEP MRA WITH MULTIPLE CONTRAST AGENT APPLICATIONS

One major problem when imaging the vasculature of the pelvis and runoff vessels is that the volume

Table 2
Review on the literature about different techniques for peripheral MRA and their contrast agent application schemes

MRA Technique	Author/Journal	Year	B_0	Gadolinium-Based Contrast Agents	Total Dose	Injection Scheme
Bolus-chase	Czum et al,[26] *Journal of Magnetic Resonance Imaging*	2000	1.5T	Gadoteridol	40 mL	20 mL @ 0.5 mL/s 20 mL @ 1.5 mL/s
Bolus-chase	Hany et al,[50] *Radiology*	2001	1.5T	Gadodiamide	40 mL	20 mL @ 1 mL/s 20 mL @ 0.5 mL/s
Bolus-chase	Kramer et al,[27] *Investigative Radiology*	2007	3.0T	Gadopentetate dimeglumine	20 mL	10 mL @ 1.5 mL/s 10 mL @ 0.8 mL/s
Bolus-chase	Maki et al,[51] *Journal of Magnetic Resonance Imaging*	2009	1.5T	Gadopentetate dimeglumine	40 mL	20 mL @ 1.8 mL/s 20 mL @ 1.4 mL/s
Bolus-chase	Maki et al,[51] *Journal of Magnetic Resonance Imaging*	2009	1.5T	Gadofosveset	0.05 mmol/kg	Calc. mL @ 0.7 mL/s
Bolus-chase	Anzidei et al,[52] *Investigative Radiology*	2011	1.5T	Gadobenate dimeglumine	15 mL	10 mL @ 2 mL/s first pass 5 mL @ 0.5 mL/s steady state
Continuous table movement	Kramer et al,[41] *Investigative Radiology*	2008	3.0T	Gadopentetate dimeglumine	15 mL	15 mL @ 1 mL/s
Continuous table movement	Voth et al,[53] *Investigative Radiology*	2009	3.0T	Gadobutrol	0.1 mmol/kg diluted 1:1 with saline	Calc. mL @ 1.5 mL/s
Hybrid MRA	Meissner et al,[32] *Radiology*	2005	1.5T	Gadopentetate dimeglumine	40 mL	15 mL @ 1.5 mL/s calf 25 mL @ 2 mL/s abdomen + thigh
Hybrid MRA	Berg et al,[34] *Investigative Radiology*	2008	3.0T	Gadodiamide	35 mL	10 mL @ 1 mL/s calf 15 mL @ 1 mL/s + 10 mL @ 0.6 mL/s abdomen + thigh
Multiple injection	Hany et al,[50] *Radiology*	2001	1.5T	Gadodiamide	38 mL	10 mL @ 2 mL/s stat. abdomen 13 mL @ 0.5 mL/s dyn. thigh 15 mL @ 0.5 mL/s dyn. calf
Multiple injection	Janka et al,[54] *Cardiovascular Interventional Radiology*	2006	1.5T	Gadopentetate dimeglumine	35 mL	10 mL @ 1.0 mL/s abdomen 15 mL @ 1.0 mL/s thigh 10 mL @ 1.0 mL/s calf

Abbreviations: calc, calculated; stat, static; dyn, dynamic.

of interest cannot be covered within a single FOV, and therefore multiple imaging acquisition stations are required. Thus, the GBCA bolus can "outrun" the ability of the MR scanner to acquire images at multiple locations, therefore risking venous enhancement that confounds image interpretation. Standard acquisition time for MRA of one FOV without any acceleration techniques at reasonable spatial resolution, anatomic coverage, and signal-to-noise ratio requires approximately 20 to 30 seconds. When injecting a standard dose of GBCA and then performing consecutive imaging of the infrarenal aorta, pelvic, thigh, and calf vessels, venous enhancement and overlay will occur, especially at the distal station (**Fig. 1**). Because of the anatomic circumstances, especially in the lower leg with 2 veins running adjacent to 1 artery, visualization of the arteries can be significantly degraded by enhancement of the veins. The easiest way to avoid this is to perform single injections for every acquired FOV and hence conduct arterial first-pass imaging in each single station as the first station after injection of the contrast bolus (**Fig. 2**).[24] Several different contrast agent injection schemes are available for this technique, the easiest of which is simply to use fluoroscopic triggering for every single station. Here,

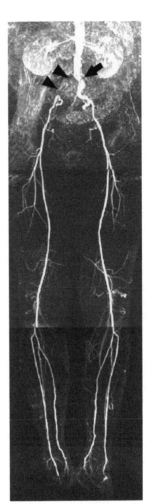

Fig. 2. Peripheral MRA acquired in 3 stations with 3 single contrast-agent administrations. Note the absence of any venous enhancement because of proper timing of contrast arrival time and image acquisition for every single station. A composite image of coronal maximum-intensity projection images from a 3-station 3-dimensional time-resolved imaging of contrast kinetics runoff in a 58-year-old male patient. A complete right common iliac occlusion (*arrowsheads*) and a stenotic left common iliac origin (*single arrow*) were confirmed on an x-ray DSA examination.

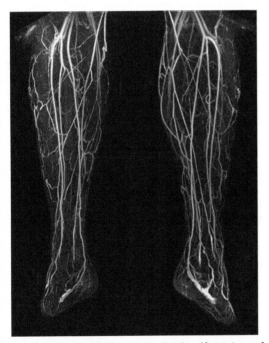

Fig. 1. Example of the most distal calf station of a bolus-chase MRA showing major venous overlay caused by long acquisition times for the more proximal abdominal and thigh vessels. Note the enhancement of venous vessels directly adjacent to the arteries, impairing the diagnostic quality of that study.

2-dimensional (2D) low-resolution gradient-echo images are acquired and monitored in real time. As soon as the contrast agent is seen in the FOV, the operator initiates acquisition of high-resolution MRA data manually. The downside of this multi-injection technique is the increasing amount of intravascular and extravascular GBCA, which influences the background signal and thus decreases the contrast-to-noise ratio in subsequent vessel territories. The presence of GBCA in the blood also causes the arrival of the new contrast bolus after injection to be very difficult to detect. The total amount of injected GBCA required for imaging also increases, which is disadvantageous, especially in patients with impaired renal function, because it places them at higher risk for developing nephrogenic systemic fibrosis. Finally, the larger amount of injected contrast material increases costs. However, this technique offers the opportunity to perform high-spatial-resolution imaging of each single station without concern about the length of the acquisition.

STEP-BY-STEP MRA WITH BOLUS CHASE

Using this technique, only one bolus of GBCA is injected and consecutive FOVs are acquired during the passage of this single bolus. To avoid the occurrence of venous enhancement in the subsequent steps, acquisition time of the earlier steps is restricted. The development of dedicated k-space sampling schemes, such as centric, elliptic centric, or other nonstandard Cartesian readout methods, and the introduction of parallel imaging helped overcome the need to shorten data acquisition through reducing spatial resolution or anatomic coverage.[25–28] The time needed to sample the most important center parts of k-space and the sequences' entire sampling time can be reduced significantly to approximately 20 seconds through implementing parallel imaging and adapting the readout to the needs of MRA while spatial resolution remains unchanged.[29–31] Through matching the contrast agents' application scheme to the imaging protocol, only one injection of standard-dose GBCA is necessary to acquire MRA data sets featuring arterial-only imaging at good image quality (**Fig. 3**). One exception to this rule is when high-spatial-resolution imaging of the distal calf and foot vessels is required. This vascular territory is often of clinical interest for therapy planning; therefore, dedicated imaging of the calf vessels can be performed with a hybrid technique, described later.

When using the bolus chase technique, data acquisition must be started in the most proximal station as early as the contrast agent bolus reaches the vessels of interest. This timing can be assured by either using a test bolus technique to estimate contrast agent arrival time or using fluoroscopic triggering, as mentioned earlier. Additionally, the injection profile should be customized to create a high initial peak bolus with an extended duration of sufficiently high concentration within the arterial vasculature. If this is done, subsequent vascular territories can be imaged in an arterial phase without venous enhancement. A way to influence the shape of the contrast agent bolus is to use a biphasic or multiphasic injection scheme in which different amounts of the bolus are injected at different flow rates, such as injecting the first half of the total volume at a high flow rate to assure a well-circumscribed and high peak maximum followed by injection of the second half of the total volume at a lower flow rate to assure a lengthened bolus.

Another option to further decrease the risk of venous contamination is to use venous compression techniques, in which a blood pressure cuff or dedicated devices are wrapped around the thighs of the patient and inflated to a pressure higher than that in the venous system but lower than that in the arterial vasculature. This method enables the inflow of contrast agent into the arteries but decreases the venous backflow and thus delays venous enhancement.

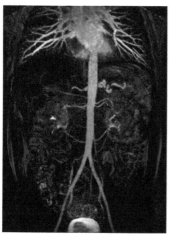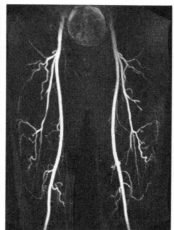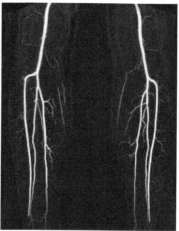

Fig. 3. Three-station bolus-chase MRA showing no venous contamination in the most distal station because of reduction of acquisition time in the more proximal stations from the use of parallel imaging techniques.

HYBRID CE-MRA

A 3-dimensional (3D) CE-MRA examination of the pelvis and lower extremities is commonly performed using a 3-station moving-table bolus chase technique. With this technique, the timing of the bolus is optimized for the first station (abdomen–pelvis), and then imaging is performed as rapidly as possible to try to keep up with the bolus of gadolinium as it passes to the feet. Although image quality is generally excellent for evaluating the first 2 stations (abdomen–pelvis and thigh), image quality of the most distal station can be inadequate for assessing the calf and foot vasculature because of venous contamination. To overcome this restriction, hybrid MRA was introduced. With this technique, the problem of venous enhancement in the most distal calf station is addressed through imaging this station first and in multiple temporal phases. Afterward, the more proximal abdominal and thigh stations are imaged with a second bolus of contrast agent (**Fig. 4**).[32–34] For an accurate assessment of bolus arrival time in the abdominal aorta and the calf, a test bolus measurement is performed at 2 different positions. For timing of data acquisition of the calf station, the arrival time of contrast agent is assessed at the level of the popliteal artery. To measure arrival time of contrast agent for the abdominal station, a region of interest is placed in the abdominal aorta at the height of the diaphragm. Acquisition of thigh MRA is directly initiated after acquisition of abdominal MRA without any additional timing bolus. With this protocol, the entire vasculature of the lower extremity, from the diaphragm down to the feet, can be imaged without any venous overlay at high spatial resolution, and dynamic information can be provided on the contrast inflow in the lower leg. These high-quality data sets are critical for treatment planning in cases with arterial occlusion when the decision is between revascularization/bypass surgery or amputation. However, this technique may be complex for those who do not perform peripheral MRA frequently, because contrast agent timing is still somewhat complicated using the 2-test-bolus approach described earlier.

TIME-RESOLVED MRA

Temporal resolution can add clinically valuable information to an examination of the peripheral arteries, including collateral flow pathways, assessment of asymmetric flow states, and visualization of arterial to venous shunting. It is suboptimal to simply repeat the standard MRA acquisition several times, because important dynamic information is lost due to the poor temporal resolution of any approach without image acceleration or view sharing. The added information from sequential standard acquisitions with an acquisition time for a single-station MRA of approximately 20 seconds is limited. Therefore, view-sharing techniques to accelerate the acquisition of 3D time-resolved MRA data sets were developed. Ordinarily, the acquisition of time-resolved MRA images requires a tradeoff between temporal and spatial resolution. View-sharing techniques, such as 3D time-resolved imaging of contrast kinetics (TRICKs), help achieve a clinically practical optimization of temporal and spatial resolution.[14,35–43] For these techniques, the center part of k-space, which encodes for contrasts in the image, is sampled more frequently than the periphery of k-space, which encodes for the details in the image. A series of time-resolved 3D data sets are re-created through sharing central and peripheral k-space data during the passage of the arterial phase of contrast enhancement. No need exists for accurate contrast agent application timing because multiple images are rapidly acquired and show the passage of contrast through the arteries of interest. Likewise, early images serve as mask images for later subtraction, creating a 3D time-resolved digital subtraction MR angiographic image. Recent developments in fat suppression also can eliminate or reduce the need for subtraction (**Fig. 5**).

The settings for spatial and temporal resolution of a time-resolved MRA acquisition should be tailored to the anatomic region and the clinical question. Generally, for dynamic imaging of a circumscribed vessel area, eg, the carotid arteries, a higher temporal resolution is needed than for dynamic imaging of the entire peripheral vasculature. Additionally, the needed temporal resolution to answer the question for collateral vessels in the case of an occluded lower leg artery is different from that needed to answer the question for a high- versus low-flow arteriovenous malformation (**Fig. 6**). When changing sequence parameters in terms of temporal resolution, adapting the contrast agent injection scheme is also recommended. Examinations with a high temporal resolution require a higher injection rate to get a well-circumscribed contrast agent bolus.

MRA WITH CONTINUOUS TABLE MOVEMENT

To compensate for the challenges associated with imaging larger anatomic areas, such as the lower extremity peripheral arteries, different multistep approaches were successfully implemented for MRA of the lower limb. Bolus chase techniques with the use of multistation table motion allow the

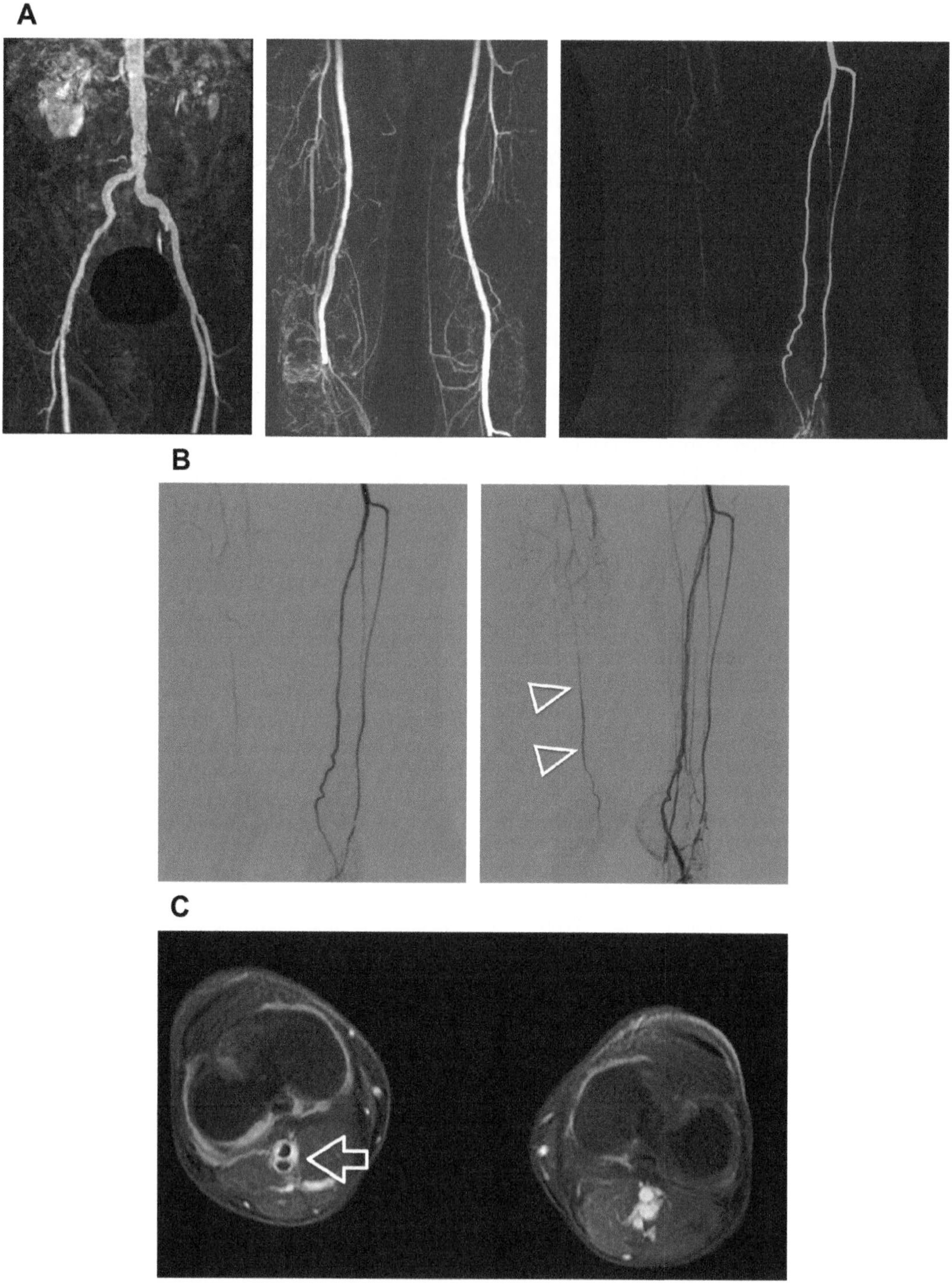

Fig. 4. Peripheral MRA using hybrid technique. (*A*) Images were acquired at 3 stations, including aorta iliac, thigh, and calf stations. The examination was performed using 2 injections of gadolinium contrast media. The calf station was acquired first, using the 3D time-resolved imaging of contrast kinetics (TRICKs) technique after injection of 10-mL gadolinium contrast. Subsequently, a 2-station MRA was performed at the aortal iliac and thigh stations using a single injection of 20-mL gadolinium contrast media and moving the table automatically between separate 3D MRA examinations at each station. (*B*) Time-resolved digital subtraction angiography of the calf station using the 3D TRICKs technique. Early 3-vessel runoff is seen on the left, and little perfusion or vessel opacification on the right. Later arterial phase shows reconstitution of flow in the right posterior tibial artery (*arrowheads*) from proximal occlusion. (*C*) Delayed, postcontrast, fat-suppressed, T1-weighted gradient-echo image showing thrombus occluding the popliteal artery and popliteal vein on the right (*arrow*), corresponding to the abrupt occlusion of the contrast column identified on the MRA image. The delayed fat-suppressed imaging is acquired with an interleaved 2D gradient-echo acquisition (TR equals 110 ms, TE equals 2 ms; 20 slices in 20 seconds). Image is acquired after a 30-mL gadobenate dimeglumine injection; the weak protein binding enhances the blood pool signal, providing excellent contrast between the vessels and surrounding tissues in steady state.

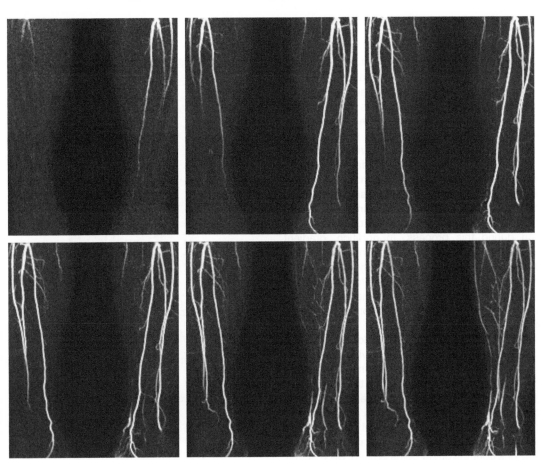

Fig. 5. Dynamic MRA using view sharing. Through compromising spatial resolution, dynamic information of up to 1 frame per approximately 1.5 seconds can be reached at reasonable image quality. Example of a dynamic MRA of the calves without stenotic disease but showing slightly delayed inflow on the right, which might cause a problem in static single-phase MRA.

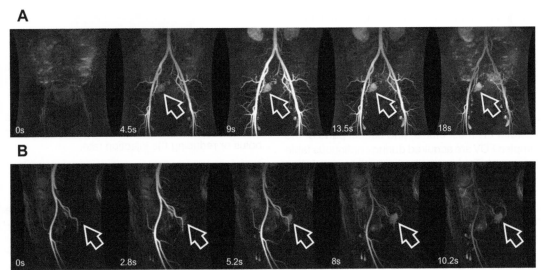

Fig. 6. Example of a dynamic MRA acquired at 2 different temporal resolutions. Set of images (*A*) shows every frame of a dynamic MRA in coronal orientation with a temporal resolution of 5.5 seconds per frame. Note the highly perfused lesion next to the patient's right internal iliac artery (IIA) showing up simultaneously with the arterial vasculature (*arrow*). (*B*) Images showing every second frame of a dynamic MRA of the same patient in sagittal orientation acquired with a temporal resolution of 1.4 seconds per frame. Note the time difference of contrast agent inflow to the IIA compared with the vascular lesion (*arrow*), making this a low-flow arteriovenous malformation.

stepwise assessment of the pelvic and runoff arteries within a single examination. Although various multistation approaches have been shown to be effective, these protocols have several inherent limitations. To cover extended anatomy with high image resolution and to stay within the arterial time window to prevent venous overlay, imaging time is restricted and data acquisition must be adapted to blood flow dynamics. Repositioning of the table between discrete stations, however, leads to a reduction in image time efficiency because of the interruption of data acquisition during this process. In addition, gradient nonlinearities at the edges of individual FOVs must be taken into account. Finally, planning and data acquisition of multiple steps for both nonenhanced and contrast-enhanced imaging are time-consuming, complicated, and prone to technical error.

These limitations have been addressed by the introduction of continuously moving table data acquisitions that provide seamless volume coverage and optimize image time efficiency (**Fig. 7**).[38,44,45] With this technique, planning and performing the examination are much easier, because only one FOV for the entire vasculature of the lower body part must be positioned and only one contrast agent bolus is used. Slice acquisition in the coronal plane is particularly beneficial for data sets in peripheral MRA, in which there is a large FOV in the *x*- (left-right) and *z*-directions (craniocaudal) but less in the *y* (anterior-posterior) plane. Before table movement is initiated in continuous-table-movement MRA, some data are acquired without moving the table to acquire the most cranial part of the FOV. Likewise, the data acquisition is prolonged for a few seconds at the end of the imaging range (ie, after the table has stopped moving) to acquire the peripheral parts of k-space in the most distal part of the acquired volume. All data referring to anatomic structures between the most cranial and caudal parts of the sampled FOV are acquired during continuous table movement. Table velocity during data acquisition is influenced by several parameters, whereas the most important ones are the acquired spatial resolution and the applied parallel imaging factor; in other words, the slower the patient table is moving, the more data are acquired. However, spatial resolution and length of FOV in head–feet direction are limited by the amount of data that can be processed by the MR system within a certain time. The contrast application scheme also must be adapted to this technique. Data acquisition can be initiated based on a test bolus or fluoroscopic triggering, as described earlier for other techniques. However, the shape of the contrast agent

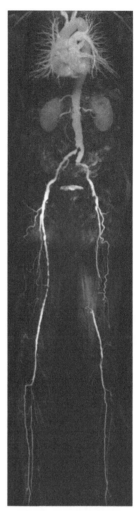

Fig. 7. Example of a peripheral MRA acquired at continuous table movement. Note the absence of any fusion-steps between the vascular levels because of one seamlessly acquired FOV in the patient's *z*-direction.

bolus must be adapted to the prolonged data acquisition, which can be done by using a biphasic bolus or reducing the injection rate.

NON–CE-MRA

The first MRI technique for imaging vasculature was a non–contrast enhanced technique (non–CE-MRA). Nowadays, contrast-enhanced techniques are the standard of reference; however, in patients with impaired renal function or allergies to GBCAs, non–CE-MRA techniques are desirable. The first non–CE-MRA technique used was time-of-flight MRA.[39–41] This technique is still used for imaging of the intracranial vasculature and, in some cases, the feet vasculature, because of its high spatial resolution (**Fig. 8**). Time-of-flight

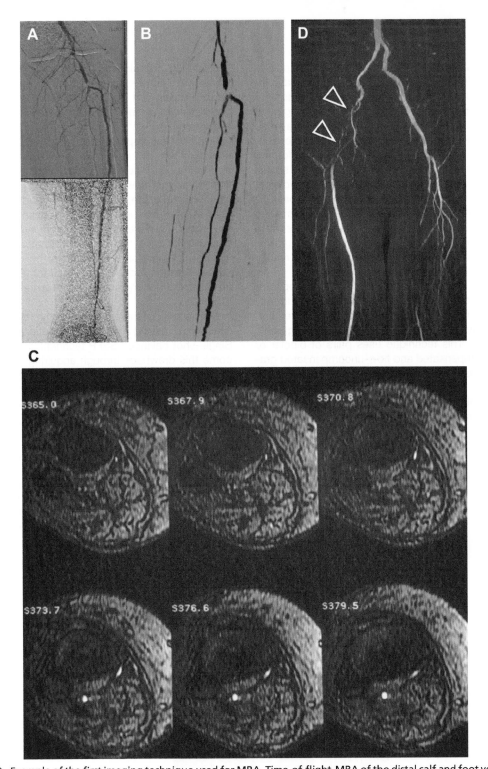

Fig. 8. Example of the first imaging technique used for MRA. Time-of-flight-MRA of the distal calf and foot vessels. Occult vessel shown using a 2D time-of-flight MRA technique. (*A*) Digital subtraction angiogram shows poor opacification of the runoff vessels, with poor visualization of the tibioperoneal trunk and anterior tibial artery. The peroneal and posterior tibial artery are not clearly shown. (*B*) Two-dimensional time-of-flight MRA shows stenosis at the distal tibioperoneal trunk, a patent anterior tibial artery, and a peroneal artery. (*C, D*) Source images and a maximum-intensity projection MRA rendering from a different 2D time-of-flight MRA of the peripheral vasculature. Note the right external iliac artery occlusion (*arrowheads*) with reconstitution of flow in the right superficial femoral artery. The flow distal to the right external iliac artery occlusion is monophasic rather than normal triphasic flow, with a high diastolic flow component, giving rise to the improved signal in the right superficial femoral artery. Retrograde flow in the occluded distal external iliac artery is not shown by the 2D time-of-flight technique because of the use of a spatial presaturation pulse to suppress venous flow. (*From* Grist TM. MRA of the abdominal aorta and lower extremities. J Magn Reson Imaging 2000;11(1):32–43; with permission.)

angiography relies on the differences in exposure to radiofrequency excitation between in-plane/in-slab stationary protons and the blood protons flowing into the section/slab. For selective imaging of arteries or veins, saturation bands can be applied to null the signal from the unwanted inflow of non-saturated protons. Acquisition can be performed using 2D or 3D methods, depending on the spatial resolution required, extent of the imaged volume, and the available imaging time. A drawback of this method was and still is the small imaging volume and the occurrence of artifacts because of slow, in-plane, or turbulent flow, impeding diagnosis and potentially causing false-positive results in terms of detecting significant stenoses.

Some of these same limitations also apply for phase-contrast imaging; this technique is currently mostly used for flow imaging and measurement, but only in rare cases for pure angiographic imaging. This technique uses pairs of bipolar or flow-compensated and flow-uncompensated gradient pulses to generate flow-sensitive phase images. Phase data can be used either to reconstruct velocity-encoded flow-quantification images or MR angiographic images.

Emerging techniques for MRA of the lower extremities are electrocardiography-gated 3D partial-Fourier fast spin echo (FSE) sequences and balanced steady-state free precession (SSFP) sequences (**Fig. 9**).[42,43,46]

Electrocardiography-gated 3D FSE imaging relies on the different flow patterns of arteries and veins. Slow-flowing blood (such as venous flow or arterial flow in diastole) has high signal, whereas modulated fast-flowing blood (arterial) shows flow voids in the systolic phase and has low signal. Data are acquired in both systolic and diastolic phases and later subtracted to get a pure high-flow arterial image of the examined region. This technique can be used for peripheral, thoracic, pulmonary, and, to some extent, carotid imaging.

A drawback of this technique is the long acquisition time, making it sensitive to motion artifacts. Single-shot balanced SSFP techniques can overcome this drawback through acquiring single 2D slices without the need for later subtraction. Quiescent-interval single-shot unenhanced MRA has proven to be a robust alternative to CE-MRA of the peripheral arteries.[47,48]

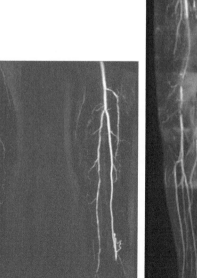
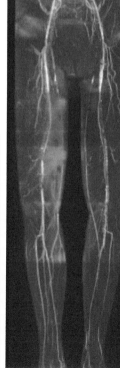

Fig. 9. Examples of advanced non-CE-MRA techniques. FSE *(A)* and SSFP *(B)* techniques both feature promising results but are prone to artifacts in severely diseased vessels with abnormal flow-patterns in the region of vascular lesions.

MR VENOGRAPHY AND HIGH-RESOLUTION STEADY-STATE IMAGING

MRA is mostly used for arterial-only imaging, and efforts are made to avoid any venous enhancement. However, dedicated clinical questions, such as evaluation of deep vein thrombosis or varicose veins, can also be answered by MRA. In the past this was mostly done using flow-dependent nonenhanced techniques. The administration of contrast agents can simplify these examinations and possibly provide additional information. When using standard contrast agents, it is possible to just perform multiphasic imaging until not only the arterial vasculature shows contrast enhancement but also the venous vessels. However, as in arterial imaging, the acquisition time frame before the contrast agent dispenses into the surrounding tissue is short. Blood pool contrast agents with a transient binding to HSA enable high-resolution steady-state imaging of the arterial and venous vasculature, allowing for evaluation of deep vein thrombosis and subtle changes of the vessel wall (**Fig. 10**).[16,49]

CLINICAL APPLICATION

The toolbox available for MRA of the peripheral vasculature makes MRA the beneficial modality for therapy planning in patients with peripheral vessel disease. It delivers excellent image quality at high spatial resolution and dynamic information without the drawbacks of competing modalities, such as ionizing radiation, user dependency, nephrotoxic contrast agents, and the absence of dynamic information. Intermittent claudication is mostly the first symptom of the manifestation of atherosclerosis and PAD, because earlier stages are often not diagnosed as PAD. A major criterion when diagnosing PAD with any imaging modality is to differentiate between a short, focal stenosis or occlusion and an occlusion over a long segment. Because of the development of collaterals if the diseased vessels narrow over a longer period, the imaging findings do not always correlate with the clinical symptoms. Critical limb ischemia with the risk of major tissue loss and amputation is one of the most severe complications in patients with PAD. Information about the extent of vascular

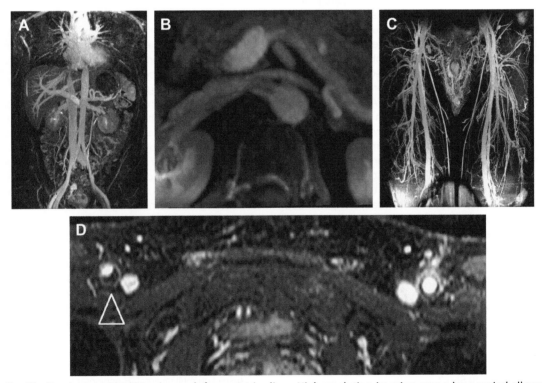

Fig. 10. Steady-state CE-MRA using gadofosveset trisodium. High-resolution imaging over a long period allows visualization of arterial and venous structures; however, venous overlay obscures arterial visualization on the maximum-intensity projection images (*A, C*). However, the high-resolution acquisition allows reconstruction of the steady-state images to show (*B*) duplicature of the right renal artery and (*D*) arterial plaque in the superficial femoral artery on the right (*arrowhead*).

lesions and the inflow and outflow segments is essential. Only invasive DSA or dynamic MRA can serve with this information for the entire peripheral vasculature. Arterial embolism leads to an acute reduction of peripheral blood supply, usually producing new or worsening symptoms and signs, and often threatening limb viability. Diagnosis of acute leg ischemia most often is based on clinical symptoms. As imaging modalities, DSA or, as a noninvasive alternative, CTA are taken into account because DSA offers the possibility of immediate intervention and CTA offers fast imaging. However, because data acquisition is getting fast and faster, MRA represents an alternative to CTA because it can add valuable dynamic information and is not impaired by calcifications, which are sometimes hard to differentiate from iodinated contrast agent in CT.

SUMMARY

Since the introduction of contrast-enhanced MRA, several different techniques for imaging the peripheral arteries have evolved. All of them provide good diagnostic image quality, whereas some older techniques suffer from drawbacks, such as long acquisition time, impaired image quality from venous enhancement, and limited spatial resolution. Most of these could be eliminated by the development of dedicated readout schemes tailored for MRA, the introduction of fast data sampling techniques, and dedicated contrast agents with characteristics beneficial for MRA. Other techniques, such as CTA, DSA, or ultrasound, are superior to MRA in terms of spatial and/or temporal resolution. However, this superiority occurs only in certain anatomic areas or under certain circumstances. MRA provides the most comprehensive modality allowing the examination to be tailored to the patient and the specific question to be answered. The drawbacks experienced at the introduction of MRA to clinical routine have largely been overcome or at least diminished, so that the benefits of MRA outbalance the limitations.

REFERENCES

1. Minino A. Death: final data for 2008. Natl Vital Stat Rep 2011;59(10):1–126.
2. Norgren L, Hiatt WR, Dormandy JA, et al. Inter-Society Consensus for the Management of Peripheral Arterial Disease (TASC II). J Vasc Surg 2007; 45(Suppl S):S5–67.
3. Weckbach S, Findeisen HM, Schoenberg SO, et al. Systemic cardiovascular complications in patients with long-standing diabetes mellitus: comprehensive assessment with whole-body magnetic

4. resonance imaging/magnetic resonance angiography. Invest Radiol 2009;44(4):242–50.
4. Dormandy J, Heeck L, Vig S. Acute limb ischemia. Semin Vasc Surg 1999;12(2):148–53.
5. Diehm C, Kareem S, Lawall H. Epidemiology of peripheral arterial disease. Vasa 2004;33(4):183–9.
6. Cowper SE. Nephrogenic systemic fibrosis: a review and exploration of the role of gadolinium. Adv Dermatol 2007;23:131–54.
7. Thomsen HS. Nephrogenic systemic fibrosis: a serious late adverse reaction to gadodiamide. Eur Radiol 2006;16(12):2619–21.
8. Green D, Parker D. CTA and MRA: visualization without catheterization. Semin Ultrasound CT MR 2003;24(4):185–91.
9. Pintaske J, Martirosian P, Graf H, et al. Relaxivity of gadopentetate dimeglumine (Magnevist), gadobutrol (Gadovist), and gadobenate dimeglumine (MultiHance) in human blood plasma at 0.2, 1.5, and 3 Tesla. Invest Radiol 2006;41(3):213–21.
10. Rohrer M, Bauer H, Mintorovitch J, et al. Comparison of magnetic properties of MRI contrast media solutions at different magnetic field strengths. Invest Radiol 2005;40(11):715–24.
11. Goyen M, Herborn CU, Vogt FM, et al. Using a 1 M Gd-chelate (gadobutrol) for total-body three-dimensional MR angiography: preliminary experience. J Magn Reson Imaging 2003;17(5):565–71.
12. Goyen M, Lauenstein TC, Herborn CU, et al. 0.5 M Gd chelate (Magnevist) versus 1.0 M Gd chelate (Gadovist): dose-independent effect on image quality of pelvic three-dimensional MR-angiography. J Magn Reson Imaging 2001;14(5):602–7.
13. Gregor M, Tombach B, Hentsch A, et al. Peripheral run-off CE-MRA with a 1.0 molar gadolinium chelate (Gadovist) with intraarterial DSA comparison. Acad Radiol 2002;9(Suppl 2):S398–400.
14. Kramer H, Michaely HJ, Requardt M, et al. Effects of injection rate and dose on image quality in time-resolved magnetic resonance angiography (MRA) by using 1.0M contrast agents. Eur Radiol 2007; 17(6):1394–402.
15. Klessen C, Hein PA, Huppertz A, et al. First-pass whole-body magnetic resonance angiography (MRA) using the blood-pool contrast medium gadofosveset trisodium: comparison to gadopentetate dimeglumine. Invest Radiol 2007;42(9):659–64.
16. Hoffmann U, Loewe C, Bernhard C, et al. MRA of the lower extremities in patients with pulmonary embolism using a blood pool contrast agent: initial experience. J Magn Reson Imaging 2002;15(4):429–37.
17. Nikolaou K, Kramer H, Grosse C, et al. High-spatial-resolution multistation MR angiography with parallel imaging and blood pool contrast agent: initial experience. Radiology 2006;241(3):861–72.
18. Tombach B, Reimer P, Bremer C, et al. First-pass and equilibrium-MRA of the aortoiliac region with

a superparamagnetic iron oxide blood pool MR contrast agent (SH U 555 C): results of a human pilot study. NMR Biomed 2004;17(7):500–6.

19. Fink C, Ley S, Schoenberg SO, et al. Magnetic resonance imaging of acute pulmonary embolism. Eur Radiol 2007;17(10):2546–53.

20. Goyen M, Debatin JF, Ruehm SG. Peripheral magnetic resonance angiography. Top Magn Reson Imaging 2001;12(5):327–35.

21. Leiner T. Magnetic resonance angiography of abdominal and lower extremity vasculature. Top Magn Reson Imaging 2005;16(1):21–66.

22. Marchal G, Michiels J, Bosmans H, et al. Contrast-enhanced MRA of the brain. J Comput Assist Tomogr 1992;16(1):25–9.

23. Bongartz GM, Boos M, Winter K, et al. Clinical utility of contrast-enhanced MR angiography. Eur Radiol 1997;7(Suppl 5):178–86.

24. Westenberg JJ, Wasser MN, van der Geest RJ, et al. Scan optimization of gadolinium contrast-enhanced three-dimensional MRA of peripheral arteries with multiple bolus injections and in vitro validation of stenosis quantification. Magn Reson Imaging 1999; 17(1):47–57.

25. Hood MN, Ho VB, Foo TK, et al. High-resolution gadolinium-enhanced 3D MRA of the infrapopliteal arteries. Lessons for improving bolus-chase peripheral MRA. Magn Reson Imaging 2002;20(7):543–9.

26. Czum JM, Ho VB, Hood MN, et al. Bolus-chase peripheral 3D MRA using a dual-rate contrast media injection. J Magn Reson Imaging 2000;12(5):769–75.

27. Kramer H, Michaely HJ, Matschl V, et al. High-resolution magnetic resonance angiography of the lower extremities with a dedicated 36-element matrix coil at 3 Tesla. Invest Radiol 2007;42(6):477–83.

28. Kramer H, Michaely HJ, Reiser MF, et al. Peripheral magnetic resonance angiography at 3.0 T. Top Magn Reson Imaging 2007;18(2):135–8.

29. Bammer R, Schoenberg SO. Current concepts and advances in clinical parallel magnetic resonance imaging. Top Magn Reson Imaging 2004;15(3):129–58.

30. Blaimer M, Breuer F, Mueller M, et al. SMASH, SENSE, PILS, GRAPPA: how to choose the optimal method. Top Magn Reson Imaging 2004;15(4):223–36.

31. Nokes SR. Elliptic centric contrast enhanced MRA provides high resolution, noninvasive evaluation of the carotid/vertebral arteries. J Ark Med Soc 2001; 98(3):83–8.

32. Meissner OA, Rieger J, Weber C, et al. Critical limb ischemia: hybrid MR angiography compared with DSA. Radiology 2005;235(1):308–18.

33. Hany TF, Pfammatter T, Debatin JF. Clinical use of contrast-enhanced MR angiography. Schweiz Med Wochenschr 1998;128(14):544–51 [in German].

34. Berg F, Bangard C, Bovenschulte H, et al. Feasibility of peripheral contrast-enhanced magnetic resonance angiography at 3.0 Tesla with a hybrid technique:

comparison with digital subtraction angiography. Invest Radiol 2008;43(9):642–9.

35. Thornton FJ, Du J, Suleiman SA, et al. High-resolution, time-resolved MRA provides superior definition of lower-extremity arterial segments compared to 2D time-of-flight imaging. J Magn Reson Imaging 2006; 24(2):362–70.

36. Carroll TJ, Korosec FR, Swan JS, et al. The effect of injection rate on time-resolved contrast-enhanced peripheral MRA. J Magn Reson Imaging 2001; 14(4):401–10.

37. Carroll TJ, Korosec FR, Swan JS, et al. Method for rapidly determining and reconstructing the peak arterial frame from a time-resolved CE-MRA exam. Magn Reson Med 2000;44(5):817–20.

38. Zenge MO, Vogt FM, Brauck K, et al. High-resolution continuously acquired peripheral MR angiography featuring partial parallel imaging GRAPPA. Magn Reson Med 2006;56(4):859–65.

39. Cronqvist M, Stahlberg F, Larsson EM, et al. Evaluation of time-of-flight and phase-contrast MRA sequences at 1.0 T for diagnosis of carotid artery disease. I. A phantom and volunteer study. Acta Radiol 1996;37(3 Pt 1):267–77.

40. Davis WL, Warnock SH, Harnsberger HR, et al. Intracranial MRA: single volume vs. multiple thin slab 3D time-of-flight acquisition. J Comput Assist Tomogr 1993;17(1):15–21.

41. Yucel EK, Kaufman JA, Geller SC, et al. Atherosclerotic occlusive disease of the lower extremity: prospective evaluation with two-dimensional time-of-flight MR angiography. Radiology 1993;187(3):637–41.

42. Miyazaki M, Lee VS. Nonenhanced MR angiography. Radiology 2008;248(1):20–43.

43. Miyazaki M, Sugiura S, Tateishi F, et al. Non-contrast-enhanced MR angiography using 3D ECG-synchronized half-Fourier fast spin echo. J Magn Reson Imaging 2000;12(5):776–83.

44. Kramer H, Zenge M, Schmitt P, et al. Peripheral magnetic resonance angiography (MRA) with continuous table movement at 3.0 T: initial experience compared with step-by-step MRA. Invest Radiol 2008;43(9):627–34.

45. Zenge MO, Ladd ME, Quick HH. Novel reconstruction method for three-dimensional axial continuously moving table whole-body magnetic resonance imaging featuring autocalibrated parallel imaging GRAPPA. Magn Reson Med 2009;61(4):867–73.

46. Kramer H, Runge VM, Morelli JN, et al. Magnetic resonance angiography of the carotid arteries: comparison of unenhanced and contrast enhanced techniques. Eur Radiol 2011;21(8):1667–76.

47. Edelman RR, Sheehan JJ, Dunkle E, et al. Quiescent-interval single-shot unenhanced magnetic resonance angiography of peripheral vascular disease: technical considerations and clinical feasibility. Magn Reson Med 2010;63(4):951–8.

48. Hodnett PA, Koktzoglou I, Davarpanah AH, et al. Evaluation of peripheral arterial disease with nonenhanced quiescent-interval single-shot MR angiography. Radiology 2011;260(1):282–93.

49. Sostman HD. MRA for diagnosis of venous thromboembolism. Q J Nucl Med 2001;45(4):311–23.

50. Hany TF, Carroll TJ, Omary RA, et al. Aorta and runoff vessels: single-injection MR angiography with automated table movement compared with multiinjection time-resolved MR angiography–initial results. Radiology 2001;221(1):266–72.

51. Maki JH, Wang M, Wilson GJ, et al. Highly accelerated first-pass contrast-enhanced magnetic resonance angiography of the peripheral vasculature: comparison of gadofosveset trisodium with gadopentetate dimeglumine contrast agents. J Magn Reson Imaging 2009;30(5):1085–92.

52. Anzidei M, Napoli A, Zaccagna F, et al. First-pass and high-resolution steady-state magnetic resonance angiography of the peripheral arteries with gadobenate dimeglumine: an assessment of feasibility and diagnostic performance. Invest Radiol 2011;46(5):307–16.

53. Voth M, Haneder S, Huck K, et al. Peripheral magnetic resonance angiography with continuous table movement in combination with high spatial and temporal resolution time-resolved MRA With a total single dose (0.1 mmol/kg) of gadobutrol at 3.0 T. Invest Radiol 2009;44(9):627–33.

54. Janka R, Wenkel E, Fellner C, et al. Magnetic resonance angiography of the peripheral vessels in patients with peripheral arterial occlusive disease: when is an additional conventional angiography required? Cardiovasc Intervent Radiol 2006;29(2):220–9.

Contrast Media in Breast Imaging

Luis F. Serrano, MD*, Brooke Morrell, MD, Andrew Mai, MD

KEYWORDS

• Angiogenesis • MRI contrast agents • Breast MRI • Enhancement • Kinetics

KEY POINTS

- Magnetic Resonance Mammography (MRM) is often the imaging modality of choice for the detection of breast cancer.
- Contrast-enhanced MRM is a noninvasive modality used in the screening of high-risk patients.
- MR mammography is also indicated for lesion characterization, contralateral evaluation in patients with biopsy-proved malignancy, and the identification of primary malignancy in patients with axillary nodal disease.

INTRODUCTION

With the exception of implant analysis for detecting rupture, the value of breast magnetic resonance (MR) imaging is centered on the use of an intravenous contrast agent. Contrast-enhanced MR mammography (MRM) significantly aids in the detection of areas of possible malignancy.[1] In addition, because breast MR technique includes the axilla, it offers the possibility of detection or confirmation of the presence of axillary metastasis.[2] With its high sensitivity and effectiveness in dense breast tissue, MR imaging is a valuable addition to the diagnostic work-up of a breast abnormality or biopsy-proved cancer. Overall, contrast-enhanced MRM provides a quantitative, noninvasive, and nondestructive means of characterizing breast tumors, both morphologically and functionally.[3] The major limitation of MRM is its low (37%) to moderate specificity, which, in combination with its high sensitivity, can lead to unnecessary biopsies, patient anxiety, and higher costs.[4,5]

The reported sensitivity of MRM for the visualization of invasive cancer has approached 100%. There are many examples in the literature of MRM demonstrating breast cancer that was clinically, mammographically, and sonographically occult.

Several protocols exist; however, a common element in contrast-enhanced breast MR imaging is acquisition of T1-weighted images before and after the administration of intravenous contrast material. The use of paramagnetic contrast agents and gradient-echo sequences, both 2-dimensional and 3-dimensional (3D), have largely replaced spin-echo sequences.[6]

MRM should be bilateral except for its use in women with a history of mastectomy or when the MR imaging is being performed expressly to further evaluate or follow findings in 1 breast. As expressed in American College of Radiology (ACR) recommendations, MRM findings should be correlated with clinical history, physical examination, mammography, and any other prior breast imaging.[7] Many published studies are concordant in finding that MRM is the most sensitive imaging technique available for preoperative breast cancer staging in both mastectomy and breast conservation candidates to define the relationship of the tumor to the fascia and its extension into pectoralis major, serratus anterior, and/or intercostal muscles[8]; however, ongoing studies are evaluating its role in improving the rate of successful breast-conserving procedures.[9] With modern, high-field MR imaging scanners and the right pulse sequences, high signal-to-noise

Disclosures: The authors have nothing to disclose.
Conflict of interest: None.
Department of Radiology, Louisiana State University Health Sciences Center, 1542 Tulane Avenue, New Orleans, LA 70112, USA
* Corresponding author.
E-mail address: monoserrano@gmail.com

Magn Reson Imaging Clin N Am 20 (2012) 777–789
http://dx.doi.org/10.1016/j.mric.2012.07.004

ratio, high spatial resolution to assess morphology, and adequate temporal resolution for optimal enhancement assessment can be achieved, with good coverage of both breasts.

ANATOMOPHYSIOLOGIC OVERVIEW OF ANGIOGENESIS

The diagnosis in dynamic contrast-enhanced MRM is based primarily on contrast enhancement velocity. Breast carcinomas generally demonstrate a faster and stronger signal intensity increase after a bolus injection of gadolinium-based contrast agent compared with most benign lesions and normal breast tissue. Increased vascularity is considered an early sign of carcinoma formation.[10,11] Contrast uptake behaves differently in breast carcinomas compared with normal breast tissue for several reasons. The blood vessels supplying the breast cancer are different than the vasculature of the normal breast parenchyma. In addition, not only does the blood supply vary, but also the vessels feeding cancers are generally increased in quantity with the formation of new capillaries. The integrity of these vessels are also diminished with defects in the basal membrane and wider interstitial spaces (**Figs. 1** and **2**). Host capillaries are dilated and hyperpermeable and exude fibrin, which releases proteases and collagenases that autodigest healthy surrounding tissues. The migration of endothelial cells is seen outside the vessels into the adjacent widened interstitial space. This process of angiogenesis begins before tumor growth and is insufficient, leading to a disorganized chaotic blood flow. There have been several proangiogenic factors described, the most potent of which is vascular endothelial growth factor. Upregulation of vascular endothelial growth factor by a tumor results in stimulation of local endothelial ingrowth into the tumor bed and recruitment of endothelial progenitor cells to travel from bone marrow to the tumor bed.[12] This results in heterogeneity of tissue oxygenation in breast cancers. Oxygenation at the tumor periphery seems to be of prognostic importance for the clinical outcome of breast cancer.[13] In addition, patients with breast carcinoma have been noted to develop arteriovenous shunts, which correlate with higher likelihood for metastatic disease and increased mortality.

MR IMAGING CONTRAST AGENTS

For virtually all breast MR imaging studies, a T1-shortening contrast agent is used to assess cross-sectional morphology, tissue perfusion, and the enhancement kinetics of breast lesions.[14] Gadolinium-based agents are the most commonly used contrast media. In its elemental state, gadolinium contains 3 unpaired outer shell electrons and is not safe for human injection.[15] Gadolinium must first undergo chelation, a process by which it is bonded with another organic compound, increasing its stability.[15,16] After chelation to a conjugate base, gadolinium can be safely injected. Patient undergoing contrast-enhanced MR imaging will receive gadolinium contrast delivered intravenously, usually at the antecubital fossa. Contrast infusion is then followed by a saline flush. According to current literature, 0.1 mmol of contrast agent per kilogram body weight is the accepted dose standard.[6] There has been only 1 small-scale study to conclude that use of a higher dose, 0.16 mmol/kg, resulted in greater conspicuity of malignant lesions.[17]

The first Food and Drug Administration (FDA)-approved gadolinium contrast agent was gadopentate dimeglumine, marketed as Magnevist (Bayer Healthcare Pharmaceuticals, Wayne, NJ), 1988.[15] There are currently 8 FDA-approved paramagnetic gadolinium-based contrast agents available in the United States.[18] **Table 1** compares physical properties of the current FDA-approved gadolinium contrast agents used in breast imaging.[15,19] Although the agents listed in **Table 1** were FDA approved initially for central nervous system imaging, and some were approved later for body applications, they are now routinely used in breast imaging when MR imaging is indicated.[15] The indications for breast MR imaging is detailed in the ACR practice guidelines for recommendations for contrast-enhanced MR imaging (**Box 1**).[4]

The cornerstone of the ability of gadolinium as a contrast agent resides in its 7 unpaired electrons, which gives it its paramagnetic property.[20] A paramagnetic metal, when placed in a magnetic field, interacts with protons within water molecules in surrounding tissues, allowing the unpaired electrons to interact with surrounding tissues, causing relaxation of T1, greater than that of T2, and identifying hypervascular lesions (**Fig. 4**).[21] Gadolinium chelates can be classified according to their physicochemical properties, as listed in **Table 1**. These unique properties affect how gadolinium-containing contrast agents react within the body. The class of

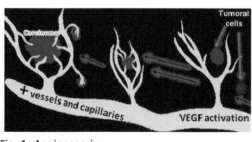

Fig. 1. Angiogenesis.

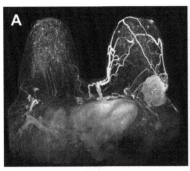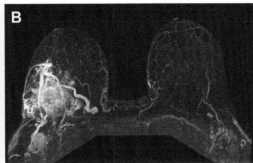

Fig. 2. (*A*) MRM, Postcontrast axial maximum intensity projection image demonstrates a large mass in the axillary tail of the left breast, consistent with known invasive carcinoma. Note the asymmetric vascular pattern caused by neovascularization. (*B*) Maximum intensity projection of an invasive carcinoma of the right breast, metastatic to the ipsilateral axilla, with extensive neovascularization process. Note the increase in vascularity with irregular vessels and arteriovenous shunts.

gadolinium chelate, linear versus macrocystic and ionic versus nonionic, affects the stability of the agent: Macrocyclic agents are more stable than linear agents, and ionic agents are more stable than nonionic agents.[22]

Future of Contrast Agents

A promising platform for MR imaging contrast agent development is nanotechnology, in which superparamagnetic iron oxide nanoparticles are tailored for MR contrast enhancement and/or for molecular imaging.[23] Studies have shown ultrasmall superparamagnetic iron oxide–enhanced MR imaging to be beneficial in demonstrating axillary lymph node metastases, which is an important determinant in the treatment of patients with breast malignancy and a vital prognostic factor.[24,25] Additionally, MR imaging contrast agents are being developed for the detection of more dynamic variables such as pH, oxygen tension, ion and metabolite concentrations, and enzyme-catalyzed reactions.[26] The *Journal of American Chemical Society* reports on research conducted from the University of Pennsylvania with glycol chitosan–coated iron oxide nanoparticles. These iron oxide nanoparticles are conjugated with glycol chitosan, a water-soluble polymer with pH-titratable charge, to generate a T2*-weighted MR contrast agent that responds to alterations in its surrounding pH via the Warburg effect.[27] The Warburg effect refers to the anaerobic pathway on which most cancer cells on to generate adenosine-5′-triphosphate.[28] In contrast to normal differentiated cells that undergo aerobic metabolism, tumor cells undergo anaerobic metabolism, producing lactic acid. Tumor cells also disrupt normal surrounding blood flow, impeding the ability of these cells to clear this acid. These processes contribute to the lower pH found in tumor cells compared with that of cells of normal tissue. The acidic environment of tumor cells attracts the sugar-based polymer, causing the nanocarrier to accumulate and become ionized in low pH, prominent on MR images.[27] The nanoparticle remains neutral in normal nonacidic tissues, further differentiating abnormal and normal tissues.[27] Researchers state that this would increase the specificity of MRM, allowing clinicians to better differentiate the benign and malignant tumors, through correlation between malignancy and pH.[27]

Dynamic contrast-enhanced breast MR imaging protocol

There are several different vendor-specific protocols for breast MR imaging: General Electric (VIBRANT [GE Healthcare, Waukesha, WI] [Volume Image Breast Assessment]), Phillips (Andover, MA) (THRIVE [T1 High-Res Isotropic Vol Excitation]), Siemens (Malvern, PA) (VIEWS [fl3d, 3D-FLASH]), Hitachi Medical (Twinsburg, OH) (TIGRE), and Toshiba America Medical Systems, (Tustin, CA) a (RADIANCE).[29,30] Although there are subtle differences and similarities among the different vendors, there are common challenges in creating an accurate and practical protocol for MRM. There are several variables to consider: signal-to-noise ratio (SNR), fat suppression, 3D-spatial resolution, temporal resolution, simultaneous coverage of the bilateral breast, and minimization of artifacts. The challenge is that SNR, spatial resolution, volume coverage, and imaging time all compete with each other, and artifact-free images may be difficult to obtain (**Box 2**).[29]

Unenhanced T1- and T2-weighted sequences

Unenhanced T1 sequence can be useful in demonstrating intralesional fat, which is a sign of benignity in a lesion of stable size. A central high

Table 1
Properties of FDA-approved gadolinium-based contrast agents

Contrast Brand Name	Contrast Generic Name	Class	Viscosity, cP, 37°C	Density, g/mL	Molecular Weight	Relaxivities, L/mmol⁻¹ T1	T2
Magnevist (Bayer Healthcare Pharmaceuticals, Wayne, NJ)	Gadopentetate dimeglumine (Gd-DTPA)	Linear, ionic	2.9	1.195	938	4.1	6.3
ProHance (Bracco Diagnostics Inc. Princeton, NJ)	Gadoteridol (Gd-HP-D03A)	Macrocytic, nonionic	1.3	1.137	559	4.1	5.3
Omniscan (GE Healthcare Inc. Princeton, NJ)	Gadodiamide (Gd-DTPA-BMA)	Linear, nonionic	1.4	1.14	574	4.3	5.1
Gadovist (Bayer Healthcare Pharmaceuticals, Wayne, NJ)	Gadobutrol dimeglumine (Gd-BTD03A)	Macrocyclic, nonIonic	4.96		605	5.6	6.5
OptiMARK (Mallinckrodt Inc. St. Louis, MO)	Gadoversetamide (Gd-DTPA-BMEA)	Linear, nonIonic	2.0	1.16	662	4.7	—
MultiHance (Bracco Diagnostics Inc. Princeton, NJ)	Gadobenate (Gd-BOPTA)	Linear, ionic	5.3	1.22	1058	6.3	12.5

Data from Bayer New Zealand Limited. Gadovist data sheet. Available at: http://www.medsafe.govt.nz/profs/datasheet/g/Gadovistinj.pdf. Accessed May 4, 2012; and Hendrick ER. Breast MRI: fundamentals and technical aspects. New York: Springer Science; 2007. p. 1–14; 113–9.

Box 1
Indications for contrast-enhanced MR imaging

- Screening of high-risk patients (>20% lifetime risk for breast cancer)
  - Carriers of BRCA mutation
  - First-degree relatives of proved BRCA mutation carriers
  - High-risk family history
  - Women with history of prior chest irradiation
  - Screening of contralateral breast in women with newly diagnosed breast malignancy
- Screening of women post augmentation limited by mammography
  - Post reconstruction
- Post free injections
- Evaluate extent of disease (Fig. 3)
- Evaluate for residual disease (post lumpectomy with positive margins)
- Monitoring response to neoadjuvant chemotherapy
- Lesion characterization

intensity signal on a T1-weighted imaging could represent an intramammary lymph node or fat necrosis.[10,31] Additionally, hamartomas can demonstrate fat. If the lesion is rapidly growing, a neoplastic process cannot be excluded.[31] A T2-weighted fat-suppressed sequence is useful because high-intensity lesions can easily be identified as a cyst.[10]

Contrast Enhancement

Lack of enhancement is one of the strongest predictors for benignity.[32] Relative enhancement of suspicious lesions results from intravenous contrast, such as gadolinium, leaking from poorly formed blood vessels within and around malignant tumors. Contrast agents shorten the relative T1 relaxation time of the lesion compared with surrounding normal tissue. Thus, provided that there is adequate SNR, suspicious lesions may seem hyperintense or enhancing on dynamic contrast-enhanced breast MR imaging.[29] There are 6 different patterns of internal enhancement: homogeneous enhancement, heterogeneous enhancement, rim enhancement, dark unenhanced septations, enhancing septations, and central enhancement.[32] Different cell types have different enhancement patterns. A time-intensity curve can be created, and the shape of the curve can be an important criterion for radiologists in differentiating between benign and malignant enhancing lesions of the breast.[33]

Spatial Resolution

High 3D spatial resolution is important in MRM, because the morphologic appearance of different lesions help radiologists differentiate certain malignant and benign lesions.[32] Diagnostic characteristics include shape, size, and margin. Irregular-shaped masses are more likely to be malignant. Certain morphologic patterns can be almost pathognomonic. For example, combined with other benign characteristics such as type I curve and nonenhancing septations, a macrolobulated mass is almost certainly a fibroadenoma.[10] Smooth margins suggest benignity, whereas spiculated margins are highly suspicious for malignancy.[34] Current ACR guidelines suggest less than 1.0 mm × 1.0 mm in plane pixel size, less than 3-mm slice thickness (with no slice gap), and not too grainy.[34]

Temporal Resolution

High temporal resolution is required not only for enhancement kinetics of a lesion but also because the early postcontrast phase is when there is lesion-to-parenchyma contrast such that an analysis of subtle morphologic features is feasible.[34] If the contrast enhanced imaging time is longer than 2 minutes and the first contrast-enhanced images are obtained too late after peak enhancement, washout may no longer be depicted in the descending part of the signal intensity–time curve.[33] A region of interest is generally determined and an enhancement kinetic curved is generated with the proper software. In dynamic contrast-enhanced breast imaging, 3 time intervals are considered: (1) a precontrast phase; (2) an early postcontrast phase (within first 2 minutes) to evaluate early peak enhancement, which is usually classified as slow, moderate, or fast; and (3) delayed enhancement is taken into consideration, which shows progressive enhancement, plateau, or washout.[35] In general, malignant breast lesions demonstrate early and abnormally increased enhancement compared with benign lesions.[6] Enhancement patterns should be assessed both in terms of quantitative approach to kinetic evaluation and qualitative evaluation of the overall shape of the enhancement curve.[29] Three patterns of intensity-time curves are used to classify lesions based on their enhancement kinetics (Fig. 5).[17] Type I, progressive enhancement, demonstrates a persistent increase in signal intensity and is associated with benign lesions (Figs. 6 and 7).[36] Type II, plateau, demonstrates a leveling-off "plateau" after reaching maximum signal intensity; more than 60% of the breast

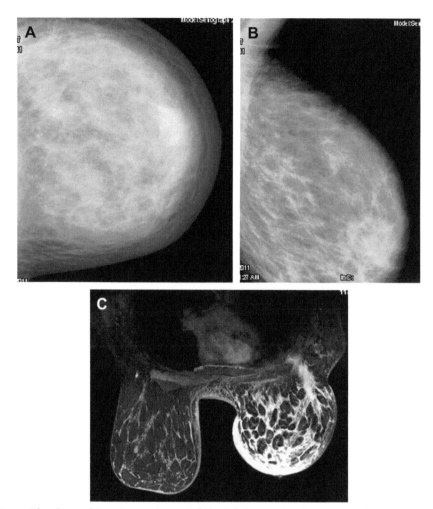

Fig. 3. Patient with advanced invasive carcinoma of the left breast. Axial, contrast-enhanced, T1-weighted MR imaging of both breasts. Invasion into the chest wall is identified; this finding is not visualized on mammogram (*A*) craniocaudal (*B*) mediolateral oblique views. (*C*) MR imaging characterizes the breast anatomy.

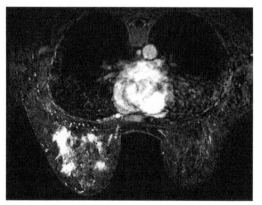

Fig. 4. Postcontrast subtracted T1-weighted dynamic protocol axial image demonstrating multiple hypervascular lesions in the right breast consistent with multicentric carcinoma.

carcinomas show this type of curve with many physicians considering this type of curve suspicious enough for biopsy (**Fig. 8**). Last, a type III curve, characterized by a rapid initial increase followed by a decrease with time (wash-in – wash-out curve), is highly suspicious for malignancy (**Fig. 9**).[15,33,37]

Spatial Resolution versus Temporal Resolution

It is widely agreed that combining morphologic features with enhancement kinetics increases the specificity of MRM.[31] High spatial resolution provides optimal evaluation of lesion morphology, including internal architecture. High temporal resolution is required not only for enhancement kinetics of a lesion, but also because the early postcontrast phase is when there is lesion-to-parenchyma contrast such that an analysis of subtle morphologic

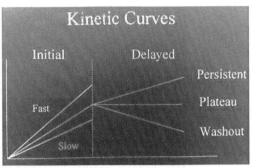

Box 2
Summary of important MR breast imaging protocol goals

Spatial resolution: Thin section acquisitions (section thickness of ≤3 mm); pixel size of <1 mm in each plane direction

Temporal resolution: Temporal resolution of <2 minutes for imaging of both breasts

Fat suppression: Homogeneous fat suppression; 3D contrast-enhanced imaging with a T1-weighted spoiled gradient-echo pulse sequence

Unenhanced T2-weighted pulse sequence to identify cysts and fibroadenomas

Bilateral: Field of view that includes images of both breasts in prone position with bilateral breast coils

Contrast enhancement: Intravenous administration of a gadolinum-based agent

Artifact minimization: Selection of a phase encoding direction other than the anteroposterior position to minimize artifacts

Fig. 5. Time-signal intensity curve types. Type I: Persistent rise (55%) corresponds to a straight line that enhancement continues during the entire dynamic study; 6% are associated with malignancy. Type II: Plateau increase (20%) with a sharp bend after the initial upstroke; 64% are associated with malignancy. Type III: Rapid initial increase (wash-in) followed by rapid washout (25%); 87% are associated with malignancy.

features is feasible.[34] However, there is a fine line in choosing the correct spatial resolution to maintain an acceptable SNR and still have adequate temporal resolution. It is generally agreed that there needs to be balance between spatial and temporal resolution, but no one has definitively drawn the line. Current ACR guidelines suggest less than 1.0 mm × 1.0 mm in plane pixel size, less than 3-mm slice thickness (with no slice gap), and not too grainy.[29,34] In the study of Kuhl and colleagues, a comparison of 1.25-mm × 1.25-mm pixel versus 0.6-mm × 0.8-mm pixels was made. Although a degree of temporal resolution for optimal enhancement kinetics was sacrificed, the change in protocol to improve spatial resolution correctly upgraded Breast Imaging-

Reporting and Data System (BI-RAD) scores of 13 of 26 cancers and downgraded 10 of 28 benign lesions.[34] There are novel techniques such as non-rectilinear k-space sampling and echo-planar imaging that may provide the ability to reduce the need for a compromise between spatial and temporal resolution by increasing speed.[38,39]

Fat Saturation

Most malignant tumors demonstrate postcontrast enhancement. Because detection of enhancement is very important, background noise must be minimized. Fatty tissue also has short T1. Breast tissue is predominantly fatty; this can create a significant amount of background noise. Thus, fat suppression is an integral part of MRM. There are several methods used for fat suppression: short tau/T1 inversion recovery, frequency selective saturation (chemical fat saturation), a combination of frequency selective and inversion recovery, phase

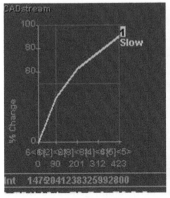

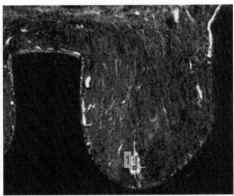

Fig. 6. Type I curve. MR imaging of the breast, axial subtracted image shows a central well-circumscribed mass, consistent with fibroadenoma (*right*). Note slowly progressive enhancement in the time course (*left*).

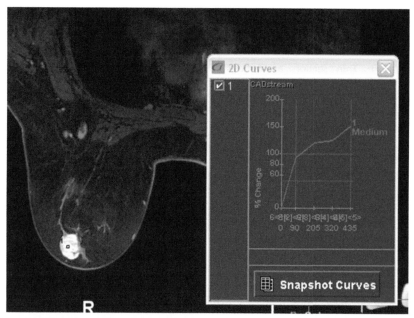

Fig. 7. Right breast MR imaging, axial subtracted image on dynamic postcontrast protocol demonstrating a large solid enhancing well-circumscribed subareolar mass in a patient with strong family history of breast cancer. Histologic correlation confirmed fibroadenoma (*left*). See type I progressive curve (*right*).

cycling, and highly water-selective binomial radiofrequency excitation.[29]

Artifact Minimization

It is also important to use a homogeneous low to intermediate field (<1.0 T); a lack of homogeneity prevents chemically selected fat suppression, which can compromise image quality.[31] Regardless of scanner performances, all protocols were designed to provide simultaneous dynamic bilateral breast imaging. The exception is in patients with a prior mastectomy.[30] Image artifacts such as cardiac motion and breathing must be minimized. Other considerations include volume wrap and nonuniform fat suppression. To minimize artifacts, a direction other than anteroposterior should be used.[40] Total section thickness should be less

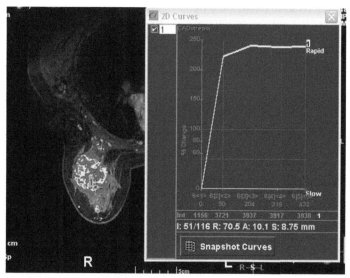

Fig. 8. Patient with proven adenocarcinoma of the right breast (*left*). Graph generated with computer-aided evaluation system (CADstream; GE Healthcare, Waukesha, WI), demonstrating type II plateau increase curve (*right*).

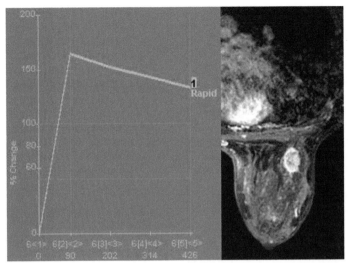

Fig. 9. MR imaging dynamic protocol after contrast injection. Axial T1 fat saturation image reveals a solid mass with heterogeneous enhancement (*right*). Ultrasound core biopsy was performed, yielding infiltrating ductal carcinoma. Note the rapid washout after the first 90 seconds, characteristic of a type III wash-in/wash-out curve (*left*).

than 3 mm, and the total acquisition time should be less than 2 minutes.[33,40]

Protocol in Summary

Proper dynamic contrast-enhanced MRM imaging protocol includes dedicated coils to provide a high SNR and simultaneous coverage of both breasts. The protocol includes a scout image, unenhanced T1 without fat saturation, T2 with fat saturation sequences, and dynamic multiphase 3D T1-weighted postcontrast sequence with fat suppression, high in-plane resolution, thin slices, and good temporal resolution (**Box 3**). Subtraction images and maximum intensity projections are then created along with software analysis providing enhancement curves.[29] While the dilemma of balancing spatial and temporal resolution will continue; the use of more novel acquisition sequences such as nonrectilinear k-space sampling and echo-planar imaging may provide the ability to reduce the need for a compromise between spatial and temporal resolutions by improving total acquisition speed.[38,39]

Breast MR imaging BI-RADS

A major goal of the American College of Radiology is to standardize breast lesion description in radiology reports. This quest has led to the BI-RADS classification system with mammography.[41–43] The ACR has also attempted to create a BI-RADS MR imaging lexicon to standardize lesion description in MRM. Enhancing lesions are divided into 3 types: mass, a 3D lesion that occupies space within the breast; focus or foci, which are enhancements

measuring less than 5 mm; and non–mass-like enhancements.[41–45] Size – According to an article published by Gutierrez and colleagues,[45] if combined with other suspicious findings, masses

---

Box 3
ACR-recommended protocol

1. Scout images (1 minute)

2. Precontrast ($\sim$5–7 minutes)

   a. T1-weighted no-fat suppressions (fat/glandular morphology)

   b. T2-weighted with fat suppression

   c. High-resolution, 3D T1-weighted fat-suppressed gradient-echo sequence (precontrast baseline image of identifying enhancing lesions)

3. Postcontrast (3–5 volume acquisitions $\sim$10 minutes)

   a. Dynamic multiphase 3D T1-weighted fat-suppressed gradient-echo sequence

4. Analysis

   a. Subtraction of precontrast and postcontrast images (identify enhancing lesions)

   b. Dynamic contrast curve evaluation (enhancement pattern assessment)

   c. Maximum intensity projection images of subtracted images (vascular bed assessment)

Data from Pulse sequences and acquisitions for breast MRI. ACR Web site. 2010. Available at: www.aapm.org/meetings/amos2/pdf/49-14409-36485-373.pdf.

> **Box 4**
> **Benign versus malignant breast mass characteristics**
>
> *Shape:* Oval masses are more likely benign; irregular masses are more likely malignant
>
> *Margin:* Irregular and spiculated margins are highly suspicious for malignancy; benign lesions usually have smooth margins
>
> *Internal enhancement:* From highly suspicious to least suspicious: rim enhancement → heterogeneous enhancement → homogeneous enhancement = heterogeneous lesions with nonenhancing internal septations

>1 cm have a significant higher probability of being malignant.

Masses are described based on internal enhancement, shape, and margins (**Box 4**) (**Fig. 10**).[41]

> *Shape* A mass can be round, oval, lobular, or irregular. Irregular-shaped lesions are most likely to be malignant, whereas oval lesions are mostly benign.[41–43]
>
> *Margins* Margins can be smooth, usually a benign characteristic, irregular, or spiculated. Irregularly margins have the highest positive predictive value for malignancy.[42] Spiculated lesions also suggest malignancy, whereas smoothly marginated lesions were almost always benign.[43]

Internal enhancement This is divided into 6 types: homogeneous enhancement, heterogeneous enhancement, rim enhancement, dark unenhanced septations within an internally enhancing lesion, enhancing septations, and central enhancement.[41] Rim enhancement has by far the highest positive predictive value for malignancy, followed by heterogeneous enhancement. Homogeneously enhancing lesions and heterogeneous lesions with nonenhancing internal septations were mostly benign, according to Sohn and colleagues.[43]

Lack of enhancement or minimal enhancement in a focus strongly suggests benignity.[44]

Non–mass-like enhancements (**Fig. 11**) are regions of enhancement that do not belong to a 3D mass.[41] They are categorized by distribution, internal enhancement, and symmetry between the 2 breasts in bilateral MR imaging studies. Non–mass-like enhancement provides a diagnostic challenge because there are a substantial number of false-positive results. In addition, the detection of ductal carcinoma in situ, which is often detected with MRM, is not considered pathologic disease in residual tumor, adding to the amount of false-positive results with MRM.[46] Nonmass lesions with ductal or segmental enhancement are highly suspicious for malignancy (**Fig. 12**).[42,45] Focal lesions were more likely benign. Rim enhancement is suspicious for malignancy. A central pattern of non–mass-like internal enhancement is suspicious

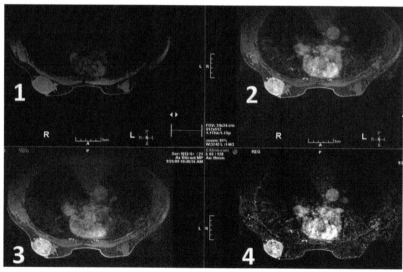

Fig. 10. MR imaging of the breast with dynamic sequential contrast protocol (VIBRANT; GE Healthcare, Waukesha, WI) in a 60-year-old male patient (1 precontrast phase). Well-circumscribed, rounded mass with heterogeneous enhancement pattern located in the central position of the right breast with skin retraction and ulceration, consistent with known invasive ductal carcinoma, grade II.

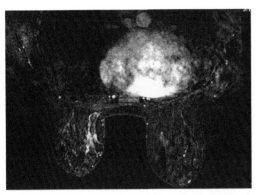

Fig. 11. Breast MR imaging with contrast. Axial subtracted image shows "non–mass-like enhancement" area with ductal distribution in the right breast at 5:00 axis, consistent with ductal carcinoma in situ with multiple foci of invasive component.

but not diagnostic of malignancy, whereas a stippled pattern of enhancement is more commonly seen in benign lesions.[42] Both malignant and benign lesions can be asymmetric; however, a symmetric pattern is a fairly reliable sign of benignity.[42] Associated findings such as skin thickening, nipple retraction, skin invasion, chest wall invasion, duct signal, and lymphadenopathy should also be mentioned (**Box 5**).

Pitfalls

Pitfalls are technical or nontechnical. Technical pitfalls relate to those patient or mechanical factors that can influence interpretation of the image. These include patient movement, metallic artifacts, and errors of postprocessing. The second group of nontechnical pitfalls refer to misinterpretation of

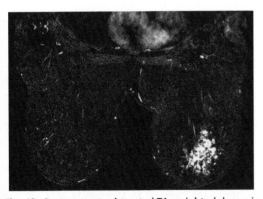

Fig. 12. Postcontrast subtracted T1-weighted dynamic protocol axial image demonstrating non–mass-like segmental. Clumped enhancement in the left breast; core biopsy was performed, yielding infiltrating ductal carcinoma.

> **Box 5**
> **Non–mass-like enhancements**
>
> *Distribution:* Ductal or segmental distribution is more likely malignant
>
> *Internal enhancement:* Rim enhancement is most suspicious for malignancy; central pattern is suspicious but not diagnostic for malignancy; a punctate pattern of enhancement is usually benign
>
> *Symmetry:* Asymmetric non–mass-like enhancement can be benign or malignant but symmetric non–mass-like patterns of enhancement are almost always benign

imaging findings in the absence of a technical problem.[47]

Benign lesions such as fibroadenoma, proliferative and nonproliferative fibrocystic change, inflammatory change, scar, sclerosing adenosis, lobular carcinoma in situ, and atypical ductal hyperplasia may seem to be strongly enhanced. False-negative findings at breast MR imaging may occur in the presence of invasive lobular carcinoma, metastatic breast masses, low-grade intraductal carcinoma, and well-differentiated invasive ductal malignancies. Furthermore, a mucinous carcinoma may lack strong enhancement secondary to the gelatinous tumor matrix, histologically represented by aggregates of cancer cells floating in extracellular pools of mucin[48]; this may replace the characteristic solid enhancing component seen in other tumors.[40] Another potential pitfall is demonstrated in cases when one or more additional nonspecific enhancing lesion is identified on MR imaging at a distance from a known primary tumor. Many of these cases require an increase in the amount of tissue excised, multiple excisions, or both. The biopsy of additional enhancing lesions that prove to be benign compromises the patient's cosmetic results following breast conservation. In addition, some patients are advised to undergo mastectomy because of MR imaging findings, despite the absence of histologic confirmation that an enhancing lesion represents multifocal breast cancer.[6]

SUMMARY

MRM has a well-established role in breast imaging, providing valuable information on staging of disease, follow-up imaging, assessment of post-treatment response, and screening of high-risk patients with genetic predispositions. Mammography and ultrasound have long been considered the core players in breast imaging; however, MRM provides a valuable adjunct, because it is more sensitive in identifying otherwise occult breast disease, detecting recurrent breast cancers, and evaluating response to therapy. Accurate interpretation is technically dependent on a finely tuned MRM protocol, which includes dedicated coils to provide a high SNR and simultaneous coverage of both breasts. Gadolinium-based agents are the most commonly used contrast media, with 8 current FDA-approved paramagnetic gadolinium-based contrast agents available in the United States. Contrast-enhanced breast MR imaging is currently considered the most sensitive imaging modality available for the detection of invasive breast malignancy. Although highly sensitive, the specificity of MRM interpretation is still low; however, new developments, such as additional MR imaging contrast agents and novel protocol modifications, are on the horizon. These evolving changes will have a positive impact, expanding the role of MRM and improving the specificity of this powerful diagnostic tool.

REFERENCES

1. Kopans D. Breast imaging. Magnetic resonance imaging of the breast. 3rd edition. Philadelphia: Lippincott Williams and Wilkins; 2007. p. 691.
2. Birdwell RL, Smith DN. MR imaging use in breast cancer staging and the assessment of treatment. Breast Imaging 2005;200 Syllabus RSNA.
3. Turetschek K, Huber S, Floyd E. MR imaging haracterization of microvessels in experimental breast tumors by using a particulate contrast agent with histopathologic correlation. Radiology 2001;218:562–9.
4. Venta L. Mammography intervention and imaging. Philadelphia: Lippincott Williams and Wilkins; 2000. p. 269.
5. Morris E, Lieberman L. Breast MRI diagnosis and intervention. New York: Springer; 2005. p. 7–8.
6. Orel SG, Schnall MD. MR imaging of the breast for the detection, diagnosis, and staging of breast cancer. Radiology 2001;220:13–30.
7. American College of Radiology. ACR practice guideline for the performance of contrast-enhanced magnetic resonance imaging (MRI) of the breast. Available at: http://www.acr.org/~/media/2A0EB28E B59041E2825179AFB72EF624.pdf. Accessed May 15, 2012.
8. Carbonaro LA, Pediconi F, Verardi N. Breast MRI using a high-relaxivity contrast agent: an overview. AJR Am J Roentgenol 2011;196:942–55.
9. Dixon JM. ABC of breast diseases. 3rd edition. Oxford (UK): BMJ Books Blackwell; 2006. p. 3.
10. Kvistad KA, Rydland J, Vainio J. MD breast lesions: evaluation with dynamic contrast-enhanced T1-weighted MR imaging and with T2*-weighted first-pass perfusion MR imaging 1. Radiology 2000;216:545–53.
11. Kaiser WA. Signs in MR-mammography. New York: Springer; 2007. p. 163.
12. Roses DF. Breast cancer. 2nd edition. Philadelphia: Elsevier Churchil Livingston; 2005. p. 37.
13. Runkel S, Wayss K, Melchert F. Angiogenesis o human breast cancers: neovascularization in xenotransplants and oxygenation in situ in patients Gynacol Geburtschilfliche Rundsch 1995;35(Suppl 1) 68–72 [in German].
14. Kuhl C. The current status of breast MR imaging part I. Choice of technique, image interpretation, diagnostic accuracy, and transfer to clinical practice. Radiology 2007;244(2):356–78.
15. Hendrick ER. Breast MRI: fundamentals and technical aspects. New York: Springer Science; 2007. p. 1–14; 113–9.
16. Bellin MF, Van Der Molen AJ. Extracellular gadolinium-based contrast media: an overview. Eur J Radiol 2008;66(2):160–7.
17. Heywang-Kobrunner SH, Haustein J, Pohl C, et al. Contrast-enhanced MR imaging of the breast: comparison of two different doses of gadopentetate dimeglumine. Radiology 1994;191(3): 639–46.
18. Food and Drug administration. FDA Drug Safety Communication: New warnings for using gadolinium-based contrast agents in patients with kidney dysfunction. Available at: http://www.fda.gov/Drugs/DrugSafety/ ucm223966.htm. Accessed May 10, 2012.
19. Bayer New Zealand Limited. Gadovist data sheet. Available at: http://www.medsafe.govt.nz/profs/ datasheet/g/Gadovistinj.pdf. Accessed May 4, 2012.
20. McRobbie DW, Moore EA, Graves J. MRI from picture to proton. Cambridge (United Kingdom): Cambridge University Press; 2003. p. 42–4.
21. Chatterji M, Mercado CL, Moy L, et al. Optimizing 1.5-tesla and 3-tesla dynamic contrast-enhanced magnetic resonance imaging of the breast. MRI Clin North Am 2010;18(2):207–24.
22. Rofsky NM, Sherry AD, Lenkinski RE. Nephrogenic systemic fibrosis: a chemical perspective. Radiology 2008;247(3):608–12.
23. Lodhia J, Mandaranol G, Ferris NJ, et al. Development and use of iron oxide nanoparticles (part 1): synthesis of iron oxide nanoparticles for MRI. Biomed Imaging Interv J 2010;6(2):12.
24. Memarsadeghi M, Riedl C, Kaneider A, et al. Axillary lymph node metastases in patients with breast carcinoma: assessment with nonenhanced versus USPIO-enhanced MR imaging. Radiology 2006;241(2): 367–77.
25. Kosaka M, Bernardo M, Mitsunga M, et al. MR and optical imaging of early micrometastases in lymph nodes: triple labeling with nano-sized agents yielding distinct signals. Contrast Media Mol Imaging 2012; 7(2):247–53.

26. Shapiroa M, Atanasijevich T. Dynamic imaging with MRI contrast agents: quantitative considerations. Magn Reson Imaging 2006;24:449–62.

27. Crayton SH, Tsourkas A. pH-titratable superparamagnetic iron oxide for improved nanoparticle accumulation in acidic tumor microenvironments. ACS Nano 2011;5(12):9592–601.

28. Vander Heiden MG, Cantley LC, Thompson CB. Understanding the Warburg effect: the metabolic requirements of cell proliferation. Science 2009; 324(5930):1029–33.

29. Ronald Price. Pulse sequences and acquisitions for breast MRI. 2010. Available at: www.aapm.org/meetings/amos2/pdf/49-14409-36485-373.pdf. Accessed May 26, 2012.

30. White DJ. Improving breast diagnosis using high-resolution MRI. Clinical Value-Breast Imaging GE Health Care MR 2006:30–2.

31. Macura K, Ouwerkerk R, Jacobs M, et al. Patterns of enhancement on breast MR images: interpretation and imaging pitfalls. Radiographics 2006;26(6): 1719–34.

32. Schnall MD, Blume J, Bluemke DA. Diagnostic architectural and dynamic features at breast MR imaging: a multicenter study. Radiology 2006;238: 42–53.

33. Kuhl CK, Mielcareck P, Klaschik S, et al. Dynamic breast MR imaging: are signal intensity time course data useful for differential diagnosis of enhancing lesions. Radiology 1999;211(1):101–10.

34. Kuhl C, Schild H, Morakkabati N. Dynamic bilateral contrast enhanced MR imaging of the breast: trade-off between spatial and temporal resolution. Radiology 2005;236:789–800.

35. Mann R, Kuhl C, Kinkel K, et al. Breast MRI: guidelines from the European Society of Breast Imaging. Eur Radiol 2008;18(7):1307–18.

36. Berg WA, Birdwell RL. Diagnostic imaging breast. 1st edition. Salt Lake City (UT): Amirsys; 2006. p. 169.

37. Jansen S, Shimauchi A, Zak L, et al. Kinetic curves of malignant lesions are not consistent across MRI systems: need for improved standardization of breast dynamic contrast-enhanced MRI acquisition. AJR Am J Roentgenol 2009;193(3):832–9.

38. Hulka CA, Smith BL, Sgroi DC, et al. Benign and malignant breast lesions: differentiation with echo-planar MR imaging. Radiology 1995;197: 33–8.

39. Hulka CA, Edmister WB, Smith BL, et al. Dynamic echo-planar imaging of the breast: experience in diagnosing breast carcinoma and correlation with tumor angiogenesis. Radiology 1997;205:837–42.

40. Rausch D, Hendrick E. How to optimize clinical breast MR imaging practices and techniques on your 1.5-T system. Radiographics 2006;26:1469–84.

41. Erguvan-Dogan B, Whitman GJ, Kushwaha A, et al. BI-RADS MRI: a primer. AJR Am J Roentgenol 2006; 187:152–60.

42. Sohns C, Scherrer M, Staab W, et al. Value of the BI-RADS classification in MR-mammography for diagnosis of benign and malignant breast tumors. Eur Radiol 2011;21:2475–83.

43. Nunes LW, Schnall MD, Orel SG, et al. Correlation of lesion appearance and histologic findings for the nodes of a breast MR imaging interpretation model. Radiographics 1999;19:79–92.

44. Nunes LW, Schnall MD, Orel SG, et al. Update of breast MR imaging architectural interpretation model. Radiology 2001;219:484–94.

45. Gutierrez RL, DeMartini WB, Eby PR, et al. BI-RADS lesion characteristics predict likelihood of malignancy in breast MRI for masses but not for non mass like enhancement. AJR Am J Roentgenol 2009;193:994–1000.

46. Monticciolo D. Magnetic resonance imaging of the breast for cancer diagnosis and staging. Semin Ultrasound CT MR 2011;32(4):319–30.

47. Coulthard A, Potterton AJ. Pitfalls of breast MRI. Br J Radiol 2000;73:665–71.

48. Cardenosa H. The core curriculum. Breast imaging. Philadelphia: Lippincott Williams and Wilkins; 2004. p. 258.

MR Imaging of the Brachial Plexus

Igor Mikityansky, MD, MPH[a],*, Eric L. Zager, MD[b],
David M. Yousem, MD, MBA[c], Laurie A. Loevner, MD[b,d]

KEYWORDS

- Brachial plexus • Root avulsion • Radiation plexopathy • Parsonage-Turner syndrome
- Brachial plexitis • Thoracic outlet syndrome • Immune mediated neuropathy • Brachial plexopathy

KEY POINTS

- Sagittal imaging should be used to assess the relationship of the plexus lesion to the plexus components and subclavian and axillary arteries.
- The coronal images with a large field of view allow for comparison of signal intensity, size, and enhancement of the affected side with the contralateral control plexus.
- The appearance and orientation of the lesion may provide valuable diagnostic hints.
- Routine use of intravenous contrast is not required.
- MR imaging after brachial plexus injury should be delayed at least 3 weeks, unless the patient develops progressive neurologic deterioration or Brown-Séquard syndrome symptoms.
- However, this is now controversial—some surgeons are recommending ultraearly plexus exploration within the first or second week when multiple root avulsions are suspected, so that nerve transfers can be done as early as possible, and to avoid operating through dense scar.
- Even in the presence of a nerve root avulsion, the residual root within the pseudomeningocele should be identified because it may allow nerve grafting.
- Involvement of C7 spinal nerve may prevent patients with C5 and C6 avulsions from undergoing an Oberlin nerve transfer procedure and should be mentioned in the report.
- Vascular evaluation should be performed in trauma cases if there is a distal pulse deficit, local hematoma, bruit, or anatomically related nerve symptoms, because of possible delay in development of pseudoaneurysm.
- In cases of direct neoplastic invasion of the brachial plexus, obliteration of the interscalene fat determines surgical candidacy.
- Unlike extrapleural lesions, the interface of the Pancoast tumor and the lung is irregular.

INTRODUCTION

The interpretation of the images of the brachial plexus may be intimidating for a general radiologist. However, knowledge of anatomy, common pathology, direct and indirect imaging signs of diseases affecting the brachial plexus, the patient's history and clinical presentation, and a systematic approach to the images will allow a radiologist to construct an anatomically correct limited differential diagnosis. Judicious use of contrast could help in classification of vascular lesions, delineation of infection, and in cases of radiation-treated tumors.

[a] Windsong Radiology Group, 55 Spindrift Drive, Williamsville, NY 14221, USA; [b] Department of Neurosurgery, Hospital of the University of Pennsylvania, 3400 Spruce Street, Philadelphia, PA 19104, USA; [c] Department of Radiology, Johns Hopkins University, 600 N. Wolfe Street, Baltimore, MD 21287, USA; [d] Department of Radiology, Hospital of the University of Pennsylvania, 3400 Spruce Street, Philadelphia, PA 19104, USA
* Corresponding author.
E-mail address: imikitya@gmail.com

Magn Reson Imaging Clin N Am 20 (2012) 791–826
http://dx.doi.org/10.1016/j.mric.2012.08.003
1064-9689/12/$ – see front matter © 2012 Elsevier Inc. All rights reserved.

ANATOMY

The brachial plexus is a neural network responsible for both sensory and motor innervation of the ipsilateral chest, shoulder, arm, and hand. It is most commonly formed by the ventral rami of C5 through T1 spinal nerves as they exit the neural foramina (**Fig. 1**). There are multiple variations in anatomy of the brachial plexus.[1] However, from the perspective of a radiologist, the detectable variations are at the level of the roots. The most common variant at this level, the prefixed brachial plexus, includes only the C4 through C7 spinal nerves. The second-most common variant at this level, the postfixed plexus, receives contributions from the C6 through T2 levels. There are also rare cases of a combination of the two, with

contributions from C4 through T2.[1] These variants are important for predisposition to certain pathologic conditions, and need to be known for surgical planning.

From the imaging perspective, the brachial plexus can be divided into the supraclavicular, retroclavicular, and infraclavicular portions. The supraclavicular plexus contains the spinal nerves (incorrectly called roots in some anatomic textbooks) and the trunks. After they exit the neural foramina, behind the vertebral arteries, the spinal nerves are located in the interscalene space (**Fig. 2**), between the anterior scalene muscle anteriorly, middle and posterior scalene muscles posteriorly, and first rib and subclavian artery inferiorly. At the lateral border of the middle scalene muscle, the C5 and C6 spinal nerves form the

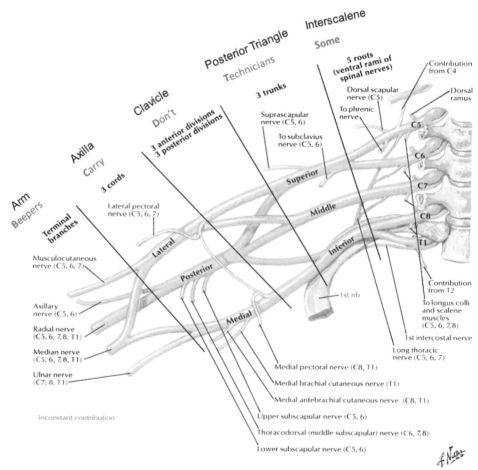

Fig. 1. Spinal nerves (sometimes incorrectly called roots), trunks, divisions, cords, and branches. To avoid including an alcoholic beverage as a part of a commonly used mnemonic of the brachial plexus components, there is an alternative mnemonic provided at the left upper aspect together with anatomic location of each component. Note that the spinal nerves and trunks could be grouped into the supraclavicular, and cords and branches into the infraclavicular brachial plexus, with the divisions representing the retroclavicular portion of the plexus. (Netter illustration from www.netterimages.com. © Elsevier Inc. All rights reserved.)

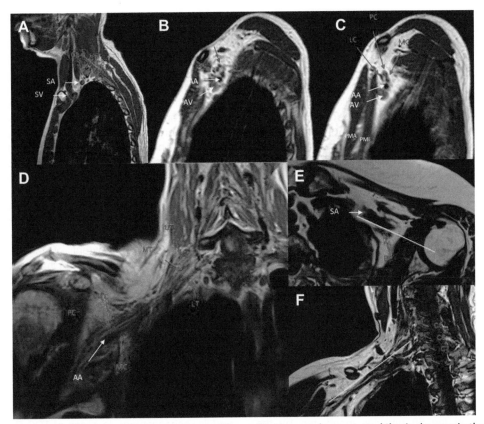

Fig. 2. MR imaging anatomy of the brachial plexus. The sagittal images demonstrate (*A*) spinal nerves in the interscalene triangle (*red arrows*), (*B*) divisions in the retroclavicular space (*red arrows*), and (*C*) cords (*red arrows*). The coronal images (*D*) demonstrate trunks just outside of the interscalene triangle, and cords surrounding the axillary artery. Note medial cord is located inferior medially to the axillary artery, whereas the lateral cord is superior lateral. The posterior cord is posterior superior and lateral. The axial images (*E*) demonstrate the relationship of the brachial plexus and the subclavian artery. The yellow line is parallel to both the brachial plexus and the subclavian artery. It represents the oblique coronal plane optimally suited for maximum visualization of the plexus. The sagittal localizing images could be used to angle the coronal plane along the posterior longitudinal ligament to align the coronal images with neural foramina. The oblique coronal T1-weighted image (*F*) demonstrates visualization of most of the roots (*red arrows*) and more distal elements of the plexus. The yellow line demarcates the oblique axial plane that could be obtained to allow for visualization of the entire plexus on a small number of the axial images. AA, axillary artery; AV, axillary vein; LC, lateral cord; LT, lower trunk; MC, medial cord; MT, middle trunk; PC, posterior cord; PMA, pectoralis major muscle; PMI, pectoralis minor muscle; SA, subclavian artery; SV, subclavian vein; UT, upper trunk.

superior trunk, C7 forms the middle trunk, and C8 and T1 form the inferior trunk. The trunks continue posterior and superior to the subclavian artery, and form anterior and posterior divisions within the posterior triangle and behind the clavicle. The costoclavicular triangle, a common location (see **Fig. 2**) of functional compression of the brachial plexus, is formed by the clavicle superiorly, the subclavius muscle anteriorly, and the first rib and middle scalene muscle posteriorly. The subclavian vein and artery are located within the inferior aspect of this space, with the former located anterior to the latter. This space contains the transition from the divisions, located in the retroclavicular space, to the cords. The infraclavicular portion of the plexus extends into the retropectoralis minor space. The anterior wall of this space is the pectoralis minor muscle, posterior and superior walls are the subscapularis muscle, and posterior and inferior walls are created by the anterior chest wall. In this space the cords are visualized posterior superior to the axillary artery (see **Fig. 2**). The medial cord, a continuation of the anterior division of the inferior trunk, in its distal portion is seen at the inferior wall of the artery. The lateral cord, receiving anterior division nerve fibers from the superior and middle trunks, is located adjacent to the anterior superior wall of the artery. The posterior cord, receiving posterior divisions' contributions from all trunks, is located superior posteriorly to the artery. The infraclavicular portion of the brachial plexus also includes five terminal branches: median, ulnar, musculocutaneous, axillary, and radial nerves (usually visualized in the lower axilla and proximal arm; see **Fig. 1**). Some of the branches originate at other zones of the brachial plexus. The latissimus dorsi, teres major, and subscapularis muscles receive their innervation from the posterior cord. The supraspinatus and infraspinatus muscles receive innervation from the upper trunk via the suprascapular nerve. The biceps and coracobrachialis muscles receive innervation from the lateral cord via the musculocutaneous nerve. The medial cord innervates cutaneous structures and the ulnar nerve. In terms of the spinal nerve innervation, C5 is responsible for supraspinatus, infraspinatus, and the deltoid; C6 for biceps; C7 for triceps and forearm extensors; and C8 and T1 for finger flexors and intrinsic muscles of the hand. On deep reflex testing, the biceps reflex is predominantly supplied by C5 spinal nerve, the brachioradialis reflex by C6, the triceps by C7, and the pectoralis by the entire plexus. Although knowing the branches, their origin, and the 59 muscles innervated by the plexus is very important for a neurosurgeon for localization of the lesions based on the symptoms caused by the affected branches, current clinical MR imaging does not allow visualization of these structures in most cases. However, direct visualization of the components of the brachial plexus on MR imaging allows for confirmation and delineation of pathologic abnormalities. It is especially valuable because the nerve conduction studies only indirectly examine the brachial plexus and the symptom-based clinical localization may be misleading in the presence of brachial plexus branching variants.

IMAGING TECHNIQUE

The imaging of the brachial plexus requires understanding of the course of its components and the best planes for their visualization. The identification of the components of the plexus and their relationship to the bony and vascular structures, and assessment of the adjacent fat planes are best done on the sagittal non–fat-suppressed T1-weighted images because this plane demonstrates the cross-section of these structures. However, most neuroradiologists are more comfortable dealing with the neural elements in the axial and coronal planes. The cords, nerve roots, and

foraminal portions of the roots are best seen on the high-resolution axial and oblique coronal images. The coronal images with a large field of view allow for comparison of signal intensity (T2-fat-suppressed imaging), size, and enhancement of the affected side with the contralateral control plexus. The unilateral coronal images are most useful for appreciation of edema, enhancement, and enlargement of the roots, trunks, divisions, and cords. The visualization of anatomic detail is variable in this plane. However, the T1-weighted images may be useful for demonstration of bony anatomy.

The use of intravenous contrast for imaging of the brachial plexus is not required on routine basis, since the fat-suppressed T2 images demonstrate the location and the extent of the common pathology, while the T1 weighted images demonstrate the relationship of an abnormality and the adjacent structures. However, the contrast administration is necessary in cases of infection, both to define the extent of the infectious process and assess for presence of adjacent drainable collections. It also could help in defining the extent of the abnormality in secondary neoplastic involvement. Futhermore, in some radiation treated tumor cases, it may differentiate tumor recurrence from radiation changes based on progression of nodular enhancement. In cases of TOS (Thoracic Outlet Syndrome) the intravenous contrast, as a part of provocative position magnetic resonance angioaphic evaluation, commonly supplemented with sagittal T1-weighted imaging in both positions, demonstrates the location and the extent of the compression as well as secondary changes in the vessel lumen. Finally, in cases presenting with vascular lesions the contrast allows for better characterization and classification of a lesion, and selection of the appropriate management.

The appearance and orientation of the lesion may provide valuable hints (**Fig. 3**).[2] The lesion centered at the interscalene triangle usually involves spinal nerves or trunks. The long axis of an oval, well-defined lesion parallel to the nerve of origin suggests a nerve sheath tumor. If such a lesion is oriented obliquely, from superomedial to inferolateral, it originates from the upper roots. If it is oriented horizontally, it originates from the inferior roots. The vertical lesion in the interscalene triangle most likely represents secondary involvement of the plexus.

Although custom tailoring each examination for the expected pathologic abnormality and lesion localization may provide the best quality of imaging examination, it is impractical in today's high-volume reading environment. The radiologist needs to separate the examinations by the

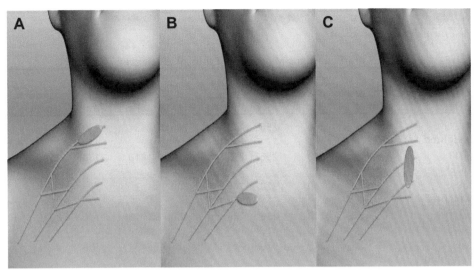

Fig. 3. Use of the orientation of the long axis of the lesion involving the spinal nerves in the interscalene triangle for determination of the origin of pathology. (*A*) inferior laterally angulated oval lesion usually originates from the superior spinal nerves. (*B*) Horizontal or minimally superior medially angulated lesion usually arises from the inferior spinal nerves. (*C*) The lesion oriented parallel to the spine usually originates outside of the brachial plexus. (*Data from* Saifuddin A. Imaging tumors of the brachial plexus. Skeletal Radiol 2003;32(7):375–87.)

pathologic categories and establish the general protocols for each category. This will allow judicious use of intravenous contrast and higher efficiency. The radiologist also has to find a comfortable balance between spatial resolution and the area of coverage based on the type of pathologic abnormality referred to the practice and adjust the MR imaging parameters, such as field of view and the matrix size, appropriately. Increased magnet strength and availability of isotropic imaging with multiplanar reconstructions may allow for a decrease in need for custom-tailored examinations and shorten overall time of the examination, especially for cooperative patients. A routine sample protocol is included in **Table 1**.

SYMPTOMS

Commonly listed brachial plexus–related symptoms are pain, paresthesias, sensory and motor deficits in the appropriate distribution, scapular winging (involvement of the spinal accessory, dorsal scapular, or long thoracic nerve), diaphragmatic paralysis (involvement of the phrenic nerve innervated by C3 and C5), and Horner syndrome (involvement of the postganglionic C8 and T1 nerve roots). However, depending on the type of pathologic abnormality, the predominant component changes (eg, motor deficits in trauma, pain in neoplasm, and sensory deficits in radiation-treated cases and some tumors).

PATHOLOGIC CONDITIONS

Brachial plexus pathologic conditions can be separated into two categories: traumatic and nontraumatic. If there is no history of trauma, then an MR imaging of the brachial plexus with contrast should be the study of choice, especially if a mass is suspected. In the setting of trauma, either CT myelography, especially for a suspected proximal injury, or brachial plexus MR imaging with T2-weighted myelography or high-resolution isotropic T2-weighted imaging could be performed.

TRAUMATIC INJURY

Trauma is the most common cause of brachial plexus symptoms. Outside of the cord, it can be subdivided into complete or partial root avulsion, stretch injury, and vascular injury. In 1985, Narakas[4] created the rule of "seven seventies" based on a series of 1068 patients, in which 70% of brachial plexopathies are caused by motor vehicle accidents, 70% of these accidents involved motorcycles or bicycles, 70% of these riders had associated multiple injuries, 70% of riders with multiple injuries had supraclavicular injuries, 70% of these supraclavicular injuries demonstrated at least one avulsed nerve root, 70% of avulsed roots involved C7 through T1, or C8 and T1, and 70% of patients with lower root avulsions had persistent pain. The more recent retrospective review of slightly more than 1000 charts of postsurgical

Table 1
Routine brachial plexus protocol

			Brachial Plexus MR Imaging Protocol (3T siemens)						
Sequence	Slice/skip (mm)	Field of view (mm)	Matrix	NEX	TE/TR	Turbo Factor	Flip Angle	Bandwidth (Hz/Px)	TI
Axial T1-weighted	4/1	240	256 × 205	2	700/9.1	3	130	271	—
Axial STIR (BLADE)	4/1	240	256 × 256	1	4500/80	16	130	362	220
Sagittal T1-weighted	4/0.8	240	320 × 240	2	700/9.4	3	150	252	—
Coronal STIR (BLADE)	4/1.2	240	256 × 256	1	4500/80	16	130	362	220
Coronal T1-weighted	4/1.2	240	320 × 240	1	625/9.6	3	150	240	—
Sagittal T1-weighted FS PRE- and POST	4/0.8	240	320 × 240	1	750/9.4	3	150	252	—
Coronal T1-weighted FS POST	4/1.2	240	320 × 240	3	650/96	3	150	240	—

Although coronal images should be obtained in the oblique plane, parallel to the subclavian artery and posterior longitudinal ligament, straight or oblique sagittal (perpendicular to the coronal plane) and axial (parallel to the C7 spinal nerve and divisions) may be used. The postcontrast images are optional except for neoplastic involvement.

Abbreviations: STIR, short tau inversion recovery; BLADE, Seimens Healthcare proprietary motion correction reconstruction technique; FS, fat-suppressed; PRE, precontrast; POST, postcontrast; NEX, number of excitations; TE, echo time; TR, repetition time; Hz/Px, Hertz per pixel; TI, inversion time.

patients reported that stretch and/or contusion (49%), laceration (7%), and gunshot wounds (12%) composed almost three-quarters of the injuries to patients. Tumors and thoracic outlet syndrome cases composed 16% each.[5]

Traumatic injuries of the brachial plexus are most commonly seen in the younger population, including neonates and adolescents. The dominant symptom is motor deficit in the appropriate distribution. In addition to motor deficits in the upper extremity, the involvement of C4 and C5 roots, which contribute to the phrenic nerve, is associated with diaphragmatic paralysis. The presence of unilateral ptosis, myosis, and anhidrosis (Horner syndrome) is seen in patients with sympathetic injury at the level of C8 and T1. The postganglionic injury, unlike the preganglionic injury, involving only the motor roots, may have associated sensory component. Although controversial, some of the investigators suggest that the involvement of C7, as demonstrated clinically by loss of sensation in the middle finger and loss of strength in triceps and wrist extensors, prevents patients with C5 and C6 avulsions from undergoing an Oberlin nerve transfer procedure (transfer

of redundant motor fascicle of the ulnar nerve to the musculocutaneous branch of the biceps muscle). Therefore, the status of the C7 should be specifically mentioned in the report.[6]

The surgeons categorize the injury by the number of involved spinal nerves (breadth), level of involvement (length), severity of involvement (depth), and time of involvement.[7] In terms of breadth of involvement, the injuries may be separated into complete brachial plexus involvement and partial injury (a single or several spinal nerves). In terms of timing, the plexus injury is divided into the following groups: immediate (less than 3 weeks), post 3 weeks (completion of Wallerian degeneration), and more than 6 months (onset of muscle degeneration).[7] The ideal window for surgical intervention for stretch and/or contusion and gunshot wounds is usually from 3 to 6 months after injury, whereas trauma by sharp mechanisms should be managed as early as possible.

During the immediate presentation, the nerve conduction studies and imaging studies may be misleading because of extensive adjacent posttraumatic changes, incomplete formation of pseudomeningoceles, and incomplete denervation.[7]

Therefore, the MR imaging after the injury is usually delayed at least 3 weeks because of the limitations of early imaging, unless the patient develops progressive neurologic deterioration (suggesting an expanding hematoma or pseudoaneurysm) or symptoms of Brown-Séquard syndrome and requires evaluation for presence of myelopathy. The imaging and nerve conduction studies become useful after completion of Wallerian degeneration, when demonstration of nerve root avulsion facilitates early intervention. On the other hand, no invasive treatment is usually performed if nerve conduction studies demonstrate signs of muscle recovery after 3 weeks.[7] Although some primary brachial plexus surgery could be performed after muscle denervation, up to 1 year after the injury, the success rate decreases every month. Tendon and free functional muscle transfers or joint fusions are commonly performed at this stage, more than 2 years after injury.[7]

The mild stretch injury (**Fig. 4**), predominantly represents neurapraxia (temporary failure of function without structural axonal injury), but includes mild cases of axonotmesis (disruption of axons without interruption of supporting structures), and presents with edema and tortuosity of the affected structures. The axonotmesis cases usually develop edema distal to the site of injury.[8] The abnormalities can be demonstrated on the fat-suppressed T2-weighted images in the oblique coronal plane.[8] Most of the cases of stretch injury improve over time.

ADULT TRAUMATIC INJURIES

The nerve root avulsions, termed neurotmesis, can be divided into the preganglionic and postganglionic categories. The latter can be subdivided into complete and partial. In adults, the avulsion injury is associated with high-impact trauma. C5 and C6

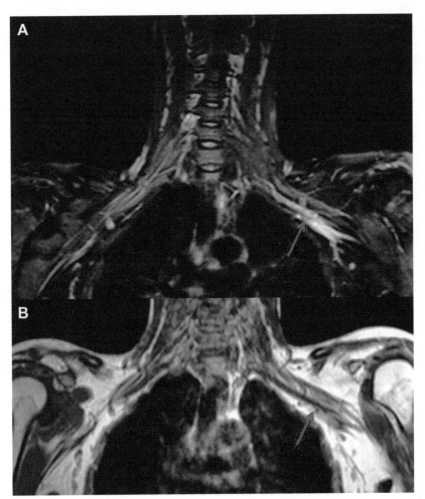

Fig. 4. The STIR (*A*) and T1-weighted (*B*) images demonstrate unilateral edema, thickening, and mild tortuosity of the left divisions and cords (*arrows*) consistent with stretch injury.

are the most commonly injured roots because of their prolonged descent in the neck and susceptibility to traction injury. Based on a series of 26 patients presenting with traction injury (**Fig. 5**), the most commonly seen abnormalities on MR imaging are (1) traumatic pseudomeningoceles (64%), (2) absence of the roots (64%), (3) lateral cord displacement (45%), (4) hemorrhage and/or

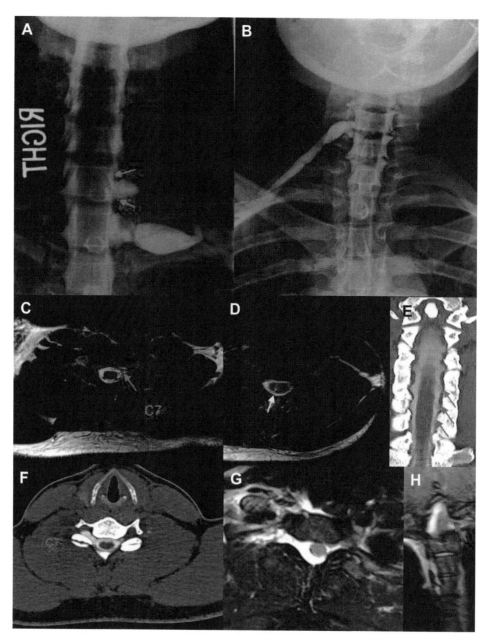

Fig. 5. The myelogram (*A*) demonstrates posttraumatic pseudomeningoceles at the left C7/T1 and T1/T2 neural foramina with residual C8 and T1 nerve roots (*red arrows*) in the canal extending to these levels. Myelogram (*B*) of a 19-year-old football player who presented with arm flaccidity after shoulder injury during a football practice demonstrates a right C6 and C7 pseudomeningocele extending to the axillary fossa. The right C7 root within the canal is not visualized. T2-weighted MR imaging (*C, D*) demonstrate complete avulsion of the right C5 and C7 nerve roots with signal changes in the right side of the cord (*yellow arrow*) and preservation of the roots on the contralateral side (*red arrow*). The CT myelogram (*E, F*) demonstrates multiple right root avulsions with preservation of the left roots (*red arrows*) and a small right C7 pseudomeningocele. The axial (*G*) and coronal (*H*) T2-weighted images demonstrate a right nerve root avulsion with associated pseudomeningocele and cord displacement to the left. There is also soft tissue edema within the right paraspinal soft tissue related to recent injury.

scarring in the canal (45%), (5) denervation of erector spinae (27%), (6) syrinx (18%), and (7) spinal cord edema (9%).[9] The CT myelogram has been used traditionally for evaluation of pregangli- onic lesions due to higher spatial resolution. However, the invasiveness of this technique is its biggest disadvantage, along with its lack of sensi- tivity for cord injuries. MR imaging using isotropic heavily T2-weighted technique (constructive inter- ference in steady state [CISS] or fast imaging employing steady-state acquisition [FIESTA]) and MR myelography, based on Sampling Perfec- tion with Application-optimized Contrasts using different flip-angle Evolutions (SPACE) sequences, is noninvasive and comparable to CT myelography in its accuracy. In many centers, this limits the use of CT myelography to patients unable to undergo MR imaging.[10] Both CT myelography and MR imaging techniques may demonstrate avulsed roots, hematomas, and (in some cases) pseudo- meningocele and displacement of the cord to the contralateral side (see **Fig. 5**).[3] The pseudome- ningoceles represent cerebrospinal fluid (CSF) leakage through the dural tear and, therefore, are seen as fluid-filled saccular dural outpouchings on MR imaging and are filled with contrast on CT myelogram.

MR imaging also allows for assessment of concomitant cord abnormalities, stretch injury, and denervation changes.[3] In some cases, it is being combined with three-dimensional (3D) MR neurography (MRN), including multiplanar recon- structions and maximum intensity projections.[11] The MRN studies are usually T2-weighted–based or diffusion-based techniques. The morphology of the neural structures is better defined by the T2-weighted–based techniques. Spectral adiabatic inversion recovery (SPAIR) is increas- ingly being used in some centers instead of short tau inversion recovery (STIR) imaging due to better signal-to-noise ratio and more favorable specific absorption rate.[12] The diffusion-weighted MRN imaging demonstrates continuity of fibers and their relationship to pathologic lesions. This not only allows for qualitative but also for quantitative assessment of the nerve signal, using apparent diffusion coefficient and fractional anisotropy values. The diffusion tensor imaging–based trac- tography demonstrates myeloradicular and spinal nerve continuity; however, it is technically difficult because of movement of the adjacent structures, need for large volume coverage, high spatial reso- lution, and presence of pulsation and susceptibility artifacts. Therefore, it is not routinely used for brachial plexus evaluation.[13] The hybrid diffusion-based MRN techniques, such as 3D diffusion-weighted reversed fast imaging with

steady-state precession (3D DW-PSIF), allow for nerve-specific imaging due to strong suppression of the adjacent vascular signal but are more commonly used for lumbar plexus, peripheral, and cranial nerves.[14]

Postganglionic injuries are usually associated with distal nerve retraction and may occasionally demonstrate mild enhancing nodular thickening known as posttraumatic neuroma. Approximately 80% of levels with nerve root avulsions develop pseudomeningoceles; about 15% of levels with pseudomeningoceles do not have an associated nerve root avulsion.[15,16] Therefore, visualization of the nerve root is of the utmost significance. Even if there is a nerve root avulsion, the residual root within the pseudomeningocele should be identified because it may allow nerve grafting. Approximately 20% of cases demonstrate cord signal abnormality on MR imaging.[17] Administra- tion of contrast may increase the conspicuity of the denervated shoulder girdle and paraspinal muscles as early as 24 hours after injury, by virtue of muscular enhancement and enhancement of the injured portion of the brachial plexus.[18]

Distinction between the preganglionic and post- ganglionic avulsions influences both management and prognosis. The postganglionic injuries are usually repaired after 3 months of observation to allow for some functional recovery, whereas the preganglionic injuries require early nerve transfers for reconstruction. In severe avulsion cases some surgeons now explore the brachial plexus within the first few weeks, and usually perform nerve transfers as a treatment. Although the procedure can be done up to 12 months after injury, the earlier transfers are performed, the better the outcome.

NEONATAL TRAUMATIC INJURIES

Neonatal injuries are seen in up to 0.5% of live births[19] and, depending on the position of the arm during the delivery, may present with superior or inferior plexus injuries. The most common neonatal plexus injury, Erb-Duchenne palsy, usually involves C5 and C6, but may also include C7 nerves. It is associated with supraspinatus, in- fraspinatus, deltoid, and bicep muscle weakness. The inferior neonatal plexus injury, Klumpke palsy, involves C8 and T1. It presents with hand inteross- eous and forearm muscle weakness. It may be associated with Horner syndrome. Rarely, there is a question of differential diagnostic consider- ations. The knowledge of fetal trauma during delivery and the expected recovery course may, in some cases, help determine the need for further evaluation. The most frequently used techniques are isotropic T2-weighted images, such as 3D CISS or 3D T2-weighted turbo spin echo, with multiplanar reconstructions. The most important preoperative question for early (3–4 months) imaging is the presence of preganglionic root avulsion in cases with insufficient recovery following partial plexus injury.[20,21]

NONTRAUMATIC PATHOLOGIC CONDITIONS

Nontraumatic pathologic conditions include these common categories: acute or chronic infectious or inflammatory brachial neuritis or neuropathy, primary or secondary benign and malignant tumors, aggressive fibromatosis, radiation-induced plexopathy, vascular abnormalities, compression of the plexus, and infection of the plexus.[3] These are better evaluated with MR imaging, except for previously treated malignant tumors in which case a PET-CT scan may be used to differentiate radiation fibrosis from the residual neoplasm.

RADIATION PLEXOPATHY

The most common nontraumatic inflammatory cause of brachial plexopathy is radiation plexitis. The plexopathy development is dose-dependent, with the risk increasing with both increase in total dose and dose per fraction.[22] Only 1.3% of patients develop radiation plexopathy when the dose is less than 50 Gy, whereas the risk increases to more than 5% when the dose is more than 50 Gy.[23] A recent report of radiation doses of 70 Gy reported 16% incidence of brachial plexopathy.[24] The peak presentation is several years after the treatment, but it has been reported as early as 1.5 months and as late as 22 years after the radiation.[23,25–30] At a total dose of 60 Gy, the risk of plexopathy increases from 3.9% at 5 years to 54% at 19 years with annual incidence for grade 1 or higher modified Late Effects Normal Tissue-Subjective, Objective, Management, Analytic (LENT-SOMA) score lesion of 2.9%.[31] The LENT-SOMA scale used for clinical grading in these cases ranges from 1 to 4, from mild sensory deficits to complete motor paresis, excruciating pain, and muscle atrophy (Table 2).[31]

Radiation plexopathy is subdivided into acute and chronic. The time threshold separating the two subtypes is 6 months. The acute radiation plexopathy is considered ischemic, whereas the chronic may be related to fibrosis.[25] There is a suggestion of genetic predisposition.[32] Radiation fibrosis is most frequently related to breast or lung cancer treatment. Use of overlapping fields and chemotherapy increases the risk of this condition.[23,33] Paresthesias and sensory loss dominate

Table 2
LENT-SOMA scale for grading the symptoms of radiation plexopathy

LENT-SOMA Scale	
Grade 1	Mild sensory deficits without pain
Grade 2	Moderate sensory deficits, tolerable pain, mild arm weakness
Grade 3	Continuous paresthesia with incomplete motor paresis
Grade 4	Complete motor paresis, excruciating pain, and muscle atrophy

Data from Stubblefield MD, O'Dell MW. Cancer rehabilitation: principle and practice. New York, NY: Demos Medical Publishing; 2009.

the symptoms; fewer patients have motor function loss.[33] Although there are reports of recovery, the disease is frequently progressive.[31] The upper trunk is more likely to be affected due to its length and absence of protection provided by the clavicle, especially in patients with axillary, infraclavicular and supraclavicular lymph node involvement. The imaging findings usually demonstrate diffuse thickening and distortion of the fibers, edema, and mild enhancement without a focal mass (Fig. 6).[25]

The differential considerations include other causes of brachial neuritis, cervical disc disease, and neoplastic and traumatic brachial plexopathy. The history is helpful in exclusion of traumatic causes. The presence of Horner syndrome and severe pain with less than 60 Gy radiation dose are more suggestive of tumor recurrence than radiation plexopathy.[34] In addition, the electromyography (EMG) finding of myokymia, or semirhythmic bursts of potentials, is the most specific finding that separates neoplastic from radiation plexopathy. However, at least 30% of patients with radiation plexopathy do not demonstrate this finding.[35–37] In radiation fibrosis, the affected area will demonstrate T1-weighted and T2-weighted hypointensity (Fig. 7). There are reports of both fibrosis and tumor demonstrating enhancement.[32] The follow-up images will be valuable in detection of enlarging masses, not seen in fibrosis. The PET scan is the best study to differentiate radiation fibrosis from neoplastic recurrence.[38,39] Biopsy may be needed to provide a definitive diagnosis.[40]

BRACHIAL PLEXITIS

Initially recognized by Spillane[41] and named "neuralgic amyotrophy" by Parsonage and Turner,[42]

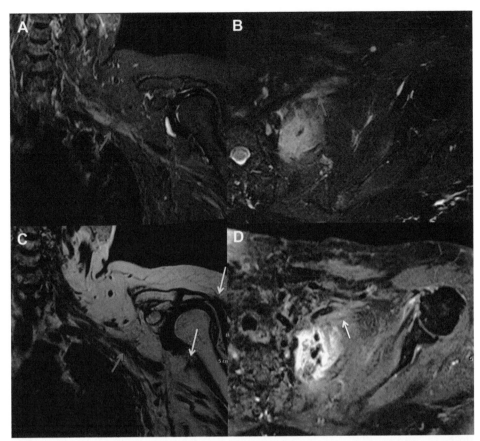

Fig. 6. Coronal STIR (*A*), axial STIR (*B*), T1-weighted (*C*) and axial post-contrast T1-weighted (*D*) images depict chronic radiation plexitis as demonstrated by thickening, edema (*red arrows*), and enhancement (*white arrow*) of the trunks, divisions and cords of the brachial plexus, as well as shoulder girdle muscle atrophy and replacement by fat (*yellow arrows*) in a patient with left upper extremity lymphedema, 8 years after radiation treatment for left breast cancer.

inflammatory brachial plexitis presents with spontaneous acute onset of severe burning shoulder pain, subsequent sensory disturbance, and delayed weakness and atrophy. This may mimic other conditions, such as cervical spondylitis, radiculitis, rotator cuff tear, shoulder impingement, and calcific tendinitis.[41–46] Although multiple dermatomal and myotomal levels of involvement, and improvement of pain before onset of the motor deficit allow for differentiation from cervical radiculitis or spondylopathy, imaging and nerve conduction studies are used for confirmation of the diagnosis and to exclude other causes.[47]

The exact causes of acute sporadic brachial plexitis are uncertain, but vaccination-related and other immune-mediated, toxin-mediated, and infectious mechanisms have been suggested in the absence of prior trauma.[46,48,49] The latter include Lyme disease, and multiple viral agents, such as cytomegalovirus, coxsackievirus, herpes zoster, Epstein-Barr, and parvovirus B19. There is also a hereditary predisposition in patients with an autosomal dominant hereditary neuralgic amyotrophy.[50] The incidence of brachial plexitis is reported to be approximately 2 to 3 per 100,000.[51,52] This condition has male predominance[43,53] and occurs at approximately 40 years of age in the sporadic form and 28 years of age the in hereditary form, with age ranges of 10 to 80 years and 3 to 56 years, respectively.[50] Slightly more than 60% of cases are initially misdiagnosed (often as spondylotic cervical radiculopathy) with median and mean time before the correct diagnosis of 11 weeks and 44 weeks, respectively.[50] Slightly more than 50% of patients have degenerative changes in the cervical spine on MR imaging.[50] The initial presentation in 96% of patients is acute onset of severe pain, which could be bilateral but is asymmetric in up to 29% of cases, and starts at night in slightly more than 60% of cases. The mean time to onset of weakness

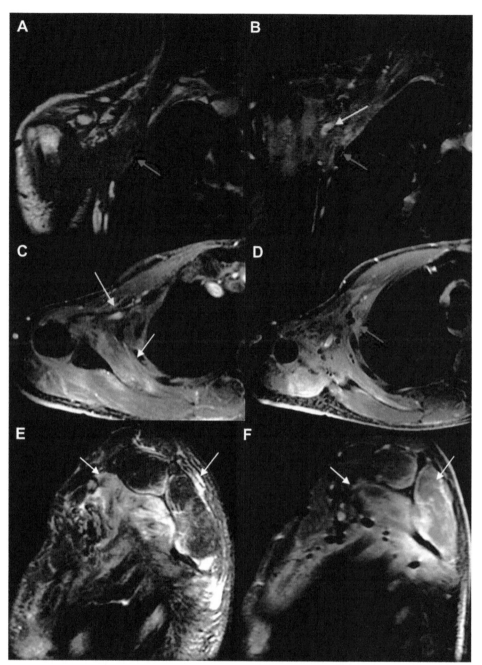

Fig. 7. T1-weighted (*A*), axial (*C* and *D*) and sagittal (*F*) fat-suppressed post-contrast T1-weighted and STIR (*B, E*) images demonstrate an ill-defined nonenhancing soft tissue mass (*red arrows*) surrounding subclavian/axillary artery (*yellow arrows*) in a patient with history of radiation treatment of metastatic basal cell carcinoma, consistent with radiation-induced fibrosis. There is edema and peripheral enhancement within the shoulder girdle muscles (*white arrows*), consistent with denervation changes.

is 2 weeks.[50] The upper part of the plexus tends to be most commonly affected.[50] Most patients have associated sensory symptoms, most commonly hypesthesias.[50]

The electrodiagnostic tests usually demonstrate changes compatible with brachial plexitis, but they vary depending on severity of injury and timing of evaluation.[50] Approximately 3 weeks after onset of symptoms, the EMG demonstrates fibrillation potentials and positive waves, suggestive of muscle denervation.[54] Three to four months after onset of symptoms, giant polyphasic potentials are seen.

Although most of the literature suggests that most commonly the condition resolves 3 to 4 months after presentation without sequelae,[44] the largest case series of 246 patients suggests that the prognosis is worse than traditionally thought, with only 25% of patients pain free and only 75% of patients able to work after 3-years follow-up.[50] The investigators attributed this discrepancy in outcomes to differences in the definition of recovery. Up to 17% of females and slightly over 3% of males had a Rankin score (Table 3) of 3 on follow-up, demonstrating need for daily assistance.[50] The results were more favorable when the patients were treated with oral steroids in an acute phase.[50] Up to 25% of sporadic and 75% of hereditary cases tend to have a recurrence of disease.[50]

MR imaging ranges from normal appearance of the plexus, to thickening and edema of the plexus components with or without enhancement (identical to the pattern with radiation plexopathy) (Fig. 8). Most cases demonstrate denervation changes in the shoulder girdle and chest musculature, with edema on water sensitive sequences, muscular enhancement in the acute phase, and atrophy and fatty replacement in subacute and chronic phases (Fig. 9).[3,44,50,55,56] This is predominantly seen in the distribution of the suprascapular and to a lesser degree axillary or long thoracic nerves or their combinations. The muscle changes are predominantly noted in the supraspinatus and infraspinatus muscles, and much less frequently in the deltoid and teres minor, followed by subscapularis, latissimus dorsi, pectoralis, and rhomboids.[55,56]

MR imaging is also useful to exclude other causes of atrophy and pain, including abnormalities of the rotator cuff, glenoid labrum, internal or external impingement, masses pressing on the brachial plexus components or branches, or presence of diffuse myopathy and/or myositis.[51] This allows patients to avoid unnecessary surgery and receive appropriate conservative therapy.[55] The treatment of this condition usually includes analgesics, frequently narcotics, immunomodulators, steroids, and physical therapy.[57] Presently, there may be a role for nerve transfers in cases that demonstrate absence of motor-function improvement beyond 6 months.

INFECTION OF THE BRACHIAL PLEXUS

Most of the viral and vector-transmitted bacterial infections of the brachial plexus fall under the Parsonage-Turner syndrome diagnosis, and present with characteristic history, following a typical prodrome. In the absence of open wound or iatrogenic introduction of bacteria, the more aggressive, frequently suppurative involvement of the brachial plexus occurs by extension from the spine osteomyelitis (Fig. 10), septic glenohumeral arthritis, empyema, or invasive infectious parenchymal lung process.[58,59] Therefore, the organisms that cause the above mentioned processes are responsible for the secondary involvement of the brachial plexus. These are *Staphylococcus aureus*, coagulase-negative staphylococci, group B streptococcus, *Mycobacterium tuberculosis*, *Nocardia*, *Cryptococcus*, *Pseudomonas*, *Pasteurella*, *Actinomycosis*, *Echinococcus*, *Aspergillus*, and *Mucor* species. The bacteria represent more than half (55%) of such infectious agents, followed by parasites (26%), and fungi (16%).[58] Aspiration is

Table 3
Modified Rankin Score is used to rate the degree of the disability and dependence on others for daily activities

	Modified Rankin Score	
0	No disability	No symptom
1	No significant disability	Able to carry out all usual activities, despite some symptoms
2	Slight disability	Able to look after own affairs without assistance, but unable to carry out all previous activities
3	Moderate disability	Requires some help, but able to walk unassisted
4	Moderately severe disability	Unable to attend to own bodily needs without assistance, or walk unassisted
5	Severe disability	Requires constant nursing care and attention, bedridden, incontinent
6	Dead	—

Data from van Swieten JC, Koudstaal PJ, Visser MC, et al. Interobserver agreement for the assessment of handicap in stroke patients. Stroke 1988;19(5):604–7.

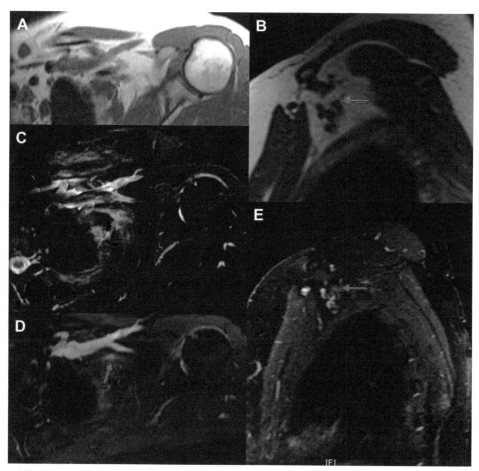

Fig. 8. Sudden onset of left upper extremity pain and mild weakness. The T1-weighted (*A, B, D*) and STIR (*C, E*) images demonstrate mild edema and enhancement (*red arrows*) in the region of the posterior cord, consistent with brachial plexitis.

usually required for both identification of the organism and determination of its sensitivities. Nevertheless, there is almost 10% mortality associated with these cases in the literature with most the deceased immunocompromised.

MALIGNANT NEOPLASMS

Secondary neoplastic involvement, by direct extension or due to metastasis, is more common than primary brachial plexus tumors and is the most common noninflammatory cause of plexopathy in middle-aged and older individuals.[3,60] The metastatic tumor frequently compresses the plexus and, in some cases, invades it. Hematogenous metastases to the plexus are rare and most commonly are caused by breast, lung, and Hodgkin's lymphoma.

The most common primary malignancies affecting the plexus are breast and lung. In the report from one of the tertiary centers on causes of nontraumatic brachial plexus lesions evaluated with MR imaging (**Fig. 11**), breast cancer was the second leading cause (24%) following radiation fibrosis (31%).[61] Similar to other secondary malignancies affecting the brachial plexus, breast cancer may involve the components of the brachial plexus via direct extension or metastasis to other adjacent structures, such as spine. Breast metastases most commonly appear as lymphadenopathy surrounding, compressing, and occasionally invading the brachial plexus.[61] The signal intensity is similar to the tumor of origin.[62] Although most of the breast metastases are hypointense on T1-weighted images and hyperintense on T2-weighted images (see **Fig. 11**), there are cases when metastatic breast disease demonstrates T2-weighted hypointense appearance, especially in desmoplastic breast cancer.[63] The patient's history allows for diagnosis in these cases.[62]

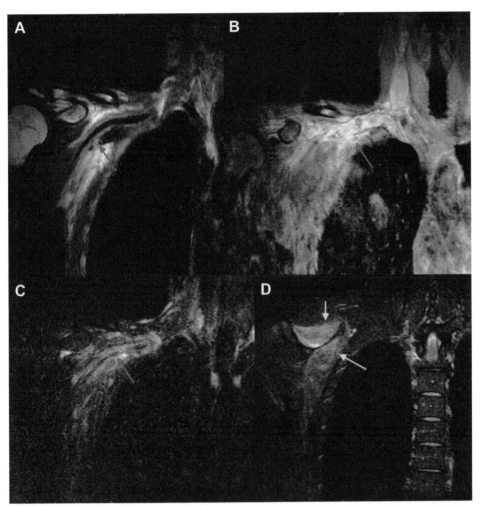

Fig. 9. T1-weighted (*A, B*) and STIR (*C, D*) images demonstrate diffuse thickening, edema, and enhancement (*red arrows*) of the right brachial plexus at the level of the divisions and cords that presented as an acute onset of pain and delayed weakness in the right upper extremity of a 35-year-old man, consistent with Parsonage-Turner syndrome. There are denervation changes in the shoulder girdle muscles (*yellow arrows*).

Lung cancer is the next most common cause, seen in 19% of cases. It involves the brachial plexus most commonly by direct extension from the superior sulcus (Pancoast tumor) but can present due to lymph node metastasis, similar to breast cancer. The Pancoast tumors (**Fig. 12**) usually are histologically non-small cell cancers, including adenocarcinoma, squamous cell, and large cell carcinomas. There is usually pain, followed by numbness and weakness involving the lower spinal nerves and inferior trunk of the brachial plexus. In up to 20% of cases, the tumor involves the sympathetic chain, resulting in Horner syndrome. Unlike extrapleural lesions, the lung interface in these cases is irregular.[64]

In cases of direct extension, the involvement of the interscalene fat pad determines whether the patient is a surgical candidate, because it suggests invasion of multiple spinal nerves of the plexus and, in some cases, vertebral involvement.[3]

Head and neck cancers may metastasize into the cervical spine or lymph nodes, resulting in either compression or invasion of the brachial plexus structures.[65] Hematologic malignancies, such as lymphoma, leukemia, and multiple myeloma, may also affect the brachial plexus, predominantly because of mass effect of the enlarged pathologic lymph nodes (**Fig. 13**).[61] Lymphoma rarely directly involves the plexus (neurolymphomatosis)[62] as

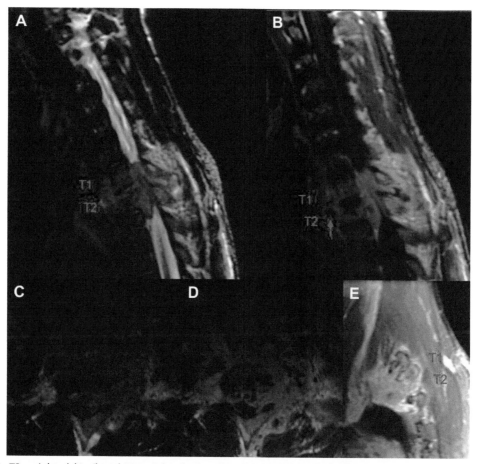

Fig. 10. T2-weighted (*A, C*) and T1-weighted contrast-enhanced (*B, D, E*) images demonstrate an expansile soft tissue mass involving the T1 and T2 vertebral bodies, sparing the disc space, and extending into the canal, left greater than right neural foramina, left posterior elements, and prevertebral soft tissues, with suggestion of a small prevertebral fluid collection (*arrow*). There is cord compression and complete obscuration of the left neural foramen. The patient was confirmed to have Pott disease (spinal tuberculosis).

a primary or systemic process.[66] The involvement is caused by B-cell lymphoma with the dominant feature of involvement of peripheral nerves. The imaging demonstrates diffuse plexus edema, distortion of fascicular morphology, and variable enhancement.[2,62]

The primary soft tissue sarcomas occurring in the area of the brachial plexus are low-grade fibrosarcoma, synovial sarcoma, and radiation-induced sarcoma.[2] The latter are most commonly seen in patients with breast cancer and occur in 0.18% of cases, usually presenting more than 6 years after the irradiation.[23] Other processes that can involve this location are mesothelioma, melanoma, gastrointestinal tumor, osteosarcoma, Ewing sarcoma (**Fig. 14**), and leiomyosarcoma metastasis. Primary vertebral lesions, such as chordoma (**Fig. 15**) or chondrosarcoma may

compress the roots and spinal nerves of the brachial plexus.

The malignant nerve sheath tumors (**Fig. 16**) are rare (14% of all neurogenic tumors of the brachial plexus) and are frequently seen after radiation treatment or in patients with neurofibromatosis (NF) type 1.[2,3] In the NF-1 patient, the presence of plexiform neurofibromas increases the patient's risk of developing malignant peripheral nerve sheath tumors (MPNST) by 20-fold, a fact that warrants close imaging and clinical follow-up.[67] The ill-defined tumor margins and invasion of adjacent structures or a combination of large size, peripheral enhancement, perilesional edema-like zone, and heterogeneity of the lesion have high specificity for malignant nerve sheath tumors on MR imaging, but the sensitivity of MR imaging remains low (43%–60%).[68–70] There are

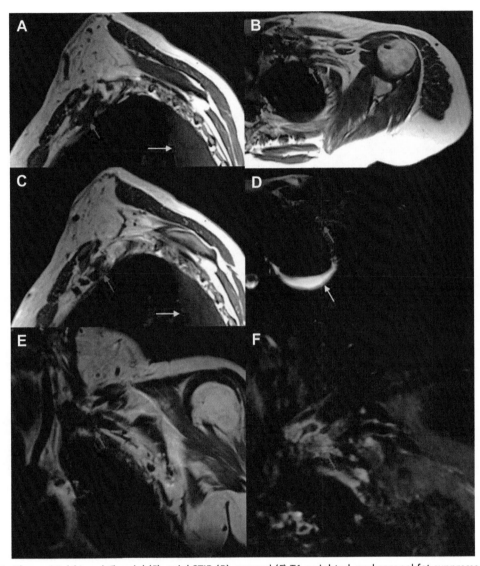

Fig. 11. The sagittal (*A* and *C*), axial (*B*), axial STIR (*D*), coronal (*E*) T1-weighted, and coronal fat-suppressed post-contrast T1-weighted (*F*) images demonstrate an ill-defined mass (*red arrows*) involving divisions and cords in a 54-year-old woman with history of breast cancer and new onset of left, upper extremity numbness and weakness, consistent with metastatic breast cancer. Note small left pleural effusion (*yellow arrows*).

reports of using gallium citrate and fluorine-18 fluorodeoxyglucose–PET to detect malignant nerve sheath tumors.[71,72] The latter has over 90% sensitivity and specificity in differentiating a neurofibroma from a malignant tumor but is less definitive in distinguishing schwannomas and MPNST.[72] The malignant nerve sheath tumors cannot be reliably distinguished from benign lesions on any single imaging study. Marked growth over time, progressive loss of function, and severe pain at rest, especially in patients with NF-1, are findings concerning for a possible malignant nerve sheath tumor and require tissue

diagnosis.[73] The MR imaging report should mention the presence of intradural extension for surgical planning and assess the need for post-surgical radiation.[2] Involvement of the vertebral artery also needs to be described and, if the vertebral artery is involved, MR angiography evaluation should be used for assessment of neck and intracranial vascular supply to the posterior fossa.[2] The criteria of resectability of the tumor with vascular sparing in cases involving less than 270°, described for the carotid artery by Yousem and colleagues,[74] could be extended to the vertebral artery in these cases.

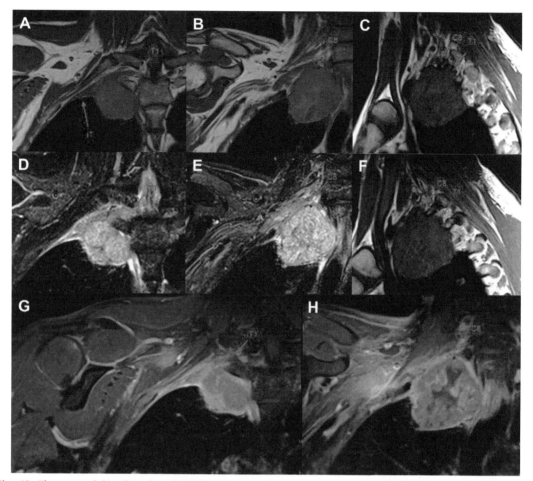

Fig. 12. The coronal (*A, B*) and sagittal (*C, F*) T1-weighted, coronal STIR (*D, E*), and coronal fat-suppressed contrast-enhanced T1-weighted (*G, H*) superior sulcus tumor involving the C8 and T1 nerves (*red arrows* with corresponding designations). IT, inferior trunk.

BENIGN MASSES

The brachial plexus can also be compressed by benign masses, such as lipoma, hemangioma, lymphangioma, ganglioneuroma, neuroblastoma, myoblastoma, branchial cleft cyst, myositis ossificans, pseudoaneurysm, fibromatosis, nodular fasciitis, and perineurioma.[3] Benign masses represent approximately 17% of cases in one large series.[61] The most common secondary process of benign cause is desmoid or aggressive fibromatosis, followed by lipoma, perineurioma, and vascular malformations.

Fibromatosis (locally aggressive extraabdominal desmoid tumor) presents with a painless mass, or occasionally with pain and neurologic dysfunction.[3] It appears as an infiltrating avidly enhancing mass with hypointense T1-weighted and heterogeneous T2-weighted signal (**Fig. 17**).[3] Occasionally, the margins are infiltrative only on the microscopic

level, and the lesion appears well-defined on imaging.[2] The treatment is resection with imaging follow-up, even if the resection margins are positive, because the tumor is expected to regress or grow slowly.[75] Use of neoadjuvant chemotherapy and/or radiation therapy is controversial. Many investigators recommend reserving adjuvant therapy for rapidly growing residual or recurrent tumor, which would require disfiguring surgery.[75–77]

Nodular and proliferative fasciitis is another fibroproliferative condition, occasionally mistaken for sarcoma. It most commonly affects the upper extremity, followed by the proximal lower extremity, head and neck, and chest. The lesions may be well-defined or infiltrative. The former is most commonly seen with the subcutaneous type. The latter is seen with fascial or intramuscular types of this process. The lesion is most common in adults and presents most commonly as a tender and rapidly growing

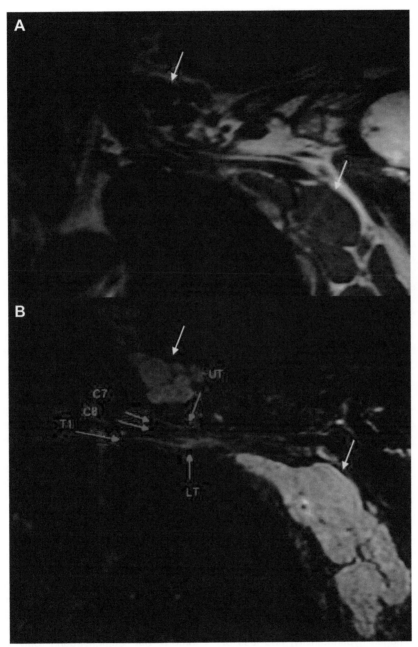

Fig. 13. Coronal T1-weighted (*A*) and STIR (*B*) images demonstrate cervical and axillary adenopathy (*yellow arrows*) with mass effect on the lower trunk and divisions in the patient with C8 and T1 radicular symptoms and history of lymphoma. The *red arrows* point to corresponding spinal nerves and trunks. *Abbreviations:* LT, lower trunk; UT, upper trunk.

mass. There are several reported cases of intraneural disease, including involvement of brachial plexus.[78] There are cases of spontaneous resolution. Surgical resection is usually curative. A CT scan may demonstrate a lesion isodense or hypodense to the muscle with rare calcifications. The lesion is usually similar to muscle on T1-weighted images and intermediate-to-high intensity compared with the muscle on T2-weighted images. There may be mild surrounding edema and mild enhancement of the lesion depending on predominance of myxoid or fibrous content.

The lipomas are easily identified based on fat signal characteristics: T1-weighted and

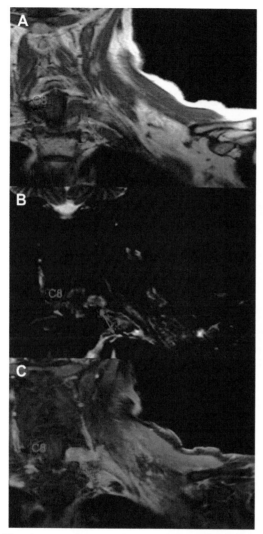

Fig. 14. Precontrast and postcontrast T1-weighted (*A, C*) and STIR (*B*) images demonstrate an enhancing mass (*arrows*) in the region of the C8 nerve root in a patient with prior resection of Ewing sarcoma, consistent with residual disease.

T2-weighted images hyperintensity, and loss of signal within fat suppression (**Fig. 18**). The differentiation of lipomas from well-differentiated liposarcomas is difficult.[2] The findings suggestive of liposarcoma are advanced age, male gender, size greater than 10 cm, presence of soft tissue nodules, or more than 25% of the mass composed of nonadipose tissue, and the presence of thick septa.[79] PET images are capable of distinguishing benign and malignant lesions. They also can identify subtypes of the liposarcomas.[80]

Nerve sheath tumors are the most common primary neoplasm involving the brachial plexus. They are most commonly seen in the neural foramina, usually ovoid, T2-weighted hyperintense, well-circumscribed, and may be associated with bony remodeling.[2] They present as painless soft tissue masses, but may be associated with a combination of paresthesias, pain, and neurologic dysfunction.[81] The physical examination usually demonstrates no significant muscle weakness or wasting, but the lesion is firm, tender, and produces a positive Tinel sign.[2] One-third of all nerve sheath tumors occur in patients with NF-1. Approximately 20% of all nerve sheath tumors occur in the brachial plexus. They include schwannomas, neurofibromas, perineuriomas, and MPNST. The neurofibromas are the most common primary tumor to affect the brachial plexus overall (50%–65%) and especially in NF.[2] They have an infiltrating pattern of growth within the nerve without a capsule and usually appear as a fusiform and longitudinally oriented lesion. They are frequently multiple and plexiform in NF-1 patients.[60] On MR imaging they are more likely than schwannomas, 58% versus 15%, to have a target sign, the central low signal with peripheral rim of T2-weighted hyperintensity (**Fig. 19**). Overall, schwannomas represent 18% to 20% of brachial plexus nerve sheath tumor.[81] However, in the absence of NF they represent over 50% of cases.[2] They grow eccentrically and are encapsulated (**Fig. 20**), making surgical excision with nerve preservation easier than neurofibroma.[2] They frequently demonstrate the fascicular sign with salt and pepper appearance on T2-weighted sequences. They are also likely to undergo "ancient" changes with cystic appearance on MR imaging. In absence of cystic degeneration, the nerve sheath tumors demonstrate avid enhancement on MR imaging.

The perineuriomas originate from the perineurium with the responsible gene located on the long arm of chromosome 22 but not at the same locus as NF-2.[82] Perineuriomas do not recur or metastasize, but can only be identified by immunohistochemistry.[82] On imaging they present as enhancing masses similar to other nerve sheath tumors but demonstrating only minimal T2-weighted hyperintensity, much lower than neurofibromas and schwannomas.[2,82]

COMPRESSIVE PLEXOPATHY

The neurogenic thoracic outlet syndrome represents greater than 95% of the thoracic outlet syndrome cases[3,83] and, most commonly, affects young women.[84] The onset of symptoms most often occurs at ages between 20 to 40 years.[85] Pain and paresthesias are the most common symptoms of neurogenic thoracic outlet syndrome,[86] with hand weakness and muscle

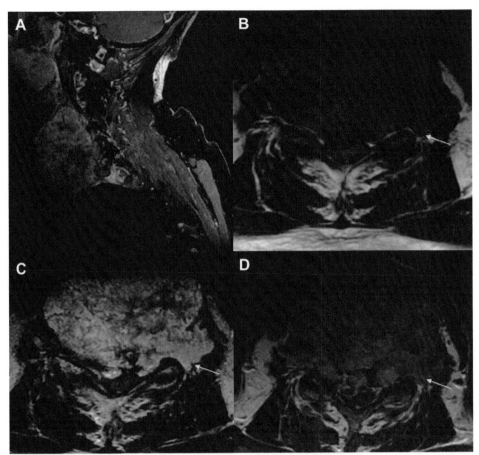

Fig. 15. Sagittal (*A*) and axial (*C*) T2-weighted, axial T1-weighted (*B*), and contrast-enhanced axial T1-weighted images (*D*) demonstrate a heterogeneous expansile vertebral body mass centered at the lower cervical spine and extending into the canal and left C6–7 neural foramen (*yellow arrows*), compressing C7 nerve root. The biopsy resulted in diagnosis of chordoma.

atrophy present in severe or mixed neurogenic and arterial ischemic cases. In 90% of cases, there is involvement of the C8 and T1 spinal nerves or the lower trunk,[86] with the patients presenting with symptoms along the medial brachial area and paresthesias in the ring and little fingers. Some patients present with neck pain, radiating to the ear and occipital region, posteriorly into the rhomboid, trapezius, and deltoid area, and anteriorly across the clavicle into the pectoral region (pseudoangina). These symptoms are usually related to upper plexus involvement, C5 and C7.[87] In some cases, there is also autonomic, predominantly vasomotor, dysfunction.[87] For example, Raynaud phenomenon is frequently seen due to overstimulation of the sympathetic fibers in the vicinity of T1 and C8 roots.[3] The cause is compression of the neurovascular bundle traversing corresponding compartments,

including the interscalene triangle, costoclavicular space, or rarely the pectoralis minor space.[87] The causes range from cervical ribs (**Fig. 21**), enlargement of the transverse process of C7 (see **Fig. 21**), scalenus, subclavius, or pectoralis muscle hypertrophy or posttraumatic fibrosis, fibrous bands, and posture.[87] Elevation of the upper extremity may exacerbate narrowing of the interscalene triangle and costoclavicular space, and reproduce a patient's symptoms.[3]

The initial step in the radiologic evaluation of suspected thoracic outlet syndrome is the cervical radiographs that may demonstrate a bony pathologic condition. However, the bony anatomy, including long transverse processes and cervical ribs, are better delineated on CT. MR imaging could be used to demonstrate muscular enlargement, presence of the fibrous bands, and deviation of the plexus and its edema. In many cases, dynamic

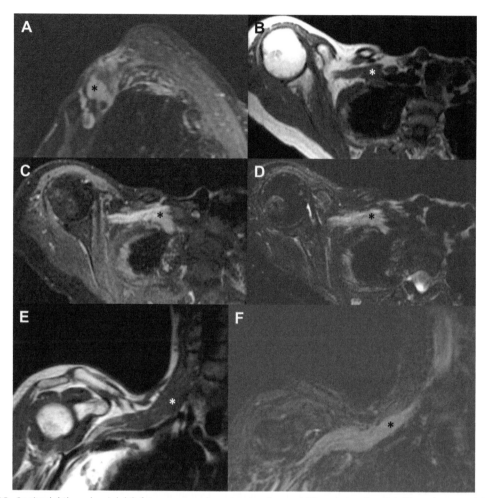

Fig. 16. Sagittal (*A*) and axial (*C*) fat-suppressed contrast enhanced T1-weighted, axial (*B*) and coronal (*E*) T1-weighted, axial (*D*) and coronal (*F*) STIR images demonstrate diffuse thickening and enhancement (*asterisk*) of the nerves, trunks, divisions, and cords of the right brachial plexus in a patient with history of remote radiation treatment of lymphoma in this area, who presents with right upper extremity polyneuropathy. The radiation-induced plexopathy, neurolymphomatosis, paraneoplastic chronic demyelinating inflammatory neuropathy were considered. The biopsy demonstrated low-grade malignant peripheral sheath tumor.

imaging is required to demonstrate compression of the brachial plexus by the adjacent structures with hyperabducted position of the arms (**Fig. 22**).[87,88] Some investigators advocate performing CT angiogram with provocative positioning. If MR imaging is used for evaluation, the sagittal followed by coronal T1-weighted sequences are the most helpful for evaluation of the relationship of the structures at the thoracic outlet.[87] Contrast-enhancement MR imaging and MR angiography may be useful in cases of suspected arterial compromise or venous thrombosis.[87] Although venous compression in the hyperabducted position can be seen in healthy volunteers, it is helpful in identifying the possible

location of the arterial and brachial plexus compressions during MR imaging evaluation.[89] The criteria for presence of neurologic compression are obscuration of the adjacent fat planes and contact with adjacent bony structures.[89]

The anterior and, in some cases, middle scalene blocks, relaxing the muscle and temporarily decompressing the thoracic outlet and improving the symptoms, are frequently used as a diagnostic study and a predictor of surgical outcome.[90] The treatment of the neurogenic thoracic outlet syndrome is based on the cause, but most commonly the initial therapy includes physical therapy, analgesic medication, muscle relaxants,

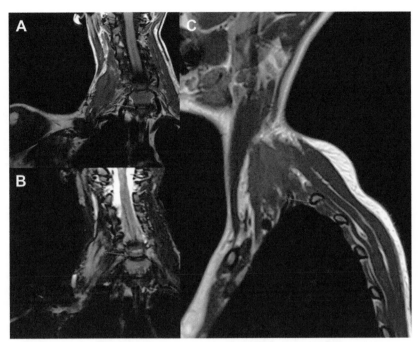

Fig. 17. Coronal (*A*), sagittal (*C*) T1-weighted, and coronal STIR (*B*) demonstrate an infiltrating soft tissue mass involving C5 and C6 nerve roots and upper trunk with mild displacement of the C7 and middle trunk (*red arrows*) in a 19-year-old woman. The biopsy demonstrated a desmoid lesion.

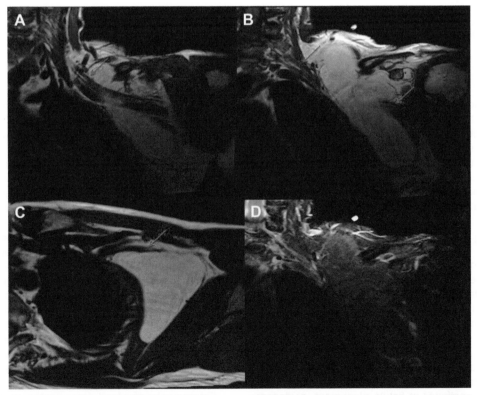

Fig. 18. Coronal (*A, B*) and axial (*C*) T1-weighted, coronal STIR (*D*) demonstrates a large circumscribed axillary mass with imaging characteristics classic for a lipoma. The lesion displaces the divisions and cords of the brachial plexus (*red arrows*).

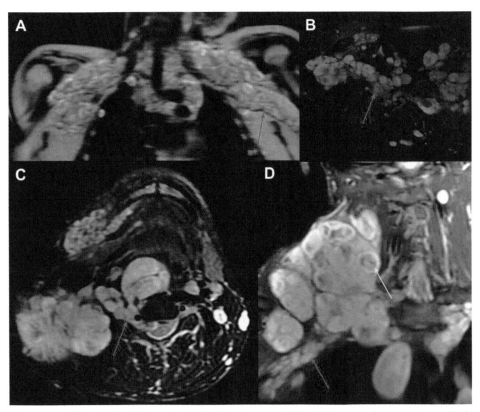

Fig. 19. The coronal T2-weighted (*A*) and axial (*B, C*) and coronal (*D*) STIR images demonstrate multiple neuro-fibromas, including plexiform (*red arrows*) lesions along the brachial plexus in the patient with history of NF-1. Note target appearance most commonly seen with neurofibromas (*yellow arrow*).

and nonsteroidal antiinflammatory medications. Recently, denervation using botulinum toxin injection into the anterior scalene muscle using CT scan, ultrasound, or fluoroscopic guidance has been used as a minimally invasive treatment option.[90] However, surgical decompression with or without sympathectomy may be needed to alleviate a patient's symptoms (**Box 1**).[87]

VASCULAR LESIONS

Other non-neoplastic compression may be caused by aneurysms, pseudoaneurysms, fistulas, and vascular malformations. The subclavian, common carotid, vertebral (**Fig. 23**), axillary arteries, and their branches have been reported as vessels of origin of the compressive vascular pathologic state. The pseudoaneurysms may be seen because of direct trauma, vascular compression, inflammation, infection, drug use, prior nerve blocks, catheter or fistula placement, or decompressive procedures (**Fig. 24**). In patients with trauma, the onset of the compressive symptoms

related to pseudoaneurysm formation may be delayed. Therefore, vascular evaluation should be performed in trauma cases if there is a distal pulse deficit, local hematoma, bruit, or anatomically related nerve symptoms. The aneurysms and/or pseudoaneurysms may demonstrate T1-weighted hyperintensity and dark signal on T2-weighted imaging (see **Fig. 23**). Laminated mixed signal may be present with partial thrombosis.[91] The pseudoaneurysm in addition may have adjacent hematoma and other evidence of bony or soft tissue injury (see **Fig. 24**).

Traumatic and iatrogenic fistulas have also been reported to cause symptomatic brachial plexus compression. In cases of suspected fistulas, ultrasound may demonstrate arterialization of the venous waveform. Time-resolved MR angiography may be used in an attempt to demonstrate location of the fistulous connection. However, conventional angiogram remains the gold standard.

Extraneural vascular lesions in the region of the brachial plexus are rare.[92] They can be isolated or associated with congenital vascular

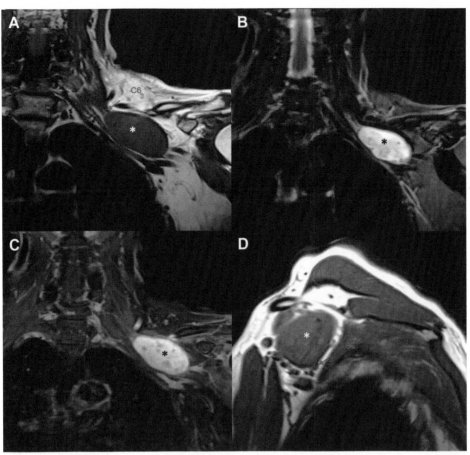

Fig. 20. Coronal (*A*) and sagittal (*D*) T1-weighted and coronal STIR (*B, C*) images demonstrate a circumscribed, avidly but heterogeneously enhancing mass (*asterisks*) associated with C6 nerve (*red arrow* in *A*), upper trunk, and divisions contributing to posterior cord (PC) (*red arrow* in *D*), with eccentric growth, consistent with a schwannoma.

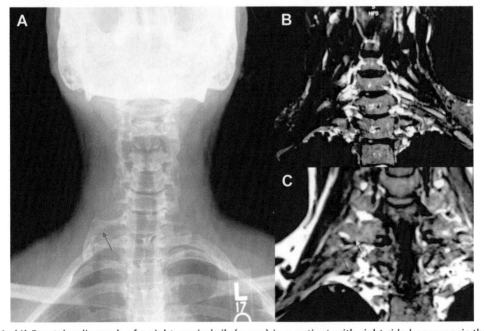

Fig. 21. (*A*) Frontal radiograph of a right cervical rib (*arrow*) in a patient with right-sided neurogenic thoracic outlet syndrome (TOS). The C7 transverse process on the left side is elongated and "beaked," a finding that has also been associated with neurogenic TOS. (*B*) Coronal STIR image demonstrates a left C7 cervical rib (*red arrow*). (*C*) The coronal T1-weighted image demonstrates an elongated right C7 transverse process (*yellow arrow*) and a rudimentary C7 rib (*red arrow*).

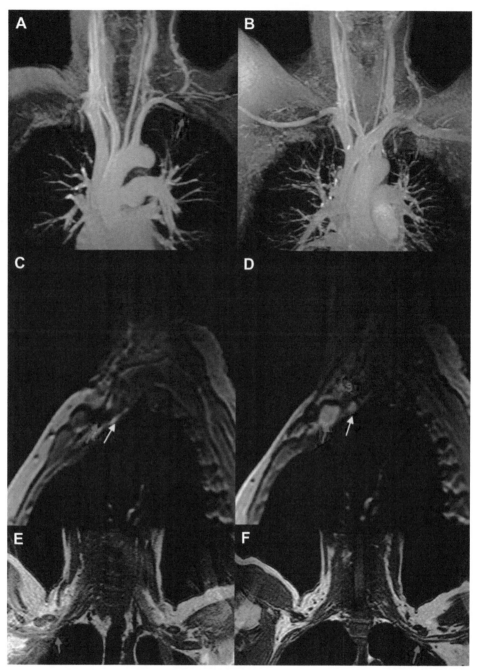

Fig. 22. Right shoulder pain, numbness, and tingling within both upper extremities with elevation of bilateral arms. The dynamic magnetic resonance angiogram with arm elevation demonstrates nonvisualization of the bilateral subclavian arteries (*arrows*) on initial images (*A*) with visualization of bilateral subclavian veins on the later images (*B*). The sagittal image with (*C*) and without (*D*) arm elevation demonstrate compression of both the subclavian artery (*yellow arrows*) and subclavian vein (*red arrows*). In addition, there is mild indentation of the bilateral divisions (*red arrows*) by the subclavius muscles with arm elevation (*E, F*). AS, anterior scalene muscle.

Box 1
Pathologic condition by age

Neonates and adolescents
- Traumatic injury

Middle-aged and older individuals
- Intrinsic and extrinsic tumors (most common cause of plexopathy)
- Radiation plexopathy
- Inflammatory plexopathy
- Cervical spondylosis
- Thoracic outlet syndrome

syndromes, such as Klippel-Trénaunay, hereditary hemorrhagic telangiectasia, PHACE (posterior fossa malformations, hemangiomas, arterial anomalies, coarctation of the aorta, cardiac defects, and eye abnormalities), and Kasabach-Merritt (see later discussion).

The 1992 classification of the vascular lesions introduced by the International Society for Study of Vascular Anomalies (ISSVA) is based on work of Mulliken and Glowacki[93] (1982) separating vascular lesions based on their biologic basis into vascular tumors and vascular malformations (**Table 4**). Most of the vascular tumors undergo involution and require no treatment, unless they cause Kasabach-Merritt syndrome (thrombocytopenia, anemia, and consumptive coagulopathy), compress vital structures,

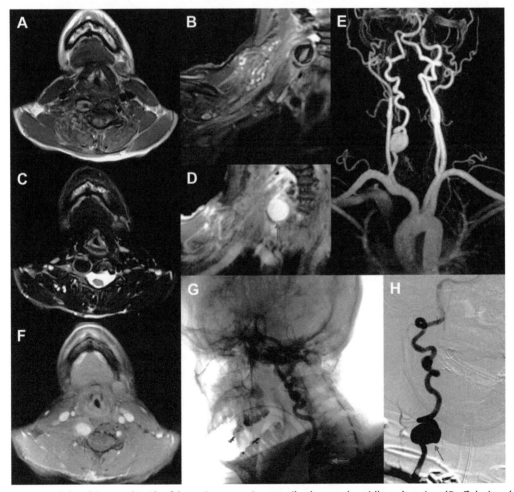

Fig. 23. T1-weighted image (*A, B*) of hyperintense, circumscribed, round, avidly enhancing (*D, F*) lesion (*red arrows*), with evidence of a flow void on T2-weighted image (*C*) within the widened right C4 and C5 neural foramen in a patient with NF1. Note absence of a separate flow void for a right vertebral artery (*red arrow* in *A*). The MR angiography (*E*) and conventional angiography (*G, H*) demonstrate a fusiform aneurysm of the right vertebral artery (*red arrows*).

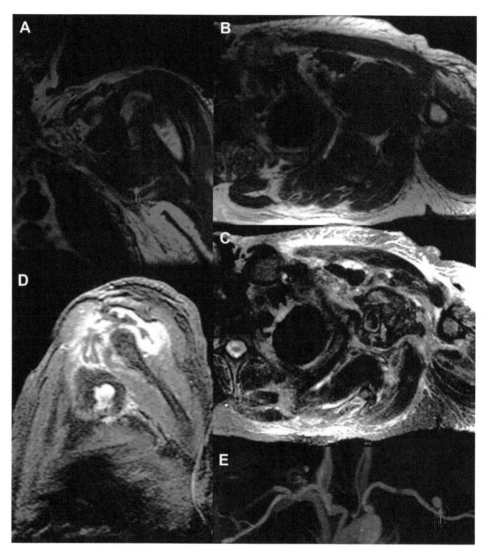

Fig. 24. Mass effect on the infraclavicular brachial plexus by a soft tissue hematoma (*red arrows*) adjacent to a humeral fracture. The hematoma is hypointense on T1-weighted images (*A, B*) and demonstrates a central circumscribed flow void on T2-weighted image (*C*) with corresponding avid central enhancement on postcontrast (*D*) images (*red arrows*). The MR angiography (*E*) demonstrates a small axillary pseudoaneurysm corresponding to the central flow void and enhancement within the hematoma (*red arrow*).

form fissures, or result in ulcerations or bleeding. Patients resistant to steroids are placed on interferon-α or vincristine sulfate or undergo resection. The vascular malformations never regress and need to be treated with percutaneous sclerosis, embolization, or resection.

Although ultrasound can be an inexpensive and readily available modality for initial evaluation, contrast-enhanced MR imaging is a preferred modality for differentiation between different types of vascular lesions. The algorithm for approach to the vascular lesions based on history and MR imaging appearance is included in **Fig. 25**. In the lesions with marked flow voids, dynamic vascular

evaluation with MR angiography can be performed for assessment of connection to the adjacent vessels, associated aneurysms, and pattern of vascular flow. In some cases, digital subtraction angiography is needed to define adjacent vascular anatomy of the feeding and draining vasculature.[94] This is extremely important for preoperative embolization of the lesion.

VASCULAR INSULTS

Plexopathy as a result of vascular insult related to systemic vasculitides, such as Churg-Strauss, polyarteritis nodosa, Wegener granulomatosis,

Table 4
Updated ISSVA classification of vascular anomalies

Vascular Tumors	Vascular Malformations
• Infantile hemangiomas	Slow-flow vascular malformations
• Congenital hemangiomas	• CM
∘ Rapidly Involuting congenital hemangioma	• VM
∘ Noninvoluting Congenital Hemangioma (NICH)	• LM
	Fast-flow vascular malformation
• Tufted angioma (± Kasabach-Merritt syndrome)	• AM
• Kaposiform hemangioendothelioma (± Kasabach-Merritt syndrome)	• AV fistula
	• AV malformation
• Spindle Cell Hemangioendothelioma	Complex combined vascular malformations
• Other, rare hemangioendotheliomas (epithelioid, composite, retiform, polymorphous, Dabska tumor, lymphangioendotheliomatosis, etc)	• CVM, CLM, LVM, LVM, CLVM, AVM-LM, CM-AVM
• Dermatologic acquired vascular tumors (pyogenic granuloma, targetoid hemangioma, glomeruloid hemangioma, microvenular hemangioma, etc.)	

Abbreviations: AV, arteriovenous; C, capillary; L, lymphatic; M, malformation; V, venous.
Data from Enjorlas O, Wassef M, Chapot R. Color Atlas of Vascular Tumors and Malformations. Cambridge, NY: Cambridge University Press; 2007.

giant cell arteritis, systemic sclerosis, collagen vascular diseases, hypersensitivity vasculitis, and Henoch-Schönlein purpura, is diagnosed based on the patient's history. The imaging is usually normal, but the brachial plexus may occasionally demonstrate mild diffuse T2-weighted hyperintensity.[3,95] The role of imaging in these cases is to exclude other lesions associated with the brachial plexus. The treatment in severe cases is prednisolone and intravenous immunoglobulin.[96]

DEMYELINATING PLEXOPATHY

The hypertrophic neuropathy family includes acquired (immune-mediated) and familial neuropathies. The patients with chronic inflammatory demyelinating polyneuropathy (CIDP), the most commonly acquired neuropathy, frequently have a history of antecedent illness. The disease is presumably autoimmune in cause and has two clinical variants: chronically progressive and

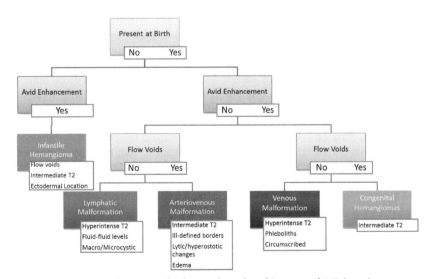

Fig. 25. The algorithm for approach to vascular lesions based on history and MR imaging appearance.

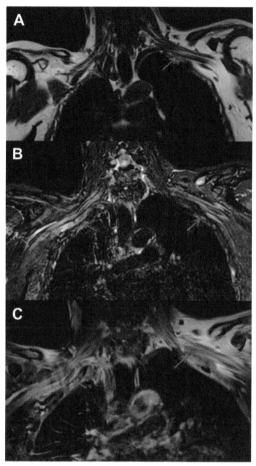

Fig. 26. Coronal T1-weighted (*A*), STIR (*B*), and fat-suppressed contrast-enhanced (*C*) T1-weighted images demonstrate mild diffuse thickening and enhancement (*red arrows*) of the bilateral brachial plexus in a patient with metastatic breast cancer and development of bilateral hand paresthesias, thought to represent a paraneoplastic chronic demyelinating neuropathy.

relapsing-remitting. It presents with bilateral muscle weakness affecting proximal and distal limbs, and less pronounced sensory loss. It predominantly affects brachial and lumbar plexus with only rare involvement of cranial and phrenic nerves. The imaging appearance is characteristic with onion bulb nerve enlargement due to proliferation of the Schwann cells and increased endoneurial collagen with preservation of axons (**Fig. 26**).[97] The clinical picture and electrophysiologic studies demonstrating a demyelinating pattern allow for diagnosis. However, MR imaging images are helpful for diagnosis, as are CSF analysis and nerve biopsies. STIR images are the mainstay of the imaging for CIDP involving the brachial plexus because this sequence has the

highest sensitivity for this pathologic state. It usually demonstrates bulb-like enlargement of the plexus and T2-weighted hyperintensity of these structures. In addition, as with other demyelinating lesions, approximately half of cases demonstrate increased diffusion and T1-weighted hyperintensity, supposedly due to increased collagen, degradation of myelin by macrophages, and uptake of lipids by Schwann cells. Only approximately 32% of cases demonstrate enhancement, likely due to disruption of the blood-nerve barrier.[97]

The imaging appearance differential considerations for CIDP are distal demyelinating polyneuropathy associated with monoclonal gammopathy (MGUS), multifocal motor neuropathy (MMN), multifocal inflammatory demyelinating neuropathy (MIDN), and hereditary motor-sensory neuropathies (HMSN), such as HMSN I (Charcot-Marie-Tooth disease [CMT1]), HMSN II [CMTII], and HMSN III [Dejerine-Sottas disease]).[98–100] They can be differentiated on the clinical basis. The patients with MIDN demonstrate asymmetric sensory loss with or without weakness.[100] The MMN is characterized by asymmetric weakness without sensory loss with usually unilateral MR imaging abnormalities.[101] The MGUS-associated polyneuropathy has predominantly sensory symptoms, demonstrates a slowly progressive course, absence of cranial nerve involvement, and absence of abnormal median nerve sensory potential. The latter is seen in CIDP, which also may have cranial nerve involvement, and motor symptom predominance.[101] The HMSN appearance most closely mimics CIDP.[97]

HEREDITARY PLEXOPATHY

The CMT encompasses a large heterogeneous group of pathologic conditions with incidence of 1 in 2500. Although the classification is complex and is undergoing frequent revisions, the grossly oversimplified summary of the categories is included in **Table 5**. The most common type, CMT1, presents with symmetric onion-bulb enlargement of the bilateral involved plexus on MR imaging related to the demyelination and remyelination within the affected structures. However, the axonal forms, for example certain phenotypes of CMT2, will not demonstrate this finding due to absence of remyelination cycles.

Dejerine-Sottas disease is very rare.[102] It is also heterogeneous genetically, but most commonly caused by a defect in chromosome 17. It presents in infancy or early childhood as hyporeflexia, nerve enlargement, delayed motor development, and progressive severe weakness of the

Table 5
Simplified classification of CMT disease

Type	Presentation	Genetics	Presentation	Nerve Conduction Velocities (NCVs)
CMT1 (classical and most common)	First decade to mid-adulthood	Autosomal dominant with more than 40 genes Most common is duplication on chromosome 17	• Lower extremities predominance • Palpable nerve enlargement • Weakness out of proportion to sensory deficits in distal extremities • Difficulty walking • No pain • Relatives with similar symptoms	Low

CMT2 (second most common)	Adulthood	Autosomal dominant with more than 11 genes Multiple mutations are de novo Some are autosomal recessive	• Phenotype 1
			  ◦ Most common
			  ◦ Similar to CMT1 but milder
			  ◦ No family history
			• Phenotype 2
			  ◦ Predominantly sensory symptoms
			  ◦ Present with complications (ulcerations, osteomyelitis, amputations)
			• Phenotype 3
			  ◦ Predominantly motor
			  ◦ Upper extremities are much more common than lower
			  ◦ Atrophy and weakness of small muscles of the hand
			  ◦ Delayed onset of distal lower extremity muscles atrophy
			  ◦ No nerve enlargement
			  ◦ Can be unilateral
			  ◦ Frequently misdiagnosed as thoracic outlet syndrome
				—

(continued on next page)

Table 5
(continued)

Type	Presentation	Genetics	Presentation	Nerve Conduction Velocities (NCVs)
CMT-DI group (Intermediate NCV)	First and second decade	Autosomal dominant, multiple genes	• Distal weakness • Mild sensory loss • Absent tendon reflexes • Slow progression	Normal to mild decreased NCV values
CMT4 (in other classifications autosomal recessive CMT1)	Early childhood	Recessive or de novo autosomal dominant, multiple genes	• Early severe motor and sensory neuropathy • Early and severe scoliosis in some subgroups	Both axonal and demyelinating range

CMT-X1	First decade in boys 20–30 years in women	X-linked Dominant	• Boys
			  ○ Severe
			  ○ Asymmetric
			  ○ Otherwise similar to classic
			  ○ Occasional transient severe ataxia and dysarthria
			• Women
			  ○ Mild
				Intermediate, but proportional to clinical severity

CMTX5 (Rosenberg-Chutorian Syndrome)	Early childhood	X-linked recessive	• Severe neuropathy • Deafness • Optic atrophy	—

Data from Reilly MM, Murphy SM, Laura M. Charcot-Marie-Tooth disease. J Peripher Nerv Syst 2011;16(1):1–14; and Banchs I, Casasnovas C, Alberti A, et al. Diagnosis of Charcot-Marie-Tooth disease. J Biomed Biotechnol 2009;2009:985415.

extremities.[103–106] Although genetic testing for hypertrophic neuropathy is widely advocated, there are challenges, including only a limited number of genes available for diagnosis and absence of specific therapy.[99] Nevertheless, in sporadic cases, genetic diagnosis will stop invasive nerve biopsies and trials of treatments with serious side effects, such as immunosuppressants.[99]

SUMMARY

MR imaging is a valuable tool for the referring physician in cases of traumatic and nontraumatic pathologic abnormalities because it frequently not only helps in localization, confirmation, and characterization of the pathologic process but also, in many cases, may significantly change choice of treatment. The key findings for each condition affecting the brachial plexus should be noted in the report, to help in clinical decision making. Optimization of the protocols based on pattern of referral and commonly seen pathologic abnormalities allows for efficient and accurate service. However, the availability of high-strength magnets and multiplanar reconstruction capabilities may allow for overall shortening of the examination time and reduction of the need for alteration of the protocol. MR neurography, diffusion tensor imaging, and diffusion weighted imaging are promising techniques that can be helpful in some cases, but are not used in everyday practice. Judicious use of contrast may be beneficial in cases of brachial plexus infections, vascular malformations, and radiation-treated tumors.

REFERENCES

1. Uysal II, Seker M, Karabulut AK, et al. Brachial plexus variations in human fetuses. Neurosurgery 2003;53(3):676–84 [discussion: 684].
2. Saifuddin A. Imaging tumours of the brachial plexus. Skeletal Radiol 2003;32(7):375–87.
3. Aralasmak A, Karaali K, Cevikol C, et al. MR imaging findings in brachial plexopathy with thoracic outlet syndrome. AJNR Am J Neuroradiol 2010;31(3):410–7.
4. Narakas AO. The treatment of brachial plexus injuries. Int Orthop 1985;9(1):29–36.
5. Kim DH, Murovic JA, Tiel RL, et al. Mechanisms of injury in operative brachial plexus lesions. Neurosurg Focus 2004;16(5):E2.
6. Oberlin C, Ameur NE, Teboul F, et al. Restoration of elbow flexion in brachial plexus injury by transfer of ulnar nerve fascicles to the nerve to the biceps muscle. Tech Hand Up Extrem Surg 2002;6(2):86–90.
7. Lim AY, Sebastin SJ. Practical management of pediatric and adult brachial plexus palsies. In: Chung K,

8. Yang LJ-S, McGillicuddy J, editors. Clinical examination and diagnosis. China: Elsevier Saunders; 2011.
8. Filler AG, Kliot M, Howe FA, et al. Application of magnetic resonance neurography in the evaluation of patients with peripheral nerve pathology. J Neurosurg 1996;85(2):299–309.
9. Hems TE, Birch R, Carlstedt T. The role of magnetic resonance imaging in the management of traction injuries to the adult brachial plexus. J Hand Surg Br 1999;24(5):550–5.
10. Gasparotti R, Garozzo D, Ferraresi S. Practical management of pediatric and adult brachial plexus palsies. In: Chung K, Yang LJ-S, McGillicuddy J, editors. Radiographic assessment of adult brachial plexus injuries. China: Elsevier Saunders; 2011.
11. Zara G, Gasparotti R, Manara R. MR imaging of peripheral nervous system involvement: Parsonage-Turner syndrome. J Neurol Sci 2012; 315(1–2):170–1.
12. Chhabra A, Lee PP, Bizzell C, et al. 3 Tesla MR neurography—technique, interpretation, and pitfalls. Skeletal Radiol 2011;40(10):1249–60.
13. Gasparotti R. New techniques in spinal imaging. Neuroradiology 2011;53(Suppl 1):S195–7.
14. Chhabra A, Subhawong TK, Bizzell C, et al. 3T MR neurography using three-dimensional diffusion-weighted PSIF: technical issues and advantages. Skeletal Radiol 2011;40(10):1355–60.
15. Smith AB, Gupta N, Strober J, et al. Magnetic resonance neurography in children with birth-related brachial plexus injury. Pediatr Radiol 2008;38(2): 159–63.
16. Carvalho GA, Nikkhah G, Matthies C, et al. Diagnosis of root avulsions in traumatic brachial plexus injuries: value of computerized tomography myelography and magnetic resonance imaging. J Neurosurg 1997;86(1):69–76.
17. Yoshikawa T, Hayashi N, Yamamoto S, et al. Brachial plexus injury: clinical manifestations, conventional imaging findings, and the latest imaging techniques. Radiographics 2006;26(Suppl 1):S133–43.
18. Hayashi N, Masumoto T, Abe O, et al. Accuracy of abnormal paraspinal muscle findings on contrast-enhanced MR images as indirect signs of unilateral cervical root-avulsion injury. Radiology 2002; 223(2):397–402.
19. Yang LJ-S, McGillicuddy JE, Chimbira W. Practical management of pediatric and adult brachial plexus palsies. In: Chung K, Yang LJ-S, McGillicuddy J, editors. Clinical presentation and considerations of neonatal brachial plexus palsy. China: Elsevier Saunders; 2011.
20. Waters PM. Update on management of pediatric brachial plexus palsy. J Pediatr Orthop B 2005; 14(4):233–44.
21. van Ouwerkerk WJ, Strijers RL, Barkhof F, et al. Detection of root avulsion in the dominant C7

obstetric brachial plexus lesion: experience with three-dimensional constructive interference in steady-state magnetic resonance imaging and electrophysiology. Neurosurgery 2005;57(5):930–40 [discussion: 930–40].

22. Wadd NJ, Lucraft HH. Brachial plexus neuropathy following mantle radiotherapy. Clin Oncol (R Coll Radiol) 1998;10(6):399–400.

23. Pierce SM, Recht A, Lingos TI, et al. Long-term radiation complications following conservative surgery (CS) and radiation therapy (RT) in patients with early stage breast cancer. Int J Radiat Oncol Biol Phys 1992;23(5):915–23.

24. Amini A, Yang J, Williamson R, et al. Dose constraints to prevent radiation-induced brachial plexopathy in patients treated for lung cancer. Int J Radiat Oncol Biol Phys 2012;82(3):e391–8.

25. Castillo M. Imaging the anatomy of the brachial plexus: review and self-assessment module. AJR Am J Roentgenol 2005;185(Suppl 6):S196–204.

26. Iyer RB, Fenstermacher MJ, Libshitz HI. MR imaging of the treated brachial plexus. AJR Am J Roentgenol 1996;167(1):225–9.

27. Hoeller U, Rolofs K, Bajrovic A, et al. A patient questionnaire for radiation-induced brachial plexopathy. Am J Clin Oncol 2004;27(1):1–7.

28. Emami B, Lyman J, Brown A, et al. Tolerance of normal tissue to therapeutic irradiation. Int J Radiat Oncol Biol Phys 1991;21(1):109–22.

29. Nich C, Bonnin P, Laredo JD, et al. An uncommon form of delayed radio-induced brachial plexopathy. Chir Main 2005;24(1):48–51 [in French].

30. Johansson S, Svensson H, Denekamp J. Dose response and latency for radiation-induced fibrosis, edema, and neuropathy in breast cancer patients. Int J Radiat Oncol Biol Phys 2002;52(5):1207–19.

31. Bajrovic A, Rades D, Fehlauer F, et al. Is there a life-long risk of brachial plexopathy after radiotherapy of supraclavicular lymph nodes in breast cancer patients? Radiother Oncol 2004;71(3):297–301.

32. Gosk J, Rutowski R, Reichert P, et al. Radiation-induced brachial plexus neuropathy - aetiopathogenesis, risk factors, differential diagnostics, symptoms and treatment. Folia Neuropathol 2007;45(1):26–30.

33. Olsen NK, Pfeiffer P, Johannsen L, et al. Radiation-induced brachial plexopathy: neurological follow-up in 161 recurrence-free breast cancer patients. Int J Radiat Oncol Biol Phys 1993;26(1):43–9.

34. Kori SH, Foley KM, Posner JB. Brachial plexus lesions in patients with cancer: 100 cases. Neurology 1981;31(1):45–50.

35. Albers JW, Allen AA 2nd, Bastron JA, et al. Limb myokymia. Muscle Nerve 1981;4(6):494–504.

36. Stohr M. Special types of spontaneous electrical activity in radiogenic nerve injuries. Muscle Nerve 1982;5(Suppl 9):S78–83.

37. Lederman RJ, Wilbourn AJ. Brachial plexopathy: recurrent cancer or radiation? Neurology 1984;34(10):1331–5.

38. Bartels AL, Zeebregts CJ, Enting RH, et al. Fluorodeoxyglucose and C-Choline positron emission tomography for distinction of metastatic plexopathy and neuritis: a case report. Cases J 2009;2:9323.

39. Ahmad A, Barrington S, Maisey M, et al. Use of positron emission tomography in evaluation of brachial plexopathy in breast cancer patients. Br J Cancer 1999;79(3–4):478–82.

40. Johansson S, Svensson H, Denekamp J. Timescale of evolution of late radiation injury after postoperative radiotherapy of breast cancer patients. Int J Radiat Oncol Biol Phys 2000;48(3):745–50.

41. Spillane JD. Localized neuritis of the shoulder girdle. A report of 46 patients in the MEF. Lancet 1943;2:532–5.

42. Parsonage MJ, Turner JW. Neuralgic amyotrophy; the shoulder-girdle syndrome. Lancet 1948;1(6513):973–8.

43. Misamore GW, Lehman DE. Parsonage-Turner syndrome (acute brachial neuritis). J Bone Joint Surg Am 1996;78(9):1405–8.

44. Helms CA, Martinez S, Speer KP. Acute brachial neuritis (Parsonage-Turner syndrome): MR imaging appearance—report of three cases. Radiology 1998;207(1):255–9.

45. Turner JW, Parsonage MJ. Neuralgic amyotrophy (paralytic brachial neuritis); with special reference to prognosis. Lancet 1957;273(6988):209–12.

46. Tsairis P, Dyck PJ, Mulder DW. Natural history of brachial plexus neuropathy. Report on 99 patients. Arch Neurol 1972;27(2):109–17.

47. Schreiber AL, Abramov R, Fried GW, et al. Expanding the differential of shoulder pain: Parsonage-Turner syndrome. J Am Osteopath Assoc 2009;109(8):415–22.

48. Magee KR, Dejong RN. Paralytic brachial neuritis. Discussion of clinical features with review of 23 cases. JAMA 1960;174:1258–62.

49. Suarez GA, Giannini C, Bosch EP, et al. Immune brachial plexus neuropathy: suggestive evidence for an inflammatory-immune pathogenesis. Neurology 1996;46(2):559–61.

50. van Alfen N, van Engelen BG. The clinical spectrum of neuralgic amyotrophy in 246 cases. Brain 2006;129(Pt 2):438–50.

51. Yanny S, Toms AP. MR patterns of denervation around the shoulder. AJR Am J Roentgenol 2010;195(2):W157–63.

52. MacDonald BK, Cockerell OC, Sander JW, et al. The incidence and lifetime prevalence of neurological disorders in a prospective community-based study in the UK. Brain 2000;123(Pt 4):665–76.

53. Turner JW. Acute brachial radiculitis. Br Med J 1944;2(4374):592–4.
54. Aymond JK, Goldner JL, Hardaker WT Jr. Neuralgic amyotrophy. Orthop Rev 1989;18(12):1275–9.
55. Gaskin CM, Helms CA. Parsonage-Turner syndrome: MR imaging findings and clinical information of 27 patients. Radiology 2006;240(2):501–7.
56. Scalf RE, Wenger DE, Frick MA, et al. MRI findings of 26 patients with Parsonage-Turner syndrome. AJR Am J Roentgenol 2007;189(1):W39–44.
57. Miller JD, Pruitt S, McDonald TJ. Acute brachial plexus neuritis: an uncommon cause of shoulder pain. Am Fam Physician 2000;62(9):2067–72.
58. White HD, White BA, Boethel C, et al. Pancoast's syndrome secondary to infectious etiologies: a not so uncommon occurrence. Am J Med Sci 2011;341(4):333–6.
59. Miron D, Bor N, Cutai M, et al. Transient brachial palsy associated with suppurative arthritis of the shoulder. Pediatr Infect Dis J 1997;16(3):326–7.
60. Lusk MD, Kline DG, Garcia CA. Tumors of the brachial plexus. Neurosurgery 1987;21(4):439–53.
61. Wittenberg KH, Adkins MC. MR imaging of nontraumatic brachial plexopathies: frequency and spectrum of findings. Radiographics 2000;20(4):1023–32.
62. Sureka J, Cherian RA, Alexander M, et al. MRI of brachial plexopathies. Clin Radiol 2009;64(2):208–18.
63. Castagno AA, Shuman WP. MR imaging in clinically suspected brachial plexus tumor. AJR Am J Roentgenol 1987;149(6):1219–22.
64. Reede DL. MR imaging of the brachial plexus. Magn Reson Imaging Clin N Am 1997;5(4):897–906.
65. Gachiani J, Kim D, Nelson A, et al. Surgical management of malignant peripheral nerve sheath tumors. Neurosurg Focus 2007;22(6):E13.
66. Suzuki M, Watanabe T, Mogi G. Primary non-Hodgkin's lymphoma of brachial plexus. Auris Nasus Larynx 1999;26(3):337–42.
67. Tucker T, Wolkenstein P, Revuz J, et al. Association between benign and malignant peripheral nerve sheath tumors in NF1. Neurology 2005;65(2):205–11.
68. Chhabra A, Soldatos T, Durand DJ, et al. The role of magnetic resonance imaging in the diagnostic evaluation of malignant peripheral nerve sheath tumors. Indian J Cancer 2011;48(3):328–34.
69. Wasa J, Nishida Y, Tsukushi S, et al. MRI features in the differentiation of malignant peripheral nerve sheath tumors and neurofibromas. AJR Am J Roentgenol 2010;194(6):1568–74.
70. Matsumine A, Kusuzaki K, Nakamura T, et al. Differentiation between neurofibromas and malignant peripheral nerve sheath tumors in neurofibromatosis 1 evaluated by MRI. J Cancer Res Clin Oncol 2009;135(7):891–900.
71. Levine E, Huntrakoon M, Wetzel LH. Malignant nerve-sheath neoplasms in neurofibromatosis: distinction from benign tumors by using imaging techniques. AJR Am J Roentgenol 1987;149(5):1059–64.
72. Benz MR, Czernin J, Dry SM, et al. Quantitative F18-fluorodeoxyglucose positron emission tomography accurately characterizes peripheral nerve sheath tumors as malignant or benign. Cancer 2010;116(2):451–8.
73. Ogose A, Hotta T, Morita T, et al. Tumors of peripheral nerves: correlation of symptoms, clinical signs, imaging features, and histologic diagnosis. Skeletal Radiol 1999;28(4):183–8.
74. Yousem DM, Hatabu H, Hurst RW, et al. Carotid artery invasion by head and neck masses: prediction with MR imaging. Radiology 1995;195(3):715–20.
75. Wang CP, Chang YL, Ko JY, et al. Desmoid tumor of the head and neck. Head Neck 2006;28(11):1008–13.
76. Dafford K, Kim D, Nelson A, et al. Extraabdominal desmoid tumors. Neurosurg Focus 2007;22(6):E21.
77. Seinfeld J, Kleinschmidt-DeMasters BK, Tayal S, et al. Desmoid-type fibromatosis involving the brachial plexus. Neurosurg Focus 2007;22(6):E22.
78. Ludemann W, Dorner L, Tatagiba M, et al. Brachial plexus palsy from nodular fasciitis with spontaneous recovery: implications for surgical management. Case illustration. J Neurosurg 2001;94(6):1014.
79. Kransdorf MJ, Bancroft LW, Peterson JJ, et al. Imaging of fatty tumors: distinction of lipoma and well-differentiated liposarcoma. Radiology 2002;224(1):99–104.
80. Suzuki R, Watanabe H, Yanagawa T, et al. PET evaluation of fatty tumors in the extremity: possibility of using the standardized uptake value (SUV) to differentiate benign tumors from liposarcoma. Ann Nucl Med 2005;19(8):661–70.
81. Binder DK, Smith JS, Barbaro NM. Primary brachial plexus tumors: imaging, surgical, and pathological findings in 25 patients. Neurosurg Focus 2004;16(5):E11.
82. Boyanton BL Jr, Jones JK, Shenaq SM, et al. Intraneural perineurioma: a systematic review with illustrative cases. Arch Pathol Lab Med 2007;131(9):1382–92.
83. Schwartzman RJ. Brachial plexus traction injuries. Hand Clin 1991;7(3):547–56.
84. van Es HW, Bollen TL, van Heesewijk HP. MRI of the brachial plexus: a pictorial review. Eur J Radiol 2010;74(2):391–402.
85. Atasoy E. Thoracic outlet compression syndrome. Orthop Clin North Am 1996;27(2):265–303.
86. Urschel HC Jr, Razzuk MA. Neurovascular compression in the thoracic outlet: changing management over 50 years. Ann Surg 1998;228(4):609–17.
87. Demondion X, Herbinet P, Van Sint Jan S, et al. Imaging assessment of thoracic outlet syndrome. Radiographics 2006;26(6):1735–50.

88. Smedby O, Rostad H, Klaastad O, et al. Functional imaging of the thoracic outlet syndrome in an open MR scanner. Eur Radiol 2000;10(4):597–600.

89. Demondion X, Bacqueville E, Paul C, et al. Thoracic outlet: assessment with MR imaging in asymptomatic and symptomatic populations. Radiology 2003;227(2):461–8.

90. Christo PJ, McGreevy K. Updated perspectives on neurogenic thoracic outlet syndrome. Curr Pain Headache Rep 2011;15(1):14–21.

91. Atlas SW, Grossman RI, Goldberg HI, et al. Partially thrombosed giant intracranial aneurysms: correlation of MR and pathologic findings. Radiology 1987;162(1 Pt 1):111–4.

92. Kim DH, Murovic JA, Tiel RL, et al. A series of 146 peripheral non-neural sheath nerve tumors: 30-year experience at Louisiana State University Health Sciences Center. J Neurosurg 2005; 102(2):256–66.

93. Enjorlas O, Wassef M, Chapot R. Color atlas of vascular tumors and malformations. Cambridge (New York): Cambridge University Press; 2007.

94. Ranalli NJ, Huang JH, Lee EB, et al. Hemangiomas of the brachial plexus: a case series. Neurosurgery 2009;65(Suppl 4):A181–8.

95. Pfadenhauer K, Roesler A, Golling A. The involvement of the peripheral nervous system in biopsy proven active giant cell arteritis. J Neurol 2007; 254(6):751–5.

96. Yilmaz C, Caksen H, Arslan S, et al. Bilateral brachial plexopathy complicating Henoch-Schonlein purpura. Brain Dev 2006;28(5):326–8.

97. Adachi Y, Sato N, Okamoto T, et al. Brachial and lumbar plexuses in chronic inflammatory demyelinating polyradiculoneuropathy: MRI assessment including apparent diffusion coefficient. Neuroradiology 2011;53(1):3–11.

98. Eurelings M, Notermans NC, Franssen H, et al. MRI of the brachial plexus in polyneuropathy associated with monoclonal gammopathy. Muscle Nerve 2001; 24(10):1312–8.

99. Reilly MM, Murphy SM, Laura M. Charcot-Marie-Tooth disease. J Peripher Nerv Syst 2011;16(1): 1–14.

100. Van den Berg-Vos RM, Van den Berg LH, Franssen H, et al. Multifocal inflammatory demyelinating neuropathy: a distinct clinical entity? Neurology 2000;54(1): 26–32.

101. Notermans NC, Franssen H, Eurelings M, et al. Diagnostic criteria for demyelinating polyneuropathy associated with monoclonal gammopathy. Muscle Nerve 2000;23(1):73–9.

102. Pearce JM. Dejerine-Sottas disease (progressive hypertrophic polyneuropathy). Eur Neurol 2006; 55(2):115–7.

103. Plante-Bordeneuve V, Said G. Dejerine-Sottas disease and hereditary demyelinating polyneuropathy of infancy. Muscle Nerve 2002;26(5):608–21.

104. Gabreels-Festen A. Dejerine-Sottas syndrome grown to maturity: overview of genetic and morphological heterogeneity and follow-up of 25 patients. J Anat 2002;200(4):341–56.

105. Maki DD, Yousem DM, Corcoran C, et al. MR imaging of Dejerine-Sottas disease. AJNR Am J Neuroradiol 1999;20(3):378–80.

106. Lynch DR, Hara H, Yum SW, et al. Autosomal dominant transmission of Dejerine-Sottas disease (HMSN III). Neurology 1997;49(2):601–3.

Index

Note: Page numbers of article titles are in **boldface** type.

Magn Reson Imaging Clin N Am 20 (2012) 827–830
http://dx.doi.org/10.1016/S1064-9689(12)00123-7
1064-9689/12/$ – see front matter © 2012 Elsevier Inc. All rights reserved.

mri.theclinics.com

United States Postal Service

Statement of Ownership, Management, and Circulation
(All Periodicals Publications Except Requestor Publications)

1. Publication Title	2. Publication Number								3. Filing Date
Magnetic Resonance Imaging Clinics of North America	0	1	1	-	9	0	0	9	9/14/12

4. Issue Frequency	5. Number of Issues Published Annually	6. Annual Subscription Price
Feb, May, Aug, Nov	4	$337.00

7. Complete Mailing Address of Known Office of Publication (Not printer) (Street, city, county, state, and ZIP+4®)

Elsevier Inc.
360 Park Avenue South
New York, NY 10010-1710

Contact Person
Stephen R. Bushing

Telephone (Include area code)
215-239-3688

8. Complete Mailing Address of Headquarters or General Business Office of Publisher (Not printer)

Elsevier Inc., 360 Park Avenue South, New York, NY 10010-1710

9. Full Names and Complete Mailing Addresses of Publisher, Editor, and Managing Editor (Do not leave blank)

Publisher (Name and complete mailing address)

Kim Murphy, Elsevier, Inc., 1600 John F. Kennedy Blvd. Suite 1800, Philadelphia, PA 19103-2899

Editor (Name and complete mailing address)

Sarah Barth, Elsevier, Inc., 1600 John F. Kennedy Blvd. Suite 1800, Philadelphia, PA 19103-2899

Managing Editor (Name and complete mailing address)

Sarah Barth, Elsevier, Inc., 1600 John F. Kennedy Blvd. Suite 1800, Philadelphia, PA 19103-2899

10. Owner (Do not leave blank. If the publication is owned by a corporation, give the name and address of the corporation immediately followed by the names and addresses of all stockholders owning or holding 1 percent or more of the total amount of stock. If not owned by a corporation, give the names and addresses of the individual owners. If owned by a partnership or other unincorporated firm, give its name and address as well as those of each individual owner. If the publication is published by a nonprofit organization, give its name and address.)

Full Name	Complete Mailing Address
Wholly owned subsidiary of	1600 John F. Kennedy Blvd., Ste. 1800
Reed/Elsevier, US holdings	Philadelphia, PA 19103-2899

11. Known Bondholders, Mortgagees, and Other Security Holders Owning or Holding 1 Percent or More of Total Amount of Bonds, Mortgages, or Other Securities. If none, check box ☐ None

Full Name	Complete Mailing Address
N/A	

12. Tax Status (For completion by nonprofit organizations authorized to mail at nonprofit rates) (Check one)
The purpose, function, and nonprofit status of this organization and the exempt status for federal income tax purposes:
☐ Has Not Changed During Preceding 12 Months
☐ Has Changed During Preceding 12 Months (Publisher must submit explanation of change with this statement)

PS Form 3526, September 2007 (Page 1 of 3 (Instructions Page 3)) PSN 7530-01-000-9931 PRIVACY NOTICE: See our Privacy policy in www.usps.com

---

13. Publication Title	14. Issue Date for Circulation Data Below
Magnetic Resonance Imaging Clinics of North America	August 2012

15. Extent and Nature of Circulation		Average No. Copies Each Issue During Preceding 12 Months	No. Copies of Single Issue Published Nearest to Filing Date
a. Total Number of Copies (Net press run)		1685	1382
b. Paid Circulation (By Mail and Outside the Mail)	(1) Mailed Outside-County Paid Subscriptions Stated on PS Form 3541. (Include paid distribution above nominal rate, advertiser's proof copies, and exchange copies)	1104	1038
	(2) Mailed In-County Paid Subscriptions Stated on PS Form 3541 (Include paid distribution above nominal rate, advertiser's proof copies, and exchange copies)		
	(3) Paid Distribution Outside the Mails Including Sales Through Dealers and Carriers, Street Vendors, Counter Sales, and Other Paid Distribution Outside USPS®	280	277
	(4) Paid Distribution by Other Classes Mailed Through the USPS (e.g. First-Class Mail®)		
c. Total Paid Distribution (Sum of 15b (1), (2), (3), and (4))	▶	1384	1315
d. Free or Nominal Rate Distribution (By Mail and Outside the Mail)	(1) Free or Nominal Rate Outside-County Copies Included on PS Form 3541	46	47
	(2) Free or Nominal Rate In-County Copies Included on PS Form 3541		
	(3) Free or Nominal Rate Copies Mailed at Other Classes Through the USPS (e.g. First-Class Mail)		
	(4) Free or Nominal Rate Distribution Outside the Mail (Carriers or other means)		
e. Total Free or Nominal Rate Distribution (Sum of 15d (1), (2), (3) and (4))	▶	46	47
f. Total Distribution (Sum of 15c and 15e)	▶	1430	1362
g. Copies not Distributed (See instructions to publishers #4 (page #3))		255	20
h. Total (Sum of 15f and g)	▶	1685	1382
i. Percent Paid (15c divided by 15f times 100)		96.78%	96.55%

16. Publication of Statement of Ownership

If the publication is a general publication, publication of this statement is required. Will be printed
in the November 2012 issue of this publication. ☐ Publication not required

17. Signature and Title of Editor, Publisher, Business Manager, or Owner

Stephen R. Bushing

Stephen R. Bushing – Inventory Distribution Coordinator

Date September 14, 2012

I certify that all information furnished on this form is true and complete. I understand that anyone who furnishes false or misleading information on this form or who omits material or information requested on the form may be subject to criminal sanctions (including fines and imprisonment) and/or civil sanctions (including civil penalties).

PS Form 3526, September 2007 (Page 2 of 3)

Moving?

Make sure your subscription moves with you!

To notify us of your new address, find your **Clinics Account Number** (located on your mailing label above your name), and contact customer service at:

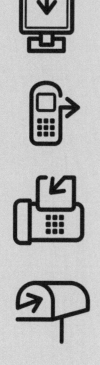

Email: journalscustomerservice-usa@elsevier.com

800-654-2452 (subscribers in the U.S. & Canada)
314-447-8871 (subscribers outside of the U.S. & Canada)

Fax number: 314-447-8029

Elsevier Health Sciences Division
Subscription Customer Service
3251 Riverport Lane
Maryland Heights, MO 63043

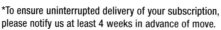

*To ensure uninterrupted delivery of your subscription, please notify us at least 4 weeks in advance of move.

Printed and bound by CPI Group (UK) Ltd, Croydon, CR0 4YY

03/10/2024

01040355-0003